PHARMACOLOGY - RESEARCH, SAFETY TESTING AND REGULATION

RECENT ADVANCES IN DRUG DELIVERY RESEARCH

PHARMACOLOGY - RESEARCH, SAFETY TESTING AND REGULATION

Additional books in this series can be found on Nova's website under the Series tab.

Additional e-books in this series can be found on Nova's website under the e-book tab.

PHARMACOLOGY - RESEARCH, SAFETY TESTING AND REGULATION

RECENT ADVANCES IN DRUG DELIVERY RESEARCH

VALERIO VOLIANI, PH.D.
EDITOR

New York

For permission to use material from this book please contact us:
Telephone 631-231-7269; Fax 631-231-8175
Web Site: http://www.novapublishers.com

NOTICE TO THE READER

Library of Congress Cataloging-in-Publication Data

ISBN: 978-1-62948-228-6

Library of Congress Control Number: 2013949354

Published by Nova Science Publishers, Inc. † New York

Contents

Preface

Recently great effort was devoted on the development of new drug delivery systems. This stems from the challenge of producing materials able to localize their effect only on the target, enhancing the therapeutical effect while reducing the side ones. The control over drug delivery improves bioavailability of the drug in the organism by preventing its premature degradation and enhancing its cellular uptake, maintains drug concentration within the therapeutic window by controlling the drug release rate, and reduces side effects by targeting to the site. Innovations in materials chemistry have fueled the development of new drug delivery systems, creating carriers that are biodegradable, biocompatible, targetable, and stimulus-responsive. Obviously, this research field is exceptionally active, and new materials/technologies showing interesting features for drug delivery are constantly developed. On this hand, "Recent advances in drug delivery research" presents a complete summary of the current progress in the field inclusive of an extensive literature.

In the first two Chapters of "Recent advances in drug delivery research" are addressed two topics required for the design of novel drug delivery systems. In Chapter 1, the origins of the observations supporting the existence of the "Enhanced Permeability and Retention" effect showed by cancerous tissues and its updated view in the context of more recent insights is presented. This is the first step in order to realize the passive ability of new nanocarriers to localize their therapeutical efficacy in a confined area of the organism. In Chapter 2, the recent advances in oral drug delivery are discussed. Indeed, the oral way for the delivery of drugs remains the most preferred administration method (about 60% of pharmaceutical products in the market), thanks to the high levels of patient acceptance and long term compliance which increased therapeutic value of the drug.

In Chapters 3-7, a wide variety of drug delivery systems are reviewed: i) pH-sensitive nanocarriers and their performance as nano-scale strategies for the efficient drug and gene delivery to the intracellular compartments and specific tissues with an acidic environment (Chapter 3), ii) self-assembled soft nanostructures called "Bio-inspired chimeric Drug Delivery nanosystems", their synthesis, structural analysis and performance (Chapter 4), iii) *in situ* gelling delivery systems and their main components, including their formation mechanisms and applications (Chapter 5), iv) solid lipid nanoparticles loaded by idebenone for the treatment of both skin oxidative damages and neurodegenerative diseases such as Parkinson's and Alzheimer diseases (Chapter 6), and v) different class of polymer-polyphenol conjugates, analyzed in terms of synthesis and biological antioxidant activity (Chapter 7).

Finally, in Chapter 8 is critically discussed with several examples the link between the planning of new drug delivery systems and their real use in clinical trial, also suggesting an approach in order to develop site-targeted drug-delivery systems.

In: Recent Advances in Drug Delivery Research
Editor: Valerio Voliani
ISBN: 978-1-62948-228-6

Chapter 1

Enhanced Permeability and Retention Effect: Insights Impacting Nanoscale Drug Delivery Systems

***S. Neslihan Alpay*[1] *and Jim Klostergaard*[2,*]**
[1]Departments of Experimental Therapeutics, The University of Texas, M. D. Anderson Cancer Center, Houston, TX, US
[2]Molecular and Cellular Oncology, The University of Texas, M. D. Anderson Cancer Center, Houston, TX, US

Abstract

The Enhanced Permeability and Retention (EPR) effect, used initially to describe the propensity for macromolecules to accumulate in solid tumors more so than low molecular weight cancer therapeutics, was first described over 25 years ago and it has helped shape much of the strategic thinking in drug delivery development since then. As we have slowly learned that the initial views on the cellular and molecular bases underlying its dynamics and that of the tumor vasculature were too simplistic and incomplete, in turn, these new insights are already having an impact on future tactics to improve current delivery approaches. This Review will revisit the origins of the observations supporting the existence of the EPR effect, and attempt to frame an updated view of the EPR effect in the context of more recent insights into the nature of the tumor vasculature and microenvironment, as well as that of nano-scale drug delivery systems.

Keywords: EPR effect, endothelial cells, pericytes, nanoparticles

* Corresponding Author: jkloster@mdanderson.org.

Abbreviations

area under the curve (AUC);
B-cell lymphoma 2 protein family (Bcl-2);
clear cell renal cell carcinoma (CCRCC);
cisplatin (CDDP);
cluster of differentiation 31 (CD31);
cluster of differentiation 44 (CD44);
maximum concentration (Cmax);
cancer stem cells (CSC);
diethylene triamine pentaacetic acid (DTPA);
doxorubicin (Dox);
docetaxel (DTXL);
dose-limiting toxicity (DLT);
endothelial cells (EC);
Enhanced Permeability and Retention (EPR);
extracellular matrix (ECM);
factor inhibiting HIF-1 (FIH);
human epidermal growth factor receptor-2 (HER-2);
anti-HER-2 MAb (Herceptin/Trastuzumab);
poly(N-(2-hydroxypropyl) methacrylamide) (HPMA);
hyaluronic Acid (HA);
hypoxia-inducing factor-1 (HIF-1α);
interstitial fluid pressure (IFP);
intraperitoneal (ip);
knock-out (KO);
lactadherin/SED1 (MFG-E8);
micellular (M);
monocloncal antibody (MAb);
mitomycin C (MMC);
mononuclear phagocyte system (MPS);
mother vessel (MV);
molecular weight (MW);
nanoparticle (NP);
octreotide (Oct);
pericytes (PC);
platelet derived growth factor (PDGF)/platelet derived growth factor receptor (PDGFR);
poly-ethylene glycol (PEG);
prostate specific membrane antigen (PSMA);
paclitaxel (PTX);
poly(vinyl alcohol) (PVA);
salinomycin (SAL);
micellular SAL (M-SAL);
smooth muscle cells (SMC);
somatostatin receptors (STTR);

transforming growth factor-beta (TGF-β);
vascular endothelial growth factor (VEGF)/vascular endothelial growth factor receptor (VEGFR);
venule basement membrane (VBM);
vesicular vacuolar organelle (VVO); X-linked inhibitor of apoptosis protein (XIAP)

Introduction

Effective drug delivery is a considered balance among competing dynamics: renal clearance/excretion, clearance by the cells of the mononuclear phagocyte system (MPS) in the liver, spleen and other organs, and uptake, retention and dispersion within the tumor microenvironment itself. Only after successful evasion of the clearance mechanisms can the Enhanced Permeability and Retention (EPR) effect even come into play. One of the increasingly clear aspects is that although the EPR effect is indeed operant in human clinical settings of malignant growth (and, e.g., inflammatory processes), it is likely to be highly heterogeneous; for a number of reasons and with few exceptions, no single histiotype of tumor will have broadly predictable responses, and no pre-clinical models will be adequately predictive of clinical outcomes. This Review will in part examine the cellular and molecular bases for this evident heterogeneity.

Materials science has recently offered almost unlimited opportunities to develop unique and multi-functional nanoparticles (NP; generally defined as structures with components < 100 nm in any dimension) supported by the concept that more complexity may lead to improved performance characteristics. However, to date the NP drug carriers which are clinically approved are few in number compared to the enormous number of early-stage candidates that may get no farther than initial *in vitro* evaluation with tumor cell lines, if even that far. Thus, a re-examination of the rationale underlying the development of these vast libraries of NP may be warranted. The bases for functionalization of these NP can be largely divided into those features associated with evasion of clearance mechanisms and those proposed to lead to receptor-specific uptake/internalization by tumor cells *in vivo*. One of the tenets that will be considered in this Review is to what extent these notions are in fact fulfilled in practice: in pre-clinical tumor models and even in the clinic.

There are clear trends in the effects of size, solution conformation, flexibility, and branching on the *in vivo* behavior of nanoscale drug carriers that reflect in part their initial interactions with these clearance mechanisms and subsequent traverse into the tumor microenvironment. 1) Increasing molecular weight generally decreases the opportunity for renal filtration, and thereby increases blood circulation time and resultant tumor accumulation, up to a threshold; 2) Increasing molecular size beyond ~100 nm typically increases clearance by the MPS, and thus decreases blood circulation time, as well as the opportunity for tumor extravasation; 3) Rigid, spherical polymers also have decreased renal filtration and longer blood circulation times compared with flexible and elongated polymers, whereas more rigid, tubular polymers can achieve higher tumor accumulation due to increased penetration of the porous tumor vasculature as an initial step in extravasation; and 4) For polymeric carriers, increasing the number of polymer arms decreases renal filtration due to decreased glomerular pore penetration and thus increases blood circulation time.

Ideally, the most suitable polymeric drug carrier will be removed from the body once it has delivered its drug payload, thus minimizing any side effects from the carrier itself.

Mechanisms Affecting NP Clearance

Renal Pathway

In order for the EPR effect to be exploited for delivery of therapeutic agents to tumors, the delivery platform must first survive various clearance mechanisms, at least for a sufficiently long time to allow opportunities for its extravasation via the tumor vasculature. In the kidney, the glomerular basement membrane and epithelial cell coat of the glomerulus consist of a matrix of collagen-like moieties and glycoproteins, which form pores with a cross-section measuring about 4 nm by 14 nm. Macromolecules with hydrodynamic radii smaller than this readily permeate those pores and are removed from the body via urine [1]. The threshold for renal filtration corresponds very roughly with molecular weights ranging from 30-50 kDa, depending on the polymer chemistry, hydrodynamic shape/conformation, and flexibility [2].

These parameters have been verified in recent studies for various NP formulations in this size range [3-6]. Once the hydrodynamic radius exceeds the renal threshold of ~ 5 nm, the filtration rate of macromolecules decreases with increasing radius, as long as other factors, such as molecular conformation and chemistry, remain constant [2]. Thus, the blood circulation t1/2, increases with increasing MW as a result of decreased filtration by the kidneys; in fact, non-degradable polymers that are too large to be excreted can be retained in the body for extended periods of time [7].

The shape and ability of a macromolecule to deform appear to impact its rate of glomerular filtration and thus blood circulation half-life. Multiple studies have compared the renal filtration rates of neutral or uncharged plasma proteins and polysaccharides. Therefore, the filtration rate of dextran, with a slightly ellipsoidal random coil conformation, is higher than that of globular proteins with equivalent hydrodynamic radii, such as horseradish peroxidase and ficoll [8-10]. A study of four differently shaped molecules with similar Stokes-Einstein radii, albumin, ficoll, hyaluronan (HA), and bikunin, also concluded that an elongated shape facilitated glomerular filtration [11]. Venturoli and Rippe have suggested that the flexibility, and hence molecular deformability, of a macromolecule plays a crucial role in the rate at which it permeates the glomerulus [12]. Their measurements showed that glomerular permeability was significantly higher when measured with flexible molecules such as dextran and ficoll than when measured with globular proteins. Cyclic polymers also have longer blood circulation in comparison to equivalent MW linear polymers. Nasongkla et al. [13] studied a family of linear and cyclic PEGylated poly-ε-caprolactones; the cyclic polymers had significantly longer blood circulation times than equivalent MW linear polymers, as a result of both the lack of a polymer chain end and an increased resistance to deformation [14], which hindered traverse through pores of the kidney.

It should be noted that many NP platforms are prepared with a coating or dispersant, in part to retain mono-dispersity in solution, which may also contribute to the net hydrodynamic volume. Further, this non-covalently bound shell is likely removed upon contact with the blood, due to proteins such as serum albumin (the most abundant) that effectively displace it [15, 16]. Thus, the NP may become buried within this protein complex, and the resulting hydrodynamic diameter markedly increased, perhaps beyond the critical 5 nm renal threshold—resulting in reduced clearance by the kidneys. These renal clearance dynamics appear to hold for NP with either positive or negative net zeta potentials.

MPS Pathway

Aside from the lower size threshold that is permissive for renal clearance, many studies including those originating in early development of liposome technology have shown that there is an upper limit for the window, as well -- ~ 100 nm -- in which NP blood circulation time and passive delivery mediated by the EPR effect are optimal; sizes greater than this increase MPS-mediated clearance [17-21]. The presence of this clearance mechanism has encouraged development of strategies to defeat or retard it, such as by interfering with plasma-derived opsonin binding to the NP [22, 23]. Opsonin proteins present in the blood bind to foreign particles to increase the probability for their detection by and binding to phagocytic cells. Aggregates or particles ≥ 200 nm diameter are readily bound with opsonin proteins and cleared by cells of the MPS, primarily resident in the liver and spleen. Opsonin proteins tend to bind and clear hydrophobic or charged polymers more readily than hydrophilic and neutral polymers, thus accelerating their removal by the liver [24]. The MPS can also degrade polymers, such as those containing peptide or ester linkages. Regarding charge characteristics, when the NP surface charges becomes strongly negative, excessive association with phagocytic cells of the MPS (principally liver Kupffer cells and splenic macrophages) also decreases circulation time [25, 26]; conversely, it has been observed that positively charged NP are cleared very rapidly due to local electrostatic interactions near the injection site [27]. Small NPs may either not be bound efficiently by plasma opsonins or by some other means evade binding by membrane receptors on Kupffer cells. Some studies have suggested that NP shape matters regarding MPS evasion and tumor delivery, and that the smallest diameter of the NP is the predominant determinant of clearance: the smaller being less-readily cleared [28, 29]. Liver clearance appears to be the predominant mechanism for larger NPs of many types [22, 30-32].

NPs that avoid initial phagocytosis by Kupffer cells then translocate through the fenestrated vascular endothelia of the liver into the Dissé spaces, where they are engulfed by hepatocytes and thus processed into the biliary canaliculi [33]. They are then subject to drainage via the biliary duct to the beginning of the small intestine and thereby excreted fecally. The charge dependence of this route appears to slightly favor positively charged NPs [34]. Overall, the trends reflect a general literature consensus: that tumor delivery correlates well with blood circulation time—longer circulation times result in improved tumor delivery--consistent with passive delivery via the dynamics of the EPR effect.

A polymer that survives both renal clearance and the MPS surveillance and is later cleared from the blood by normal tissues passes through the intercellular junctions in the post-capillary fenestrae and discontinuous capillaries in the vasculature. The major mechanism of transport into the interstitium is diffusion through small (~2-6 nm) gaps in the endothelial wall in normal vasculature, as well as passing the glycocalyx on endothelial cells (EC).

Extracellular fluid and solutes in the interstitium are drained by developed lymphatics in normal tissues and then returned to the blood [35].

Cellular and Biophysical Parameters Contributing to Heterogeneity of EPR Effect

Diverse Nature of Originating Vessels

One of the first levels at which the variability in the expression of the EPR effect is manifest lies in the diverse nature of the vessels that constitute the tumor vasculature, including mother vessels (MV), capillaries, glomeruloid microvascular proliferations, and vascular malformations [36]. The first of the developing blood vessel types is the MV [37, 38] that arises largely from pre-existing venules, which are characterized as large, hyperpermeable sinusoids. MV formation occurs via degradation of venule basement membranes (VBM), rigid structures that normally limit the expansion of the microvasculature [39], whereas MVs have lumens that are several-fold larger than those of the normal vessels from which they arise: hence, the need for VBM degradation to overcome this constraint. This process is regulated by both cathepsins and matrix metalloproteases [40]. VBM degradation both sheds pericyte (PC) coverage, due to the latter having lost their previous substrate, and results in a thinner endothelium, as an expanded surface area must be covered. There is some evidence that these different vessel types have differential responses to vascular endothelial growth factor (VEGF) that might account for differences in vessel permeability [41].

Pores in Vasculature

Another and perhaps more obvious source of heterogeneity in the EPR effect is the size distribution of the pores of various types in the tumor vasculature and the resultant hyper-permeability. As with the pores that form the basis for glomerular filtration in the kidney and with the mechanism for particle opsonization by the MPS, there is an inter-dependent relationship between parameters of particle size and the tumor vasculature pores. Being a key and complex issue for understanding tumor physiology, some studies date back more than 25 years.

Trans-endothelial cell fenestrations, caveolae, and unique vesicular vacuolar organelle (VVO) structures are present more frequently than inter-endothelial cell gaps in the tumor vasculature, and differ greatly in size distribution [42-44]. In solid tumors, the anatomic pore sizes of trans-endothelial cell fenestrations, caveolae and VVOs have been estimated by electron microscopy and differential permeability to macromolecular solutes to range from 40-200 nm [44-46], whereas the sizes of inter-endothelial cell gaps range widely, with estimates between 100 nm and 4700 nm [44, 47, 48]: another potential basis for marked variability in vessel permeability. This hyperpermeable nature of solid tumors allows particles smaller than the upper limits to extravasate into the tumor interstitium [49]. In contrast, adjacent normal vessels have a pore cutoff size generally indistinguishable from that of normal tissue.

Maeda and colleagues are credited with first recognizing the phenomenon they termed the *EPR effect* during studies of a conjugate of neocarzinostatin in the mid-1980's [50]; it was observed to accumulate in tumor tissue at much higher levels than in normal tissue. Due to the typically chaotic neovascularization of tumors and resultant architectural defects, the tumor vasculature is more permeable to macromolecules than is normal vasculature. The lymphatic system is also defective or even essentially nonexistent in tumor tissue, causing increased retention of macromolecules [47, 51]. These factors, combined with the interstitial volume of tumors typically being larger than for normal tissues [50], allows in totality for increased uptake and retention of macromolecules by tumors.

NP Structural Features

Murakami et al. studied the relationship between tumor accumulation and molecular weight (MW) using different MW poly-ethylene glycol (PEG) formulations in Meth-A fibrosarcomas [52]. For six different sized polymers, ranging from ~ 31 to ~ 200 kDa, they observed an increase in tumor accumulation correlating with an increase in MW. However, for polymers with MW greater than 215 kDa, they saw a decrease in tumor accumulation. Seymour et al. [53] measured higher levels of accumulation of 297 and 556 kDa poly(N-(2-hydroxypropyl)methacrylamide) (HPMA) in Sarcoma 180 tumors than accumulation of 778 kDa HPMA, suggesting a different upper limit in this model. While studying the pharmacokinetics and tumor accumulation of poly-vinyl alcohol (PVA), Tabata et al. observed an increase in the tumor accumulation after three hours for polymers having a hydrodynamic diameter of up to 60 nm; above this, accumulation levels decreased [54].

The importance of both shape and flexibility in dictating tumor uptake is exemplified when examining rigid and elongated polymers. A flexible, loosely coiled polymer could readily deform to pass through a pore in the tumor vasculature. Given that branching decreases the ability to deform, they should be filtered less readily by the renal glomerulus and circulate in the blood compartment longer. Polymers with less flexible, elongated conformations, or "rigid rod" conformations, have shown higher tumor accumulation than more flexible, elongated polymers. A study of poly-L-lysine conjugated with DTPA-Gd[29] [55] showed that at conjugation levels of ~ 90%, the polymer assumed an extended rigid rod conformation, leading to significantly higher signal enhancement than observed with randomly coiled, lesser conjugated polymer and albumin-DTPA-Gd controls. In addition, a larger signal was observed in the interior of the tumor than at its periphery, suggesting that the extended polymer was able to more effectively penetrate through the tumor interstitium.

High tumor accumulation of a rigid rod polymer was also observed [56] in the study of the pharmacokinetics and biodistribution of dendronized linear poly(4-hydroxystyrene), with some of the highest values for tumor accumulation being in the murine C26 colon carcinoma tumor model. Various *in vitro* and *in vivo* studies have shown greater diffusion coefficients for linear macromolecules than for globular macromolecules with equivalent radii [51]. It has been suggested that the extended conformation of rigid rod polymers enables them to more easily traverse openings in the tumor vasculature and through the tumor extracellular matrix (ECM), since they are less likely to entangle with the ECM.

PEG functionalization has long been of interest to create proteins and agents with prolonged circulation half-lives. A library of PEGylated polyester "bow-tie" dendrimers [57] established the relationship between branching and blood circulation time [57-59]. For a series of bow-ties with equivalent MW (about 40 kDa), there was an increase in t1/2, from ~ 1.4 h for the two-arm dendrimer, essentially a linear polymer, to ~ 26 h for the four-arm dendrimer, and finally to ~ 31 h for the eight-arm dendrimer [59]. Corresponding biodistribution studies in healthy mice showed no significant variation in tissue uptake among the three polymers and there was decreased polymer excreted in the urine with increased branching. Given that the blood circulation half-life increased with the number of arms while polymer excreted in the urine decreased, the slower rates of renal filtration for bow-ties with more arms may have resulted from a hindered ability to move through the glomerular pores. This polymer drug carrier studied in C26 colon carcinoma-bearing mice showed long blood circulation times and remarkable efficacy in delivering doxorubicin (Dox) to tumors, leading to their complete eradication, in sharp contrast to the ineffectiveness of free Dox [60].

In a related finding, Gerber and Radke [61] have separated star and linear polymers by 2D chromatography on the basis of their number of arms. Although their observations did not involve compounds with strictly equivalent MW, Bowen et al. observed [62] that proteins PEGylated with branched PEG chains also showed prolonged blood circulation half-lives and activities when compared with proteins PEGylated with a single PEG chain. This relationship between the number of branches and t1/2 also applies when branched polymers are compared with linear polymers. When PEGylated bow-tie dendrimers are compared with similar MW linear PEG, the dendrimer with linear PEG has a shorter blood circulation time [60, 63].

In an over-arching comparison of families of PEGylated dendrimers that did not possess either the same chemistry or the same branched architecture, Lim et al. [64] suggested that the most important parameter for determining blood circulation t1/2 of branched polymers was the number of arms and not their MW, chemistry, or branched architecture. Comparing their PEGylated triazine dendrimers with the PEGylated bow-tie dendrimers, they observed an increase in blood circulation t1/2 with an increase in the number of PEG chains. It has been noted that these triazine dendrimers may self-orient and aggregate in solution, and their hydrodynamic diameters should be measured before fully accepting this as a general conclusion.

Contrary to the view that the EPR effect is mostly dependent on Enhanced Permeability of the leaky tumor vasculature, Noguchi et al. proposed that it results primarily from prolonged Retention [65]. Using radiolabeled HPMA of MW broadly ranging from 4,500 to 800, 000 Da, they observed that all polymers were taken up into tumor tissue at approximately the same rate; however, polymers at the higher end of the size spectrum were unable to diffuse out of the tissue as rapidly as the smaller ones, presumably due to poor lymphatic activity.

VEGF Signaling

Another possible source of heterogeneity in manifestation of the EPR effect may reside in expression of vascular endothelial growth factor (VEGF) and its receptors (VEGF-R) in tumors, which have been found to vary spatially and temporally [66-70]. Hypoxia, hypoglycemia, and low pH have all been shown to up-regulate VEGF expression [71-73], and tumor interstitial pO_2 and pH are themselves both known to be spatially and temporally heterogeneous in distribution [74]. Thus, this complex and diverse pattern of expression in the VEGF pathway may contribute to heterogeneity in vascular permeability. Further, EC phenotypes and CD31 expression may be distinct in newly forming, remodeling, and regressing tumor vessels [75], as will be discussed more next.

Pericyte/Mural Cell Coverage, Post-Vessel Stroma and Extracellular Matrix (ECM)

Normal blood vessels are typically composed of two distinct cell types: endothelial cells (EC) which form the channels through which blood flows in the lumen, and mural cells, including pericytes (PC) and smooth muscle cells (SMC), which serve to support and stabilize the endothelium (Figure 1). In tumors, sprouting microvessels establish a plexus that keeps all tumor cells within a distance of 100–200 μm from their necessary blood supply [76]. During tumor growth, the vasculature develops as the angiogenic switch is intermittently turned on and off [77]. The imbalance between tumor cell growth and vascular formation may cause a collapse of tumor cells as well as the new vasculature. Resultant hypoxic areas exist heterogeneously in the majority of human solid cancer tissues [78].

This new tumor vascular architecture is considered "immature" and differs from normal (or mature) vascular structures in many ways. Immature vessels lack distinct vascular organization and hierarchy and are unevenly distributed within tumor tissue. They are frequently irregularly shaped, tortuous and dilated. As a result of impaired cell-to-cell attachment, abnormal basement membranes, and increased permeability, these new microvessels are typically leaky and unable to sustain balanced intravascular pressure gradients, which can lead to interstitial hypertension. ECs in the tumor vasculature are dependent on cell survival factors, in contrast to ECs in the mature vasculature of normal tissues [79]. PCs help to mediate EC survival and maturation in normal vasculature, but are abnormal in the tumor vasculature [80] (Figure 2).

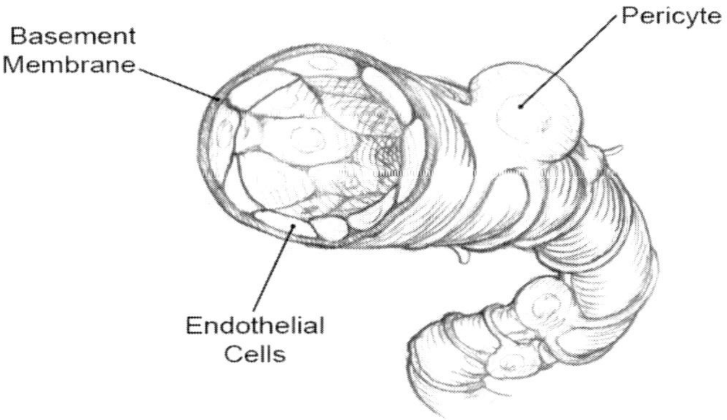

Figure 1. Depiction of cellular and structural features of blood vessel in normal tissue. A channel lined with a basement membrane (BM) is encased with pericytes (PC) and other mural cells; PC serves to constrain and regulate normal vessel outgrowth and provide physical support to the vessel. The lumen of the vessel is lined with endothelial cells (EC), which are closely spaced with gap junctions that serve to control fluid and solute movement from the lumen to the extra-vascular tissue.

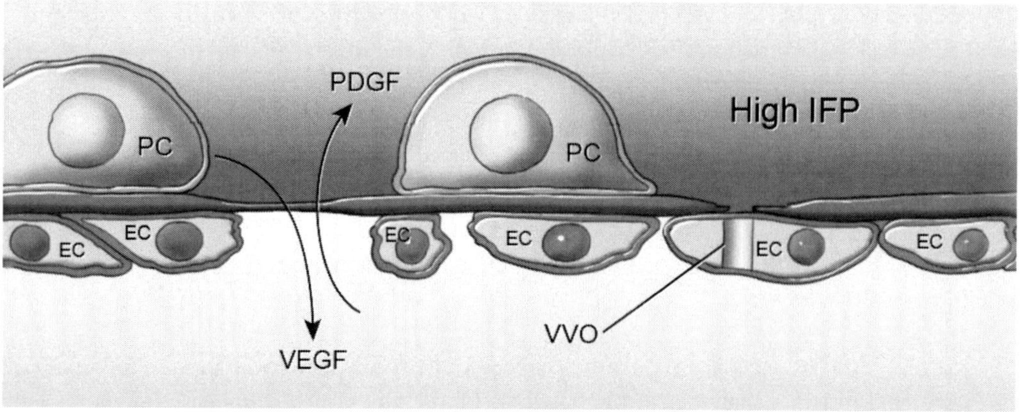

Figure 2. Schematic of cross-section of tumor vessel, showing intercellular communication pathways and structural features that regulate NP extravasation. ECs in the immature tumor vasculature are usually dependent on a continuous source of VEGF, unlike mature vasculature; PC, though generally less abundant than with normal vessels, may contribute VEGF in a paracrine manner; in turn, EC may support PC by paracrine release of PDGF. Sections of the vessel denuded of EC on the luminal aspect--and thereby incapable of sustaining normal gap junctions, thin or fenestrated BM, and transcytosis through vesicular vacuolar organelles (VVO) in EC, are examples of exploitable opportunities for NP extravasation, although resisted by high interstitial fluid pressure (IFP), in part due to inadequate lymphatic function.

Most functional studies have focused on the responses of ECs to pro-angiogenic stimuli; indeed, there is mounting evidence that the supporting mural cells, particularly PCs, may play key regulatory roles in both promoting vessel growth as well as in terminating vessel growth to generate a mature, quiescent normal vasculature. However, tumor vessels are characterized by numerous structural and functional abnormalities, including altered EC/PC associations. These dysfunctional, unstable vessels contribute to hypoxia, increased interstitial fluid pressure (IFP), and enhanced susceptibility to metastatic invasion. PCs are usually absent in the tumor vasculature or have only loose associations with ECs, leaving most of the tumor microvessels immature. In normal blood vessels, PCs and ECs are surrounded by a basement membrane (BM) that contains laminin, collagen type IV, nidogen, and heparin sulfate proteoglycans, and which is a source of growth factors for both ECs and PCs [81-83]. In tumor vessels, this (BM) has defects in its structure and composition and can provide a productive environment for metastatic malignant epithelial cells and proliferating ECs [84]. Increasing evidence points to PCs as critical regulators of endothelial activation and subsequent vessel development, stability, and function.

The molecular crosstalk between PCs and ECs during angiogenesis is not well understood. Activated ECs sprout and form an endothelial tube, a lumen with an EC lining. These ECs stop proliferating and secrete platelet-derived growth factor (PDGF) to recruit PCs and progenitor PCs (e.g., from the bone marrow), which express PDGF receptors (PDGF-Rs) [85]. Recruited PCs proliferate and encapsulate these new channels. Newly-formed vessels that are enveloped with PCs mature and stop remodeling [86]. PCs react to PDGF-β secreted by EC tip cells at newly formed vascular sprouts by first migrating along the PDGF-β gradient, and then by proliferating [87, 88]. In turn, PCs increase expression of cell-bound VEGF-α during maturation and recruitment into newly formed vessels [89] (Figure 2). PCs produce VEGF-α that acts in a paracrine fashion combined with autocrine expression of

VEGF-α by tumor ECs [90]. Recruitment of PCs to angiogenic sprouts is closely correlated to enhanced BM production [91]. In normal tissues, PCs must be in apposition to ECs to confer induction of VEGF-α and Bcl-ω, possibly because of the requirement to deposit BM products within close range of the EC (Figure 1); however, this may not be needed in the case of tumor angiogenesis, where PCs are frequently loosely attached to the vasculature [92].

Stimulation of ECs by extracellular VEGF-α induces several anti-apoptotic signaling proteins, including Bcl-2, survivin and XIAP [93, 94]. The primary cell-autonomous function of VEGF-α in ECs is thought to be promotion of survival, although the molecular mechanism has not been fully explored [95]. Autocrine VEGF-α from PCs leads to induction of the anti-apoptotic protein, Bcl-ω.

Based on these insights regarding EC/PC relationships, some pre-clinical studies have begun to probe the role of PC coverage of tumor vasculature on uptake of nanoscale drug delivery systems [96, 97] and to characterize histopathological sections of human tumors to ascertain the clinical relevance of the pre-clinical models. There was a general trend for therapeutically-resistant tumors to have greater PC coverage than those that were sensitive [98]. These Investigators proposed transforming growth factor-beta (TGF-β) inhibitors to be used in conjunction with nanoscale delivery systems as a means to reduce PC coverage [99] and increase NP accumulation in stroma-rich tumor models [100-102].

Taking this approach further, the clinical relevance of PC coverage in terms of prognosis has come under investigation [98]. For example, in clear cell renal cell carcinoma (CCRCC), it has been demonstrated that higher values of PC coverage were associated with higher tumor grades, higher tumor stages, higher necrosis rates, and an unfavorable prognosis, and that vessels resistant to anti-angiogenic therapy were mainly those supported by PC [103]. These Investigators noted an uneven distribution of differentiated vessels, as well as reduced density of differentiated vessels in the tumor interior, suggesting that some of the inner vessels may have disappeared as the tumor invaded surrounding tissues. Also, the higher PC value for inner tumor vessels suggests that those surviving vessels rely more on PCs to resist the microenvironment. This finding is very different from a report in breast cancer, in which poor PC coverage coupled with higher expression of the met proto-oncogene (hepatocyte growth factor receptor) was correlated with a worse prognosis [104, 105].

Hypoxia is a common feature of many solid tumors leading to hypoxia-inducing factor-1 (HIF-1) stabilization, which in turn stimulates the growth of new blood vessels, facilitates the adaptation of tumor cells to changes in the microenvironment and promotes their invasion and survival [106-110]. Many experimental studies support the hypothesis that HIF-1 acts as a tumor promotor, although in certain models, the opposite effect has been observed [111, 112]. Factor inhibiting HIF-1 (FIH) is expressed in certain malignancies, like human renal cell carcinoma, follicular lymphoma, non-small cell lung carcinomas and invasive breast cancer [113-115]. The signaling pathways that are activated in FIH-overexpressing tumor cells are sufficient to stimulate the recruitment of immature PCs that are associated with enhanced tumor growth [116], but fail to induce a more mature PC phenotype. Nevertheless, alpha-smooth muscle actin (α-SMA) positive mural cells were able to reduce vessel leakiness, since dextran could no longer extravasate from α-SMA-(+) vessels. Moreover, FIH overexpression reduced the overall percentage of leaky vessels in the tumors. Therefore, enhanced vessel maturation in these tumors led to a reduction in overall vessel leakiness, consequently facilitating delivery of oxygen and nutrients to the tumor tissue and finally resulting in increased tumor growth.

MFG-E8 (also called lactadherin and SED1) is a glycoprotein that has multiple domains and binds to multiple ligands [117-120], and PDGFR-β(+) PCs, PC precursors, or both are a major source. MFG-E8 accumulation in tumors was primarily perivascular and MFG-E8 staining co-localized with PCs more than with ECs [121]. Assessment of vascular structures in B16 melanomas in control and MFG-E8 KO mice revealed significant differences that were consequential; vessel density and PC coverage were reduced, and vascular permeability was increased in tumors in MFG-E8 KO mice. These alterations were associated with decreased malignant cell proliferation and delayed tumor growth.

Interstitial Fluid Pressure (IFP)

Only a minor fraction of systemically-administered NP end up in tumors; NP do not have any inherent host propulsive forces driving them out of circulation and into a tumor target [122], To the contrary, elevated tumor interstitial fluid pressure (IFP) is a hindrance to drug delivery due to weakening of fluid pressure gradients that normally would produce rapid, flow-based convective penetration into tumors [123]; the result is diffusion-limited, random distribution and restriction of transvascular drug transport across vessel walls into tumors and through the tumor interstitium [28].

The IFP remains at elevated levels due to both high vascular permeability and poor lymphatic development and only decreases at the tumor periphery. This elevated IFP not only results in diminished NP extravasation, but even in outward interstitial fluid movement at the tumor periphery; the net outcome is poor delivery of drugs to the tumor interior and even drug egress. This outward interstitial fluid movement has been estimated to be ~ 0.1–0.2 μm/s for a 1 cm isolated tumor [51].

Vascular normalization in response to anti-angiogenic therapies can remodel tumor vessel abnormalities, such as the large heterogeneous pores that underlie leakiness [124, 125]. Effects on the delivery of slowly-diffusing nano-scale therapeutics, following vessel normalization induced by anti-VEGF-receptor-2 (VEGFR2) antibody, due to the competing dynamics of reducing IFP vs. increasing hydrodynamic steric hindrance from pore size reduction were analyzed [126]. In an orthotropic breast tumor model, therapeutics in the 1–12 nm range had the most rapid tumor penetration, whereas larger therapeutics (125–250 nm) extravasated poorly. Convection was observed to predominate at smaller vascular pore sizes, whereas increasing the pore size beyond ~140 nm hindered delivery due to rising IFP and possibly interaction with the intra-tumoral ECM: thus, leading to limited convection and rendering diffusion alone dominant.

The therapeutic relevance of these modulations was then further characterized using two clinically-approved nanoscale drugs: Doxil, with a diameter of ~100 nm, and Abraxane, which although formulated at ~130 nm achieves a size of only ~10 nm upon dilution in plasma. In an orthotopic breast xenograft model, both Doxil and Abraxane arms induced similar growth delays; however, vascular normalization with anti-VEGFR2 antibody only enhanced the effectiveness of the smaller Abraxane, but not that of the larger Doxil. Since physical principles dictate that both diffusive and convective penetration are favored for smaller particles [127-130], the latter (Abraxane) may best take advantage of the EPR effect responsible for the improved toxicity profiles for nanomedicines [131]. In this manner, the outcomes for therapeutics functionalized with either vascular-targeted tumor-penetrating ligands—to enhance nanoparticle penetration—or tumor cell-targeting ligands--to improve cellular uptake—may be constrained, since they cannot overcome barriers exacerbated by increasingly larger size [28].

It is also known that the IFP in tumor tissue is higher in the interior than at the periphery, and while convective flow out of the tumor has been suggested but never directly measured, the outward driving force of pressure may decrease the ability of larger polymers to pass deeper into the tumor tissue [123, 124]. Thus, accumulation in the tumor initially increases with increasing MW; however, this trend can reverse at very high MWs.

Evidence for and Against Benefit of Active Targeting Post-EPR-mediated Uptake

Once the nanoscale drug delivery platform has run the gauntlet from its point of injection, traversed through the bloodstream—avoiding both renal and MPS-mediated clearance, and diffused into and taken up residence within the tumor interstitial volume via the EPR effect, what may occur next is also complex. NP internalization has been demonstrated, at least in *in vitro* settings, with many cell types, including non-phagocytic cells [132, 133]. Polymer molecules in the interstitial space of healthy tissue and tumor tissue can be taken up by cells via endocytosis at rates that are dependent on the affinity of the polymer for the cell surface. It has long been thought that most inert synthetic polymers can be internalized by fluid-phase pinocytosis [7]. Once in the cell, polymeric carriers are generally trafficked to late endosomes and lysosomes for degradation. Nevertheless, many synthetic polymers may not be degraded by the lysosomal environment and instead accumulate in vesicles within the cell, which may have longer-term toxic consequences.

To attempt to separate and establish the relative contributions to tumor targeting of those features of NPs that are linked to the EPR effect vs. those that are linked to specific, receptor-mediated internalization, the results from a number of drug delivery systems will be presented here; these include those targeting the cell-surface proteoglycan family, CD44, somatostatin receptors (STTR), human epidermal growth factor receptor-2 (HER-2), and prostate specific membrane antigen (PSMA), all extra-cellular determinants.

CD44

HA-modified Liposomes

Peer and Margilit developed liposomes that were modified by covalent anchoring of hyaluronan (HA), the natural ligand for CD44, to their surface [134]. It had been shown *in vitro* that these liposomes bound with high affinity to cells and to ECM via specific recognition sites [135-140]. They hypothesized that surface-bound HA may serve two roles: the hydrophilic coat could promote long circulation by interference with opsonization, thereby better exploiting the EPR effect; and HA could also act as a specific CD44-targeting agent. To test this hypothesis, they examined both the biodistribution and the anti-tumor activity of mitomycin C (MMC) encapsulated in small unilamellar liposomes with HA bound to their surface (termed tHA-LIP).

Formulating MMC in liposomes extended its clearance time compared to free MMC, both for non-targeted liposomes (termed nt-LIP) and much more so for tHA-LIP, with AUC ratios for tHA-LIP/nt-LIP and tHA-LIP/free MMC approaching ~1 $\log_{10}$ and ~2 $\log_{10}$, respectively. This strongly supported a predominantly stealthing function of the HA coating, since one would expect that targeting HA receptors (e.g., on the ECM) would reduce rather than increase plasma circulation time. Regarding tissue distribution, at the single 6 hr time-point examined, the rank order of MMC uptake was free drug > nt-LIP > tHA-LIP; in liver and spleen, encapsulation in the tHA-LIP lowered MMC uptake significantly compared to both free drug and to MMC in nt-LIP. This order was inverted for MMC uptake into tumor: ~ four-fold and 30-fold higher for tHA-LIP compared to nt-LIP and to free MMC, respectively. Examination at an additional later time-point would have allowed direct assessment of whether sustained retention was lower for the free vs. the liposomal MMC, as expected for EPR dynamics with small molecules.

This biodistribution profile generally predicted anti-tumor efficacy observed in mice bearing B16F10.9 syngeneic melanoma, which develop a lung metastatic burden reflected in increased lung weights. Only treatment with the MMC-loaded tHA-LIP reduced the metastatic burden significantly, i.e., only a modest increase in lung weight and a concomitant small number of lung metastasis. This was also reflected in the survival data; treatment with MMC-loaded tHA-LIP generated a significant increase in survival compared to either free MMC or to MMC-loaded nt-LIP. In a C57BL/6 mouse model bearing D122-derived lung metastases from the HA-receptor-over-expressing Lewis Lung Carcinoma [141], survival trends were also similar; survival in groups treated with saline, free MMC or MMC-loaded nt-LIP was poor, whereas treatment with MMC-loaded tHA-LIP was quite effective.

Overall, in these models, the anti-tumor effects of the HA-decorated, MMC-bearing liposomes were consistently superior to those of the non-targeted liposomes and certainly to those for free MMC. The biodistribution data alone suggest that most of this was likely due to the hydrophilic nature of the HA coating, serving to impede opsonization and allow greater exploitation of the EPR effect; however, post-EPR effects occurring within the tumor interstitium may also have been enhanced by HA-mediated, receptor-specific internalization of the tHA-LIP by tumor cells, as the *in vitro* results would suggest. However, a more definitive control to settle this question, beyond the intent of the original investigation, would have been to coat MMC-containing liposomes with a non-specific polymeric sugar, to impart hydrophilicity without a specific targeting component.

In a subsequent study [142], these Investigators made related observations using Doxorubicin (Dox)-loaded liposomes, with an important additional Doxil control that allowed them to indirectly address the mechanistic question raised in the preceding section. Regarding pharmacokinetics, as with free MMC, free Dox was removed rapidly from the systemic circulation, but clearance was prolonged by liposomal encapsulation, the retardation being least for the nt-LIP, but more significant for both Doxil and tHA-LIP. As they noted, "...both Doxil and tHA-LIP probably benefited from their combination of small sizes and hydrophilic coats": thus, supporting the previous conjecture regarding the role of a hydrophilic coat and de-emphasizing the role of HA-specific interactions.

Biodistribution studies revealed that when delivered as a tHA-LIP formulation, Dox accumulation in the tumor was 30-fold higher than when the drug was administered in free form, about seven-fold higher than when delivered through nt-LIP, and about three-fold higher when delivered with Doxil. It is tempting to speculate that this edge over Doxil may have been due to CD44 targeting. This possibility could be assessed by pre-blocking with free HA or by use of CD44(-) tumor models. These Investigators went on to demonstrate that Dox encapsulated in tHA-LIP generated significant improvements in several parameters of anti-tumor activity in both syngeneic mouse tumor models and in human tumor xenografts, with the commonality among them being over-expression of HA receptors [142-144].

HA-backbone Drug Conjugate

Multiple randomized trials have demonstrated that intraperitoneal (ip) therapy with cisplatin (CDDP) and paclitaxel (PTX) can improve survival in patients with optimally debulked advanced ovarian cancer [145-152]. The key pharmacologic principle underlying this approach is that when these drugs are administered by the ip route, they are delivered to peritoneal tumor nodules both via capillary flow (systemically) as well as by free surface diffusion within the peritoneum. To better target CDDP to CD44(+) ovarian cancer cells, large nano- or micron-sized particles were generated by co-incubating CDDP and HA under stoichiometrically-controlled conditions resulting in cross-linking between the free HA carboxyl groups and the chloride groups of the CDDP, a ligand replacement reaction, generating Hyplat [153]. Hyplat could still bind strongly to and kill CD44(+) human ovarian carcinoma cell lines, but not CD44(-) UCI101 cells. In pharmacokinetic studies, free CDDP was rapidly cleared from the peritoneal cavity and the plasma levels also peaked rapidly; Hyplat was cleared substantially more slowly from the peritoneal cavity and its plasma Cmax occurred later and levels were slower to fall, as expected since it has been shown that particle size is an important determinant of peritoneal clearance [154]. Mice that received Pt-equivalent ip doses of free CDDP or Hyplat were studied for tissue distribution. Free CDDP Pt levels rose rapidly in all tested organs, particularly high levels being in the kidneys; the rate of renal elimination of Pt was much slower for Hyplat than for free CDDP. Nude mice implanted ip with human ovarian carcinoma cells were subsequently injected with either CDDP or Hyplat at their respective MTDs. The Pt levels in the CD44(+) tumor nodules were two- to three-fold higher following Hyplat administration compared to CDDP; no significant difference was found in the CD44(-) tumor model: suggesting HA-mediated specific uptake. For equivalent levels of renal accumulation of Pt, the site of dose-limiting toxicity (DLT) for CDDP, Hyplat delivered three-fold more Pt to the tumor. The overall survival on day 100 for untreated, CDDP-treated and Hyplat-treated mice was 10%, 42.9% and 85.7%, respectively. The enhanced delivery of Pt to the tumor and resultant survival benefit may be due to both the prolonged exposure of Hyplat in the peritoneal cavity and the ability of Hyplat to target to CD44; the relative contributions cannot currently be distinguished.

STTR

Somatostatin receptors (SSTR) have been investigated as potential tumor targets since they are overexpressed in most neuroendocrine tumors and many other tumors compared to normal tissues [155, 156]. Octreotide (Oct) is an octapeptide analog of endogenous SST and mainly binds to STTR [157], making Oct a potential ligand for targeted delivery to SSTR(+) tumors. Salinomycin (SAL), a polyether antibiotic, has recently been shown to have antitumor properties, owing to its ability to reduce the proportion of cancer stem cells (CSC) by >100 fold relative to PTX [158]. However, SAL has poor aqueous solubility and nanoscale delivery systems loaded with anti-CSC drugs improved solubility and were more effective than the free drugs [159].

To explore this approach, polymeric micelles were developed to both overcome the solubility limitation as well as to improve the biodistribution of SAL [160].In an MCF-7 human breast cancer xenograft model, a significantly enhanced anti-tumor effect was observed with combination therapy of Oct-modified micelles bearing PTX (Oct-M-PTX) plus micellular Sal (M-SAL) over either of the monotherapy groups. The antitumor effect of Oct-M-PTX was much stronger than the non-targeted micellular formulation, M-PTX, or Taxol, suggesting a combined effect of passive targeting via the EPR effect and enhanced intracellular delivery via STTR-mediated targeting. M-SAL alone produced significant tumor inhibition, while free SAL showed only slight tumor inhibition. Compared to free SAL, M-SAL was more effective in suppressing breast CSC, attributed to exploiting passive targeting via the EPR effect [45, 161].

HER-2

Since the introduction of human epidermal growth factor receptor-2 (HER-2) targeted therapeutic agents, including the MAb, Herceptin/Trastuzumab, and HER-2 kinase inhibitors, the prognosis of HER-2(+) breast cancer patients has markedly improved [Reviewed in [162]], although not without controversy [163, 164]. Different modes of administration, duration, and combinations with chemotherapy have been evaluated. Currently one year of trastuzumab in combination with or after chemotherapy is standard adjuvant therapy; in the neoadjuvant setting, the addition of this MAb to chemotherapy has resulted in a significantly higher activity compared to the latter alone.

These clinical results have continued the interest in pre-clinical development of HER-2-targeted chemotherapeutics. One study of liposome targeting demonstrated that anti-HER-2 MAb tethered to the liposome surface failed to increase accumulation to HER-2(+) tumor tissue compared to control; the pharmacokinetic profiles were essentially indistinguishable [165]. In another similar study, HER-2-MAb coated poly(DL-lactic acid) NP and control NP were also indistinguishable in terms of biodistribution [166]. These studies supported the notion that initial extravasation and successful exploitation of the EPR effect is an over-riding determinant compared to ligand-mediated tumor uptake.

PSMA

Prostate-specific membrane antigen (PSMA) is a Type II transmembrane glycoprotein enzyme with an extracellular domain bearing defined epitopes; it is over-expressed on the surface of prostate cancer cells and in the neovasculature in most solid tumors [167]. Using an anti-PSMA aptamer [168], an aptamer-directed NP encapsulating docetaxel (DTXL) and based on a platform selected from a library of over 100 compositions of approved biomaterials with varied parameters of size, surface hydrophilicity, targeting ligand density, drug loading, and drug release was synthesized and evaluated for biodistribution and antitumor efficacy [169]. Circulating NPs had a plasma half-life of ~24 hour in rats, reflecting retarded clearance via the MPS and successful incorporation of stealthing characteristics. Compared to free DTXL, encapsulation in NP greatly retarded DTXL distribution from the plasma, as expected.

Efficacy studies in mice bearing PSMA(+) human LNCaP prostate carcinoma xenografts revealed that treatment with PSMA-targeted DTXL-loaded NPs resulted in tumor regression superior to that from treatment with the non-targeted DTXL-loaded NPs or with free DTXL [168]. It is interesting to note that the separation in the tumor growth curves took several weeks after the end of the four-dose regiment to become significant. The two NP formulations were essentially indistinguishable in efficacy when evaluated in PSMA(-) xenograft models, again supporting a role and benefit to molecular targeting with this NP construct.

These Investigators stated: "The similar effects of targeted and nontargeted NPs in non–PSMA-expressing tumors were presumably due to increased tumor drug accumulation by means of the EPR effect." Conversely, absent direct measurement of tumor drug levels in the PSMA(+) model, the possible inference that the targeted NP DTXL formulation achieved higher levels in the tumors than the non-targeted may not be a correct attribution. Only comparisons of free DTXL and the PSMA-targeted NP-DTXL in the PSMA(+) LnCAP model were reported. One might expect that initial uptake via the EPR effect would be very similar for both the targeted and non-targeted NP---and the early anti-tumor effects are consistent with that; perhaps the longer-term benefit observed is attributable solely to post-EPR intracellular uptake in this model.

Conclusion

This Review has attempted to take a global and bottom-up approach to a deeper understanding of each of the multitude of major factors that underlie and contribute to the EPR effect. As each of the individual factors contributes its own inherent variability to the integrated whole, a recurring theme that strongly emerges can be summarized in one word: heterogeneity---heterogeneity borne of the chaos associated with tumor growth. With that realization also comes a sense that the current quest for ever-more complex NP structures and their subsequent functionalizations, particularly with regard to targeting moieties, may be somewhat over-zealous and misguided. As noted, some evidence does exist that active targeting, defined typically as invoking affinity-based interactions to specifically bind to a cancer-relevant molecular determinant such as a receptor, provides at least some advantage over NP delivery systems that are without such targeting. Nevertheless, the major issues remain most pertinent to tumor localization and delivery: surviving both renal and MPS-mediated clearance mechanisms and staying in circulation long enough to complete the traverse from the plasma through the pores in the tumor vascular BM, EC/PC and ECM barriers—and doing so without the benefit of convective forces and against the tumor IFP gradient. Only after successfully running this gauntlet would the capability of receptor-mediated internalization likely demonstrate any benefit in terms of higher delivered tumor drug levels and resultant greater anti-tumor efficacy. Some of these issues and their impact on the EPR effect have been broached in recent excellent reviews [170-172].

We live in an age where cost-containment of medical care is an unavoidable and vexing issue. Every aspect of health care delivery is undergoing increased scrutiny for demonstration of benefit, including the very drugs used in such care, and the associated costs of bringing new therapeutics through regulatory approval. To that end, the hope is that this Review will be thought provoking on a number of fronts. First, nanotechnology as applied to cancer medicine should increasingly disengage the bench-centric mindset that NP formulation has endless possibilities; rather, exploitation of the EPR effect remains the foremost goal, secondary targeting and intracellular distribution playing roles of lesser significance, as recently noted [173]. Secondly, although additional NP functionalization may be feasible and justifiable under some circumstances, the impact on final NP production costs and the potential for added complexities for subsequent regulatory approval must be justified by intended benefit to patient outcomes. Finally, given the emerging realization that EPR dynamics are expressed in a heterogeneous fashion, varying not only across tumor histiotypes, but also from patient-to-patient, and likely even within the same host harboring multiple tumors, strategies to better align those patients likely to benefit most from NP-based drug delivery need to be developed. If informed *a priori* patient selection could be conducted based on the demonstrated existence of adequate EPR responses for current nanoscale drug formulations as well as for those in the approval pipeline, patients could be spared from therapies unlikely to benefit them, and those new drug candidates most likely to advance to further clinical evaluation could be more rapidly identified. In this light, assessment of the EPR effect might become as significant a component of patient profiling and informed treatment planning as the current "omics"-oriented assessments.

Acknowledgments

The Authors wish to thank Amy Sisson, M.L.S., for expert assistance with manuscript preparation.

References

[1] M. A. Venkatachalam, H. G. Rennke, The structural and molecular basis of glomerular filtration, *Circulation research*, 43 (1978) 337-347.

[2] R. Duncan, The dawning era of polymer therapeutics, Nature reviews. *Drug discovery*, 2 (2003) 347-360.

[3] H. S. Choi, W. Liu, F. Liu, K. Nasr, P. Misra, M. G. Bawendi, J.V. Frangioni, Design considerations for tumour-targeted nanoparticles, *Nature nanotechnology*, 5 (2010) 42-47.

[4] H. S. Choi, W. Liu, P. Misra, E. Tanaka, J. P. Zimmer, B. Itty Ipe, M. G. Bawendi, J. V. Frangioni, Renal clearance of quantum dots, *Nature biotechnology*, 25 (2007) 1165-1170.

[5] J. F. Hainfeld, D. N. Slatkin, T. M. Focella, H. M. Smilowitz, Gold nanoparticles: a new X-ray contrast agent, *The British journal of radiology*, 79 (2006) 248-253.

[6] H. Kobayashi, S. Kawamoto, S. K. Jo, H. L. Bryant, Jr., M. W. Brechbiel, R. A. Star, Macromolecular MRI contrast agents with small dendrimers: pharmacokinetic differences between sizes and cores, *Bioconjugate chemistry*, 14 (2003) 388-394.

[7] R. Duncan, J. Kopeček, Soluble synthetic polymers as potential drug carriers, in: *Polymers in Medicine*, Springer, 1984, pp. 51-101.

[8] D. Asgeirsson, D. Venturoli, E. Fries, B. Rippe, C. Rippe, Glomerular sieving of three neutral polysaccharides, polyethylene oxide and bikunin in rat. Effects of molecular size and conformation, *Acta physiologica*, 191 (2007) 237-246.

[9] M. P. Bohrer, W. M. Deen, C. R. Robertson, J. L. Troy, B. M. Brenner, Influence of molecular configuration on the passage of macromolecules across the glomerular capillary wall, *The Journal of general physiology*, 74 (1979) 583-593.

[10] H. G. Rennke, M. A. Venkatachalam, Glomerular permeability of macromolecules. Effect of molecular configuration on the fractional clearance of uncharged dextran and neutral horseradish peroxidase in the rat, *The Journal of clinical investigation*, 63 (1979) 713-717.

[11] M. Ohlson, J. Sorensson, K. Lindstrom, A. M. Blom, E. Fries, B. Haraldsson, Effects of filtration rate on the glomerular barrier and clearance of four differently shaped molecules, American journal of physiology. *Renal physiology*, 281 (2001) F103-113.

[12] D. Venturoli, B. Rippe, Ficoll and dextran vs. globular proteins as probes for testing glomerular permselectivity: effects of molecular size, shape, charge, and deformability, American journal of physiology. *Renal physiology*, 288 (2005) F605-613.

[13] N. Nasongkla, B. Chen, N. Macaraeg, M. E. Fox, J. M. Frechet, F. C. Szoka, Dependence of pharmacokinetics and biodistribution on polymer architecture: effect of cyclic versus linear polymers, *Journal of the American Chemical Society*, 131 (2009) 3842-3843.

[14] W. Burchard, Theory of cyclic macromolecules, in: *Cyclic polymers*, Springer, 1986, pp. 43-84.

[15] Y. Pan, A. Leifert, D. Ruau, S. Neuss, J. Bornemann, G. Schmid, W. Brandau, U. Simon, W. Jahnen-Dechent, Gold nanoparticles of diameter 1.4 nm trigger necrosis by oxidative stress and mitochondrial damage, *Small*, 5 (2009) 2067-2076.

[16] C. Rocker, M. Potzl, F. Zhang, W. J. Parak, G. U. Nienhaus, A quantitative fluorescence study of protein monolayer formation on colloidal nanoparticles, *Nature nanotechnology*, 4 (2009) 577-580.

[17] W. S. Enochs, G. Harsh, F. Hochberg, R. Weissleder, Improved delineation of human brain tumors on MR images using a long-circulating, superparamagnetic iron oxide agent, Journal of magnetic resonance imaging: *JMRI*, 9 (1999) 228-232.

[18] S. E. McNeil, Nanotechnology for the biologist, *Journal of leukocyte biology*, 78 (2005) 585-594.

[19] A. Moore, E. Marecos, A. Bogdanov, Jr., R. Weissleder, Tumoral distribution of long-circulating dextran-coated iron oxide nanoparticles in a rodent model, *Radiology*, 214 (2000) 568-574.

[20] C. Zimmer, R. Weissleder, K. Poss, A. Bogdanova, S. C. Wright, Jr., W. S. Enochs, MR imaging of phagocytosis in experimental gliomas, *Radiology*, 197 (1995) 533-538.

[21] C. Zimmer, S. C. Wright, Jr., R. T. Engelhardt, G. A. Johnson, C. Kramm, X. O. Breakefield, R. Weissleder, Tumor cell endocytosis imaging facilitates delineation of the glioma-brain interface, *Experimental neurology*, 143 (1997) 61-69.

[22] W. H. De Jong, W. I. Hagens, P. Krystek, M. C. Burger, A. J. Sips, R. E. Geertsma, Particle size-dependent organ distribution of gold nanoparticles after intravenous administration, *Biomaterials*, 29 (2008) 1912-1919.

[23] J. V. Jokerst, T. Lobovkina, R. N. Zare, S.S. Gambhir, Nanoparticle PEGylation for imaging and therapy, *Nanomedicine*, 6 (2011) 715-728.

[24] D. E. Owens, 3rd, N. A. Peppas, Opsonization, biodistribution, and pharmacokinetics of polymeric nanoparticles, *International journal of pharmaceutics*, 307 (2006) 93-102.

[25] S. M. Moghimi, S. S. Davis, Innovations in avoiding particle clearance from blood by Kupffer cells: cause for reflection, *Critical reviews in therapeutic drug carrier systems*, 11 (1994) 31-59.

[26] S. M. Moghimi, A. C. Hunter, J. C. Murray, Long-circulating and target-specific nanoparticles: theory to practice, *Pharmacological reviews*, 53 (2001) 283-318.

[27] C. Chouly, D. Pouliquen, I. Lucet, J. J. Jeune, P. Jallet, Development of superparamagnetic nanoparticles for MRI: effect of particle size, charge and surface nature on biodistribution, *Journal of microencapsulation*, 13 (1996) 245-255.

[28] V. P. Chauhan, T. Stylianopoulos, Y. Boucher, R. K. Jain, Delivery of molecular and nanoscale medicine to tumors: transport barriers and strategies, *Annual review of chemical and biomolecular engineering*, 2 (2011) 281-298.

[29] K. S. Chu, W. Hasan, S. Rawal, M. D. Walsh, E. M. Enlow, J. C. Luft, A. S. Bridges, J. L. Kuijer, M. E. Napier, W. C. Zamboni, J. M. Desimone, Plasma, tumor and tissue pharmacokinetics of Docetaxel delivered via nanoparticles of different sizes and shapes in mice bearing SKOV-3 human ovarian carcinoma xenograft, *Nanomedicine*, 9 (2013) 686-693.

[30] S. K. Balasubramanian, J. Jittiwat, J. Manikandan, C. N. Ong, L. E. Yu, W. Y. Ong, Biodistribution of gold nanoparticles and gene expression changes in the liver and spleen after intravenous administration in rats, *Biomaterials*, 31 (2010) 2034-2042.

[31] N. E. Saterborg, The distribution of 198Au injected intravenously as a colloid and in solution, *Acta radiologica: therapy, physics, biology*, 12 (1973) 509-528.

[32] G. S. Terentyuk, G. N. Maslyakova, L. V. Suleymanova, B. N. Khlebtsov, B. Y. Kogan, G. G. Akchurin, A. V. Shantrocha, I. L. Maksimova, N. G. Khlebtsov, V. V. Tuchin, Circulation and distribution of gold nanoparticles and induced alterations of tissue morphology at intravenous particle delivery, *Journal of biophotonics*, 2 (2009) 292-302.

[33] H. J. Johnston, G. Hutchison, F. M. Christensen, S. Peters, S. Hankin, V. Stone, A review of the in vivo and in vitro toxicity of silver and gold particulates: particle attributes and biological mechanisms responsible for the observed toxicity, *Critical reviews in toxicology*, 40 (2010) 328-346.

[34] L. Balogh, S. S. Nigavekar, B. M. Nair, W. Lesniak, C. Zhang, L. Y. Sung, M. S. Kariapper, A. El-Jawahri, M. Llanes, B. Bolton, F. Mamou, W. Tan, A. Hutson, L. Minc, M. K. Khan, Significant effect of size on the in vivo biodistribution of gold composite nanodevices in mouse tumor models, *Nanomedicine*, 3 (2007) 281-296.

[35] H. Maeda, J. Wu, T. Sawa, Y. Matsumura, K. Hori, Tumor vascular permeability and the EPR effect in macromolecular therapeutics: a review, *Journal of controlled release : official journal of the Controlled Release Society*, 65 (2000) 271-284.

[36] H. F. Dvorak, V. M. Weaver, T.D. Tlsty, G. Bergers, Tumor microenvironment and progression, *Journal of surgical oncology*, 103 (2011) 468-474.

[37] S. Paku, N. Paweletz, First steps of tumor-related angiogenesis, Laboratory investigation; *a journal of technical methods and pathology*, 65 (1991) 334-346.

[38] A. Pettersson, J. A. Nagy, L. F. Brown, C. Sundberg, E. Morgan, S. Jungles, R. Carter, J. E. Krieger, E. J. Manseau, V. S. Harvey, I. A. Eckelhoefer, D. Feng, A. M. Dvorak, R. C. Mulligan, H. F. Dvorak, Heterogeneity of the angiogenic response induced in different normal adult tissues by vascular permeability factor/vascular endothelial growth factor, Laboratory investigation; *a journal of technical methods and pathology*, 80 (2000) 99-115.

[39] G. T. Swayne, L. H. Smaje, D. H. Bergel, Distensibility of single capillaries and venules in the rat and frog mesentery, *International journal of microcirculation, clinical and experimental* / sponsored by the European Society for Microcirculation, 8 (1989) 25-42.

[40] S. H. Chang, K. Kanasaki, V. Gocheva, G. Blum, J. Harper, M. Moses, S. C. Shih, J. A. Nagy, J. Joyce, M. Bogyo, R. Kalluri, H. F. Dvorak, VEGF-A induces angiogenesis by perturbing the cathepsin-cysteine protease inhibitor balance in venules, causing basement membrane degradation and mother vessel formation, *Cancer research*, 69 (2009) 4537-4544.

[41] S. C. Shih, A. Zukauskas, D. Li, G. Liu, L. H. Ang, J. A. Nagy, L. F. Brown, H. F. Dvorak, The L6 protein TM4SF1 is critical for endothelial cell function and tumor angiogenesis, *Cancer research*, 69 (2009) 3272-3277.

[42] D. Feng, J. A. Nagy, A. M. Dvorak, H. F. Dvorak, Different pathways of macromolecule extravasation from hyperpermeable tumor vessels, *Microvascular research*, 59 (2000) 24-37.

[43] W. G. Roberts, G. E. Palade, Neovasculature induced by vascular endothelial growth factor is fenestrated, *Cancer research*, 57 (1997) 765-772.

[44] N. A. Vick, D. D. Bigner, Microvascular abnormalities in virally-induced canine brain tumors. Structural bases for altered blood-brain barrier function, *Journal of the neurological sciences*, 17 (1972) 29-39.

[45] H. Hashizume, P. Baluk, S. Morikawa, J. W. McLean, G. Thurston, S. Roberge, R. K. Jain, D. M. McDonald, Openings between defective endothelial cells explain tumor vessel leakiness, *The American journal of pathology*, 156 (2000) 1363-1380.

[46] K. E. Schlageter, P. Molnar, G. D. Lapin, D. R. Groothuis, Microvessel organization and structure in experimental brain tumors: microvessel populations with distinctive structural and functional properties, *Microvascular research*, 58 (1999) 312-328.

[47] A. M. Dvorak, S. Kohn, E. S. Morgan, P. Fox, J. A. Nagy, H. F. Dvorak, The vesiculo-vacuolar organelle (VVO): a distinct endothelial cell structure that provides a transcellular pathway for macromolecular extravasation, *Journal of leukocyte biology*, 59 (1996) 100-115.

[48] R. K. Jain, Transport of molecules across tumor vasculature, *Cancer metastasis reviews*, 6 (1987) 559-593.

[49] S. K. Hobbs, W. L. Monsky, F. Yuan, W. G. Roberts, L. Griffith, V. P. Torchilin, R. K. Jain, Regulation of transport pathways in tumor vessels: role of tumor type and microenvironment, *Proceedings of the National Academy of Sciences of the United States of America*, 95 (1998) 4607-4612.

[50] Y. Matsumura, H. Maeda, A new concept for macromolecular therapeutics in cancer chemotherapy: mechanism of tumoritropic accumulation of proteins and the antitumor agent smancs, *Cancer research*, 46 (1986) 6387-6392.
[51] R. K. Jain, Transport of molecules in the tumor interstitium: a review, *Cancer research*, 47 (1987) 3039-3051.
[52] Y. Murakami, Y. Tabata, Y. Ikada, Tumor accumulation of poly (ethylene glycol) with different molecular weights after intravenous injection, *Drug Delivery*, 4 (1997) 23-31.
[53] L. W. Seymour, Y. Miyamoto, H. Maeda, M. Brereton, J. Strohalm, K. Ulbrich, R. Duncan, Influence of molecular weight on passive tumour accumulation of a soluble macromolecular drug carrier, *European journal of cancer*, 31A (1995) 766-770.
[54] Y. Tabata, Y. Murakami, Y. Ikada, Tumor accumulation of poly(vinyl alcohol) of different sizes after intravenous injection, *Journal of controlled release : official journal of the Controlled Release Society*, 50 (1998) 123-133.
[55] E. Uzgiris, The role of molecular conformation on tumor uptake of polymeric contrast agents, *Investigative radiology*, 39 (2004) 131-137.
[56] C. C. Lee, M. Yoshida, J. M. Frechet, E. E. Dy, F. C. Szoka, In vitro and in vivo evaluation of hydrophilic dendronized linear polymers, *Bioconjugate chemistry*, 16 (2005) 535-541.
[57] E. R. Gillies, J. M. Frechet, Designing macromolecules for therapeutic applications: polyester dendrimer-poly(ethylene oxide) "bow-tie" hybrids with tunable molecular weight and architecture, *Journal of the American Chemical Society*, 124 (2002) 14137-14146.
[58] O. P. De Jesus, H. R. Ihre, L. Gagne, J. M. Frechet, F. Szoka, Polyester dendritic systems for drug delivery applications: in vitro and in vivo evaluation, *Bioconjugate chemistry*, 13 (2002) 453-461.
[59] E. R. Gillies, E. Dy, J. M. Frechet, F. C. Szoka, Biological evaluation of polyester dendrimer: poly(ethylene oxide) "bow-tie" hybrids with tunable molecular weight and architecture, *Molecular pharmaceutics*, 2 (2005) 129-138.
[60] C. C. Lee, E. R. Gillies, M. E. Fox, S. J. Guillaudeu, J. M. Frechet, E. E. Dy, F. C. Szoka, A single dose of doxorubicin-functionalized bow-tie dendrimer cures mice bearing C-26 colon carcinomas, *Proceedings of the National Academy of Sciences of the United States of America*, 103 (2006) 16649-16654.
[61] J. Gerber, W. Radke, Topological separation of linear and star-shaped polystyrenes by off-line 2D chromatography. Stars having high molar mass arms and quantification of the star fraction, *Polymer*, 46 (2005) 9224-9229.
[62] S. Bowen, N. Tare, T. Inoue, M. Yamasaki, M. Okabe, I. Horii, J. F. Eliason, Relationship between molecular mass and duration of activity of polyethylene glycol conjugated granulocyte colony-stimulating factor mutein, *Experimental hematology*, 27 (1999) 425-432.
[63] T. Yamaoka, Y. Tabata, Y. Ikada, Distribution and tissue uptake of poly(ethylene glycol) with different molecular weights after intravenous administration to mice, *Journal of pharmaceutical sciences*, 83 (1994) 601-606.
[64] J. Lim, Y. Guo, C.L. Rostollan, J. Stanfield, J.T. Hsieh, X. Sun, E.E. Simanek, The role of the size and number of polyethylene glycol chains in the biodistribution and tumor localization of triazine dendrimers, *Molecular pharmaceutics*, 5 (2008) 540-547.

[65] Y. Noguchi, J. Wu, R. Duncan, J. Strohalm, K. Ulbrich, T. Akaike, H. Maeda, Early phase tumor accumulation of macromolecules: a great difference in clearance rate between tumor and normal tissues, *Japanese journal of cancer research: Gann*, 89 (1998) 307-314.
[66] H. F. Dvorak, T. M. Sioussat, L. F. Brown, B. Berse, J. A. Nagy, A. Sotrel, E. J. Manseau, L. Van de Water, D. R. Senger, Distribution of vascular permeability factor (vascular endothelial growth factor) in tumors: concentration in tumor blood vessels, *The Journal of experimental medicine*, 174 (1991) 1275-1278.
[67] D. Feng, J. A. Nagy, J. Hipp, H. F. Dvorak, A. M. Dvorak, Vesiculo-vacuolar organelles and the regulation of venule permeability to macromolecules by vascular permeability factor, histamine, and serotonin, *The Journal of experimental medicine*, 183 (1996) 1981-1986.
[68] H. Qu, J. A. Nagy, D. R. Senger, H. F. Dvorak, A. M. Dvorak, Ultrastructural localization of vascular permeability factor/vascular endothelial growth factor (VPF/VEGF) to the abluminal plasma membrane and vesiculovacuolar organelles of tumor microvascular endothelium, *The journal of histochemistry and cytochemistry : official journal of the Histochemistry Society*, 43 (1995) 381-389.
[69] W. G. Roberts, G. E. Palade, Increased microvascular permeability and endothelial fenestration induced by vascular endothelial growth factor, *Journal of cell science*, 108 (Pt 6) (1995) 2369-2379.
[70] K. Weindel, J. R. Moringlane, D. Marme, H. A. Weich, Detection and quantification of vascular endothelial growth factor/vascular permeability factor in brain tumor tissue and cyst fluid: the key to angiogenesis?, *Neurosurgery*, 35 (1994) 439-448; discussion 448-439.
[71] T. Alon, I. Hemo, A. Itin, J. Pe'er, J. Stone, E. Keshet, Vascular endothelial growth factor acts as a survival factor for newly formed retinal vessels and has implications for retinopathy of prematurity, *Nature medicine*, 1 (1995) 1024-1028.
[72] D. Shweiki, A. Itin, G. Neufeld, H. Gitay-Goren, E. Keshet, Patterns of expression of vascular endothelial growth factor (VEGF) and VEGF receptors in mice suggest a role in hormonally regulated angiogenesis, *The Journal of clinical investigation*, 91 (1993) 2235-2243.
[73] K. Xie, S. Huang, L. Xu, I. J. Fidler, Molecular mechanisms for the regulation of vascular endothelial growth factor by extracellular and intracellular pH, in: American Association of Cancer Research, 1998.
[74] G. Helmlinger, F. Yuan, M. Dellian, R. K. Jain, Interstitial pH and pO2 gradients in solid tumors in vivo: high-resolution measurements reveal a lack of correlation, *Nature medicine*, 3 (1997) 177-182.
[75] G. Thurston, A. L. Baldwin, Endothelial actin cytoskeleton in rat mesentery microvasculature, *The American journal of physiology*, 266 (1994) H1896-1909.
[76] D. Marmé, N. E. Fusenig, Tumor Angiogenesis: Basic Mechanisms and Cancer Therapy, Springer-Verlag Berlin Heidelberg, 2008.
[77] S. Toffoli, A. Roegiers, O. Feron, M. Van Steenbrugge, N. Ninane, M. Raes, C. Michiels, Intermittent hypoxia is an angiogenic inducer for endothelial cells: role of HIF-1, *Angiogenesis*, 12 (2009) 47-67.
[78] R. J. Gillies, P. A. Schornack, T. W. Secomb, N. Raghunand, Causes and effects of heterogeneous perfusion in tumors, *Neoplasia*, 1 (1999) 197-207.

[79] Z. Zhang, K. G. Neiva, M. W. Lingen, L. M. Ellis, J. E. Nor, VEGF-dependent tumor angiogenesis requires inverse and reciprocal regulation of VEGFR1 and VEGFR2, *Cell death and differentiation*, 17 (2010) 499-512.
[80] A. Raza, M. J. Franklin, A. Z. Dudek, Pericytes and vessel maturation during tumor angiogenesis and metastasis, *American journal of hematology*, 85 (2010) 593-598.
[81] A. Armulik, A. Abramsson, C. Betsholtz, Endothelial/pericyte interactions, *Circulation research*, 97 (2005) 512-523.
[82] L. Diaz-Flores, R. Gutierrez, J. F. Madrid, H. Varela, F. Valladares, E. Acosta, P. Martin-Vasallo, L. Diaz-Flores, Jr., Pericytes. Morphofunction, interactions and pathology in a quiescent and activated mesenchymal cell niche, *Histology and histopathology*, 24 (2009) 909-969.
[83] K. Gaengel, G. Genove, A. Armulik, C. Betsholtz, Endothelial-mural cell signaling in vascular development and angiogenesis, *Arteriosclerosis, thrombosis, and vascular biology*, 29 (2009) 630-638.
[84] R. Kalluri, Basement membranes: structure, assembly and role in tumour angiogenesis, Nature reviews. *Cancer*, 3 (2003) 422-433.
[85] C. Lamagna, G. Bergers, The bone marrow constitutes a reservoir of pericyte progenitors, *Journal of leukocyte biology*, 80 (2006) 677-681.
[86] G. Bergers, S. Song, The role of pericytes in blood-vessel formation and maintenance, *Neuro-oncology*, 7 (2005) 452-464.
[87] H. Gerhardt, M. Golding, M. Fruttiger, C. Ruhrberg, A. Lundkvist, A. Abramsson, M. Jeltsch, C. Mitchell, K. Alitalo, D. Shima, C. Betsholtz, VEGF guides angiogenic sprouting utilizing endothelial tip cell filopodia, *The Journal of cell biology*, 161 (2003) 1163-1177.
[88] P. Lindblom, H. Gerhardt, S. Liebner, A. Abramsson, M. Enge, M. Hellstrom, G. Backstrom, S. Fredriksson, U. Landegren, H. C. Nystrom, G. Bergstrom, E. Dejana, A. Ostman, P. Lindahl, C. Betsholtz, Endothelial PDGF-B retention is required for proper investment of pericytes in the microvessel wall, *Genes & development*, 17 (2003) 1835-1840.
[89] D. C. Darland, L. J. Massingham, S. R. Smith, E. Piek, M. Saint-Geniez, P. A. D'Amore, Pericyte production of cell-associated VEGF is differentiation-dependent and is associated with endothelial survival, *Developmental biology*, 264 (2003) 275-288.
[90] K. D. Barlow, A. M. Sanders, S. Soker, S. Ergun, L. J. Metheny-Barlow, Pericytes on the tumor vasculature: jekyll or hyde?, *Cancer microenvironment: official journal of the International Cancer Microenvironment Society*, 6 (2013) 1-17.
[91] A. N. Stratman, K. M. Malotte, R. D. Mahan, M. J. Davis, G. E. Davis, Pericyte recruitment during vasculogenic tube assembly stimulates endothelial basement membrane matrix formation, *Blood*, 114 (2009) 5091-5101.
[92] S. Morikawa, P. Baluk, T. Kaidoh, A. Haskell, R. K. Jain, D. M. McDonald, Abnormalities in pericytes on blood vessels and endothelial sprouts in tumors, *The American journal of pathology*, 160 (2002) 985-1000.
[93] H. P. Gerber, V. Dixit, N. Ferrara, Vascular endothelial growth factor induces expression of the antiapoptotic proteins Bcl-2 and A1 in vascular endothelial cells, *The Journal of biological chemistry*, 273 (1998) 13313-13316.
[94] J. Tran, J. Rak, C. Sheehan, S. D. Saibil, E. LaCasse, R. G. Korneluk, R. S. Kerbel, Marked induction of the IAP family antiapoptotic proteins survivin and XIAP by VEGF

in vascular endothelial cells, *Biochemical and biophysical research communications*, 264 (1999) 781-788.

[95] S. Lee, T. T. Chen, C. L. Barber, M. C. Jordan, J. Murdock, S. Desai, N. Ferrara, A. Nagy, K. P. Roos, M. L. Iruela-Arispe, Autocrine VEGF signaling is required for vascular homeostasis, *Cell*, 130 (2007) 691-703.

[96] M. R. Kano, Y. Bae, C. Iwata, Y. Morishita, M. Yashiro, M. Oka, T. Fujii, A. Komuro, K. Kiyono, M. Kaminishi, K. Hirakawa, Y. Ouchi, N. Nishiyama, K. Kataoka, K. Miyazono, Improvement of cancer-targeting therapy, using nanocarriers for intractable solid tumors by inhibition of TGF-beta signaling, *Proceedings of the National Academy of Sciences of the United States of America*, 104 (2007) 3460-3465.

[97] M. R. Kano, Y. Komuta, C. Iwata, M. Oka, Y. T. Shirai, Y. Morishita, Y. Ouchi, K. Kataoka, K. Miyazono, Comparison of the effects of the kinase inhibitors imatinib, sorafenib, and transforming growth factor-beta receptor inhibitor on extravasation of nanoparticles from neovasculature, *Cancer science*, 100 (2009) 173-180.

[98] Y. Cao, Z. L. Zhang, M. Zhou, P. Elson, B. Rini, H. Aydin, K. Feenstra, M. H. Tan, B. Berghuis, R. Tabbey, J. H. Resau, F. J. Zhou, B. T. Teh, C. N. Qian, Pericyte coverage of differentiated vessels inside tumor vasculature is an independent unfavorable prognostic factor for patients with clear cell renal cell carcinoma, *Cancer*, 119 (2013) 313-324.

[99] H. Cabral, Y. Matsumoto, K. Mizuno, Q. Chen, M. Murakami, M. Kimura, Y. Terada, M. R. Kano, K. Miyazono, M. Uesaka, N. Nishiyama, K. Kataoka, Accumulation of sub-100 nm polymeric micelles in poorly permeable tumours depends on size, *Nature nanotechnology*, 6 (2011) 815-823.

[100] M. Kumagai, M. R. Kano, Y. Morishita, M. Ota, Y. Imai, N. Nishiyama, M. Sekino, S. Ueno, K. Miyazono, K. Kataoka, Enhanced magnetic resonance imaging of experimental pancreatic tumor in vivo by block copolymer-coated magnetite nanoparticles with TGF-beta inhibitor, *Journal of controlled release : official journal of the Controlled Release Society*, 140 (2009) 306-311.

[101] K. Miyata, M. Oba, M. R. Kano, S. Fukushima, Y. Vachutinsky, M. Han, H. Koyama, K. Miyazono, N. Nishiyama, K. Kataoka, Polyplex micelles from triblock copolymers composed of tandemly aligned segments with biocompatible, endosomal escaping, and DNA-condensing functions for systemic gene delivery to pancreatic tumor tissue, *Pharmaceutical research*, 25 (2008) 2924-2936.

[102] R. A. Weinberg, The biology of cancer, *Garland Science*, 2007.

[103] D. Huang, Y. Ding, Y. Li, W. M. Luo, Z. F. Zhang, J. Snider, K. Vandenbeldt, C. N. Qian, B. T. Teh, Sunitinib acts primarily on tumor endothelium rather than tumor cells to inhibit the growth of renal cell carcinoma, *Cancer research*, 70 (2010) 1053-1062.

[104] V. G. Cooke, V. S. LeBleu, D. Keskin, Z. Khan, J. T. O'Connell, Y. Teng, M. B. Duncan, L. Xie, G. Maeda, S. Vong, H. Sugimoto, R. M. Rocha, A. Damascena, R. R. Brentani, R. Kalluri, Pericyte depletion results in hypoxia-associated epithelial-to-mesenchymal transition and metastasis mediated by met signaling pathway, *Cancer cell*, 21 (2012) 66-81.

[105] L. Qin, J. L. Bromberg-White, C. N. Qian, Opportunities and challenges in tumor angiogenesis research: back and forth between bench and bed, *Advances in cancer research*, 113 (2012) 191-239.

[106] G. Breier, S. Blum, J. Peli, M. Groot, C. Wild, W. Risau, E. Reichmann, Transforming growth factor-beta and Ras regulate the VEGF/VEGF-receptor system during tumor angiogenesis, *International journal of cancer. Journal international du cancer*, 97 (2002) 142-148.

[107] J. P. Duffy, G. Eibl, H. A. Reber, O. J. Hines, Influence of hypoxia and neoangiogenesis on the growth of pancreatic cancer, *Molecular cancer*, 2 (2003) 12.

[108] K. H. Plate, G. Breier, H. A. Weich, W. Risau, Vascular endothelial growth factor is a potential tumour angiogenesis factor in human gliomas in vivo, *Nature*, 359 (1992) 845-848.

[109] H. E. Ryan, J. Lo, R. S. Johnson, HIF-1α is required for solid tumor formation and embryonic vascularization, *The EMBO journal*, 17 (1998) 3005-3015.

[110] P. Vaupel, The role of hypoxia-induced factors in tumor progression, *The oncologist*, 9 Suppl 5 (2004) 10-17.

[111] T. Acker, A. Diez-Juan, J. Aragones, M. Tjwa, K. Brusselmans, L. Moons, D. Fukumura, M. P. Moreno-Murciano, J. M. Herbert, A. Burger, J. Riedel, G. Elvert, I. Flamme, P. H. Maxwell, D. Collen, M. Dewerchin, R. K. Jain, K. H. Plate, P. Carmeliet, Genetic evidence for a tumor suppressor role of HIF-2alpha, *Cancer cell*, 8 (2005) 131-141.

[112] P. Carmeliet, Y. Dor, J. M. Herbert, D. Fukumura, K. Brusselmans, M. Dewerchin, M. Neeman, F. Bono, R. Abramovitch, P. Maxwell, C. J. Koch, P. Ratcliffe, L. Moons, R. K. Jain, D. Collen, E. Keshert, Role of HIF-1alpha in hypoxia-mediated apoptosis, cell proliferation and tumour angiogenesis, *Nature*, 394 (1998) 485-490.

[113] K. Dagnon, E. Pacary, F. Commo, M. Antoine, M. Bernaudin, J. F. Bernaudin, P. Callard, Expression of erythropoietin and erythropoietin receptor in non-small cell lung carcinomas, *Clinical cancer research: an official journal of the American Association for Cancer Research*, 11 (2005) 993-999.

[114] E. J. Soilleux, H. Turley, Y. M. Tian, C. W. Pugh, K. C. Gatter, A. L. Harris, Use of novel monoclonal antibodies to determine the expression and distribution of the hypoxia regulatory factors PHD-1, PHD-2, PHD-3 and FIH in normal and neoplastic human tissues, *Histopathology*, 47 (2005) 602-610.

[115] E. Y. Tan, L. Campo, C. Han, H. Turley, F. Pezzella, K. C. Gatter, A. L. Harris, S. B. Fox, Cytoplasmic location of factor-inhibiting hypoxia-inducible factor is associated with an enhanced hypoxic response and a shorter survival in invasive breast cancer, *Breast cancer research: BCR*, 9 (2007) R89.

[116] P. Nasarre, M. Thomas, K. Kruse, I. Helfrich, V. Wolter, C. Deppermann, D. Schadendorf, G. Thurston, U. Fiedler, H. G. Augustin, Host-derived angiopoietin-2 affects early stages of tumor development and vessel maturation but is dispensable for later stages of tumor growth, *Cancer research*, 69 (2009) 1324-1333.

[117] M. H. Andersen, L. Berglund, J. T. Rasmussen, T. E. Petersen, Bovine PAS-6/7 binds alpha v beta 5 integrins and anionic phospholipids through two domains, *Biochemistry*, 36 (1997) 5441-5446.

[118] K. Ogura, K. Nara, Y. Watanabe, K. Kohno, T. Tai, Y. Sanai, Cloning and Expression of cDNA for< i> O</i>-Acetylation of GD3 Ganglioside, *Biochemical and biophysical research communications*, 225 (1996) 932-938.

[119] C. Shao, V. A. Novakovic, J. F. Head, B. A. Seaton, G. E. Gilbert, Crystal structure of lactadherin C2 domain at 1.7A resolution with mutational and computational analyses

of its membrane-binding motif, *The Journal of biological chemistry*, 283 (2008) 7230-7241.

[120] J. D. Stubbs, C. Lekutis, K. L. Singer, A. Bui, D. Yuzuki, U. Srinivasan, G. Parry, cDNA cloning of a mouse mammary epithelial cell surface protein reveals the existence of epidermal growth factor-like domains linked to factor VIII-like sequences, *Proceedings of the National Academy of Sciences of the United States of America*, 87 (1990) 8417-8421.

[121] S. Motegi, W. W. Leitner, M. Lu, Y. Tada, M. Sardy, C. Wu, T. Chavakis, M. C. Udey, Pericyte-derived MFG-E8 regulates pathologic angiogenesis, *Arteriosclerosis, thrombosis, and vascular biology*, 31 (2011) 2024-2034.

[122] P. Ruenraroengsak, J. M. Cook, A. T. Florence, Nanosystem drug targeting: Facing up to complex realities, *Journal of controlled release: official journal of the Controlled Release Society*, 141 (2010) 265-276.

[123] R. K. Jain, L. T. Baxter, Mechanisms of heterogeneous distribution of monoclonal antibodies and other macromolecules in tumors: significance of elevated interstitial pressure, *Cancer research*, 48 (1988) 7022-7032.

[124] R. T. Tong, Y. Boucher, S. V. Kozin, F. Winkler, D. J. Hicklin, R. K. Jain, Vascular normalization by vascular endothelial growth factor receptor 2 blockade induces a pressure gradient across the vasculature and improves drug penetration in tumors, *Cancer research*, 64 (2004) 3731-3736.

[125] F. Winkler, S. V. Kozin, R. T. Tong, S. S. Chae, M. F. Booth, I. Garkavtsev, L. Xu, D. J. Hicklin, D. Fukumura, E. di Tomaso, L. L. Munn, R. K. Jain, Kinetics of vascular normalization by VEGFR2 blockade governs brain tumor response to radiation: role of oxygenation, angiopoietin-1, and matrix metalloproteinases, *Cancer cell*, 6 (2004) 553-563.

[126] V. P. Chauhan, T. Stylianopoulos, J. D. Martin, Z. Popovic, O. Chen, W. S. Kamoun, M. G. Bawendi, D. Fukumura, R. K. Jain, Normalization of tumour blood vessels improves the delivery of nanomedicines in a size-dependent manner, *Nature nanotechnology*, 7 (2012) 383-388.

[127] P. M. Bungay, H. Brenner, The motion of a closely fitting sphere in a fluid filled tube, *International Journal of Multiphase Flow*, 1 (1973) 25-56.

[128] W. Deen, Hindered transport of large molecules in liquid-filled pores, *AIChE Journal*, 33 (1987) 1409-1425.

[129] R. K. Jain, T. Stylianopoulos, Delivering nanomedicine to solid tumors, Nature reviews. *Clinical oncology*, 7 (2010) 653-664.

[130] D. Peer, J. M. Karp, S. Hong, O. C. Farokhzad, R. Margalit, R. Langer, Nanocarriers as an emerging platform for cancer therapy, *Nature nanotechnology*, 2 (2007) 751-760.

[131] E. Ruoslahti, S. N. Bhatia, M. J. Sailor, Targeting of drugs and nanoparticles to tumors, *The Journal of cell biology*, 188 (2010) 759-768.

[132] E. Frohlich, The role of surface charge in cellular uptake and cytotoxicity of medical nanoparticles, *International journal of nanomedicine*, 7 (2012) 5577-5591.

[133] J. A. Kim, C. Åberg, A. Salvati, K. A. Dawson, Role of cell cycle on the cellular uptake and dilution of nanoparticles in a cell population, *Nature nanotechnology*, 7 (2011) 62-68.

[134] D. Peer, R. Margalit, Loading mitomycin C inside long circulating hyaluronan targeted nano-liposomes increases its antitumor activity in three mice tumor models, International journal of cancer. *Journal international du cancer*, 108 (2004) 780-789.
[135] R. Margalit, Liposome-mediated drug targeting in topical and regional therapies, *Critical reviews in therapeutic drug carrier systems*, 12 (1995) 233-261.
[136] R. Margalit, Bioadhesive Liposomes for Topical Treatment of Wounds, *Drugs and the pharmaceutical sciences*, 77 (1996) 425-462.
[137] R. Margalit, M. Okon, N. Yerushalmi, E. Avidor, Bioadhesive liposomes as topical drug delivery systems: molecular and cellular studies, *Journal of controlled release*, 19 (1992) 275-287.
[138] N. Yerushalmi, A. Arad, R. Margalit, Molecular and cellular studies of hyaluronic acid-modified liposomes as bioadhesive carriers for topical drug delivery in wound healing, *Archives of biochemistry and biophysics*, 313 (1994) 267-273.
[139] N. Yerushalmi, R. Margalit, Bioadhesive, collagen-modified liposomes: molecular and cellular level studies on the kinetics of drug release and on binding to cell monolayers, *Biochimica et biophysica acta*, 1189 (1994) 13-20.
[140] N. Yerushalmi, R. Margalit, Hyaluronic acid-modified bioadhesive liposomes as local drug depots: effects of cellular and fluid dynamics on liposome retention at target sites, *Archives of biochemistry and biophysics*, 349 (1998) 21-26.
[141] M. Hofmann, C. Fieber, V. Assmann, M. Gottlicher, J. Sleeman, R. Plug, N. Howells, O. von Stein, H. Ponta, P. Herrlich, Identification of IHABP, a 95 kDa intracellular hyaluronate binding protein, *Journal of cell science*, 111 (Pt 12) (1998) 1673-1684.
[142] D. Peer, R. Margalit, Tumor-targeted hyaluronan nanoliposomes increase the antitumor activity of liposomal Doxorubicin in syngeneic and human xenograft mouse tumor models, *Neoplasia*, 6 (2004) 343-353.
[143] V. Abetamann, H. F. Kern, H. P. Elsasser, Differential expression of the hyaluronan receptors CD44 and RHAMM in human pancreatic cancer cells, *Clinical cancer research: an official journal of the American Association for Cancer Research*, 2 (1996) 1607-1618.
[144] I. Rivkin, K. Cohen, J. Koffler, D. Melikhov, D. Peer, R. Margalit, Paclitaxel-clusters coated with hyaluronan as selective tumor-targeted nanovectors, *Biomaterials*, 31 (2010) 7106-7114.
[145] D. S. Alberts, P. Y. Liu, E. V. Hannigan, R. O'Toole, S. D. Williams, J. A. Young, E. W. Franklin, D. L. Clarke-Pearson, V. K. Malviya, B. DuBeshter, Intraperitoneal cisplatin plus intravenous cyclophosphamide versus intravenous cisplatin plus intravenous cyclophosphamide for stage III ovarian cancer, *The New England journal of medicine*, 335 (1996) 1950-1955.
[146] D. K. Armstrong, B. Bundy, L. Wenzel, H. Q. Huang, R. Baergen, S. Lele, L. J. Copeland, J. L. Walker, R. A. Burger, G. Gynecologic Oncology, Intraperitoneal cisplatin and paclitaxel in ovarian cancer, *The New England journal of medicine*, 354 (2006) 34-43.
[147] E. de Bree, P. A. Theodoropoulos, H. Rosing, J. Michalakis, J. Romanos, J. H. Beijnen, D. D. Tsiftsis, Treatment of ovarian cancer using intraperitoneal chemotherapy with taxanes: from laboratory bench to bedside, *Cancer treatment reviews*, 32 (2006) 471-482.

[148] A. Gadducci, F. Carnino, S. Chiara, I. Brunetti, L. Tanganelli, A. Romanini, M. Bruzzone, P. F. Conte, Intraperitoneal versus intravenous cisplatin in combination with intravenous cyclophosphamide and epidoxorubicin in optimally cytoreduced advanced epithelial ovarian cancer: a randomized trial of the Gruppo Oncologico Nord-Ovest, *Gynecologic oncology*, 76 (2000) 157-162.

[149] M. Markman, B. N. Bundy, D. S. Alberts, J. M. Fowler, D. L. Clark-Pearson, L. F. Carson, S. Wadler, J. Sickel, Phase III trial of standard-dose intravenous cisplatin plus paclitaxel versus moderately high-dose carboplatin followed by intravenous paclitaxel and intraperitoneal cisplatin in small-volume stage III ovarian carcinoma: an intergroup study of the Gynecologic Oncology Group, Southwestern Oncology Group, and Eastern Cooperative Oncology Group, *Journal of clinical oncology : official journal of the American Society of Clinical Oncology*, 19 (2001) 1001-1007.

[150] A. Polyzos, N. Tsavaris, C. Kosmas, L. Giannikos, M. Katsikas, N. Kalahanis, G. Karatzas, K. Christodoulou, K. Giannakopoulos, D. Stamatiadis, N. Katsilambros, A comparative study of intraperitoneal carboplatin versus intravenous carboplatin with intravenous cyclophosphamide in both arms as initial chemotherapy for stage III ovarian cancer, *Oncology*, 56 (1999) 291-296.

[151] J. L. Walker, D. K. Armstrong, H. Q. Huang, J. Fowler, K. Webster, R. A. Burger, D. Clarke-Pearson, Intraperitoneal catheter outcomes in a phase III trial of intravenous versus intraperitoneal chemotherapy in optimal stage III ovarian and primary peritoneal cancer: a Gynecologic Oncology Group Study, *Gynecologic oncology*, 100 (2006) 27-32.

[152] M. S. Yen, C. M. Juang, C. R. Lai, G. C. Chao, H. T. Ng, C. C. Yuan, Intraperitoneal cisplatin-based chemotherapy vs. intravenous cisplatin-based chemotherapy for stage III optimally cytoreduced epithelial ovarian cancer, *International journal of gynaecology and obstetrics*: the official organ of the International Federation of Gynaecology and Obstetrics, 72 (2001) 55-60.

[153] S. D. Li, S. B. Howell, CD44-targeted microparticles for delivery of cisplatin to peritoneal metastases, *Molecular pharmaceutics*, 7 (2010) 280-290.

[154] M. Tsai, Z. Lu, J. Wang, T. K. Ych, M. G. Wientjes, J. L. Au, Effects of carrier on disposition and antitumor activity of intraperitoneal Paclitaxel, *Pharmaceutical research*, 24 (2007) 1691-1701.

[155] V.D. Corleto, S. Nasoni, F. Panzuto, S. Cassetta, G. Delle Fave, Somatostatin receptor subtypes: basic pharmacology and tissue distribution, *Digestive and liver disease: official journal of the Italian Society of Gastroenterology and the Italian Association for the Study of the Liver*, 36 Suppl 1 (2004) S8-16.

[156] I. Virgolini, M. Leimer, H. Handmaker, S. Lastoria, C. Bischof, P. Muto, T. Pangerl, D. Gludovacz, M. Peck-Radosavljevic, J. Lister-James, G. Hamilton, K. Kaserer, P. Valent, R. Dean, Somatostatin receptor subtype specificity and in vivo binding of a novel tumor tracer, 99mTc-P829, *Cancer research*, 58 (1998) 1850-1859.

[157] T. Hoelting, Q. Y. Duh, O. H. Clark, C. Herfarth, Somatostatin analog octreotide inhibits the growth of differentiated thyroid cancer cells in vitro, but not in vivo, *The Journal of clinical endocrinology and metabolism*, 81 (1996) 2638-2641.

[158] P. B. Gupta, T. T. Onder, G. Jiang, K. Tao, C. Kuperwasser, R. A. Weinberg, E. S. Lander, Identification of selective inhibitors of cancer stem cells by high-throughput screening, *Cell*, 138 (2009) 645-659.

[159] Y. Liu, W. L. Lu, J. Guo, J. Du, T. Li, J. W. Wu, G. L. Wang, J. C. Wang, X. Zhang, Q. Zhang, A potential target associated with both cancer and cancer stem cells: a combination therapy for eradication of breast cancer using vinorelbine stealthy liposomes plus parthenolide stealthy liposomes, *Journal of controlled release : official journal of the Controlled Release Society*, 129 (2008) 18-25.

[160] Y. Zhang, H. Zhang, X. Wang, J. Wang, X. Zhang, Q. Zhang, The eradication of breast cancer and cancer stem cells using octreotide modified paclitaxel active targeting micelles and salinomycin passive targeting micelles, *Biomaterials*, 33 (2012) 679-691.

[161] H. Maeda, The enhanced permeability and retention (EPR) effect in tumor vasculature: the key role of tumor-selective macromolecular drug targeting, *Advances in enzyme regulation*, 41 (2001) 189-207.

[162] V. Guarneri, E. Barbieri, M. V. Dieci, F. Piacentini, P. Conte, Anti-HER2 neoadjuvant and adjuvant therapies in HER2 positive breast cancer, *Cancer treatment reviews*, 36 Suppl 3 (2010) S62-66.

[163] J. Gabe, K. Chamberlain, P. Norris, K. Dew, H. Madden, D. Hodgetts, The debate about the funding of Herceptin: a case study of 'countervailing powers', *Social science & medicine*, 75 (2012) 2353-2361.

[164] A. A. Joy, J. R. Mackey, Adjuvant trastuzumab: progress, controversies, and the steps ahead, *Current oncology*, 13 (2006) 8-13.

[165] D. B. Kirpotin, D. C. Drummond, Y. Shao, M. R. Shalaby, K. Hong, U. B. Nielsen, J. D. Marks, C. C. Benz, J. W. Park, Antibody targeting of long-circulating lipidic nanoparticles does not increase tumor localization but does increase internalization in animal models, *Cancer research*, 66 (2006) 6732-6740.

[166] A. Cirstoiu-Hapca, F. Buchegger, N. Lange, L. Bossy, R. Gurny, F. Delie, Benefit of anti-HER2-coated paclitaxel-loaded immuno-nanoparticles in the treatment of disseminated ovarian cancer: Therapeutic efficacy and biodistribution in mice, *Journal of controlled release: official journal of the Controlled Release Society*, 144 (2010) 324-331.

[167] A. K. Rajasekaran, G. Anilkumar, J. J. Christiansen, Is prostate-specific membrane antigen a multifunctional protein?, *American journal of physiology. Cell physiology*, 288 (2005) C975-981.

[168] O. C. Farokhzad, J. Cheng, B. A. Teply, I. Sherifi, S. Jon, P. W. Kantoff, J. P. Richie, R. Langer, Targeted nanoparticle-aptamer bioconjugates for cancer chemotherapy in vivo, *Proceedings of the National Academy of Sciences of the United States of America*, 103 (2006) 6315-6320.

[169] J. Hrkach, D. Von Hoff, M. Mukkaram Ali, E. Andrianova, J. Auer, T. Campbell, D. De Witt, M. Figa, M. Figueiredo, A. Horhota, S. Low, K. McDonnell, E. Peeke, B. Retnarajan, A. Sabnis, E. Schnipper, J. J. Song, Y. H. Song, J. Summa, D. Tompsett, G. Troiano, T. Van Geen Hoven, J. Wright, P. LoRusso, P. W. Kantoff, N. H. Bander, C. Sweeney, O. C. Farokhzad, R. Langer, S. Zale, Preclinical development and clinical translation of a PSMA-targeted docetaxel nanoparticle with a differentiated pharmacological profile, *Science translational medicine*, 4 (2012) 128ra139.

[170] D. J. Crommelin, A. T. Florence, Towards more effective advanced drug delivery systems, *International journal of pharmaceutics*, (2013).

[171] T. Lammers, F. Kiessling, W. E. Hennink, G. Storm, Drug targeting to tumors: principles, pitfalls and (pre-) clinical progress, *Journal of controlled release : official journal of the Controlled Release Society*, 161 (2012) 175-187.
[172] V. Torchilin, Tumor delivery of macromolecular drugs based on the EPR effect, *Advanced drug delivery reviews*, 63 (2011) 131-135.
[173] Z. Cheng, A. Al Zaki, J. Z. Hui, V. R. Muzykantov, A. Tsourkas, Multifunctional nanoparticles: cost versus benefit of adding targeting and imaging capabilities, *Science*, 338 (2012) 903-910.

In: Recent Advances in Drug Delivery Research
Editor: Valerio Voliani
ISBN: 978-1-62948-228-6

Chapter 2

Recent Advances in Oral Drug Delivery Systems

Tolulope O. Ajala, Olufunke D. Akin-Ajani and Oluwatoyin A. Odeku *
Department of Pharmaceutics and Industrial Pharmacy,
University of Ibadan, Nigeria

Abstract

Oral drug delivery systems remain the most preferred form of drug delivery due to its ease of administration, high levels of patient acceptance and long term compliance which increases the therapeutic value of the drug. It accounts for about 60% of pharmaceutical products in the market. However, not all drugs could be administered via the oral route due to enzymatic degradation and first pass effects which has led to the increase in the frequency of dosing. During the past three decades, numerous oral controlled release formulation have been developed for drugs that are easily absorbed from the gastrointestinal tract but are quickly eliminated from the blood circulation due to their short half-life. Recent advances in oral drug delivery systems have been aimed at providing an increase in bioavailability of drug, reduction in the frequency of administration, prolong duration of action due to a reduction in the fluctuation of peak trough concentration and drug targeting. They are designed to achieve a prolonged therapeutic effect by continuously releasing medication over an extended period of time after administration of a single dose. Such advances include the use of oral extended release dosage forms, mucoadhesive dosage forms, pulsatile delivery systems, floating gastroretentive drug delivery systems, oral fast disintegrating/dissolving tablets films and pulsatile drug delivery system. This chapter provides a review of these technologies and their potential application as novel drug carriers.

Keywords: Oral drug delivery, controlled release, pulsatile delivery, gastroretentive drug delivery, disintegrating tablets, mucoadhesive dosage form

---

* Corresponding author: E -mail: pejuodeku@yahoo.com; o.odeku@mail.ui.edu.ng; Tel: +234 8057320466.

Abbreviations

controlled release drug delivery system (CRDDS);
gastric residence time (GRT);
gastrointestinal (GI);
active pharmaceutical ingredient (API);
hydroxypropylmethylcellulose (HPMC);
mucoadhesive drug delivery systems (MDDS);
oral fast disintegrating/dissolving tablets (ODT);
oral fast disintegrating/dissolving films (OFDF);
floating drug delivery systems (FDDS);
gastroretentive time (GRT)

Introduction

The oral route is generally considered as the model, most natural, uncomplicated, safe, convenient and most desired route for the administration of drugs [1]. This is because of its ease of administration, cost- effective manufacturing process, high levels of patient acceptance and long term compliance which increases the therapeutic value of the drug [2]. It is also the oldest delivery system and accounts for about 60% of pharmaceutical products in the market [3]. Most commercially available dosage forms for oral drug administration are tablets and capsules and are mostly for immediate release of drugs which guarantees rapid absorption [4]. Some precincts of these immediate release dosage forms include [5, 6]:

1. Drugs with small therapeutic index are prone to precipitating opposing effects due to fluctuating drug levels
2. The achievement of steady state condition is difficult because the usual peak-valley plasma concentration-time profile is obtained
3. The possibility of under or over-medication is high because of unavoidable oscillations in drug concentration
4. Drugs with short half-life requires frequent administration and this increases the chance of poor compliance by patients
5. They do not generally enable site-specific or rate-controlled release
6. The gastrointestinal (GI) transit time of most drugs is brief and this hinders the formulation of single daily dosage forms
7. It is estimated that 50% of the population have problems swallowing conventional capsules/tablets due to dysphagia or other reasons [7]. Generally, the higher the dose, the larger the tablet and the greater the difficulty in swallowing.

During the past three decades, numerous oral controlled release formulation have been developed for drugs that are easily absorbed from the gastrointestinal tract but are quickly eliminated from the blood circulation due to their short half-life. The most important objective of controlled release drug delivery system (CRDDS) is the elongation of gastric residence time (GRT) which is believed to prolong duration of drug action [8, 9]. Other important objectives of CRDDS include reduction in the fluctuation of peak trough concentration with attended possible improvement in specific drug distribution, increased bioavailability and reduction of side effects [10]. The system utilizes an extended period of time for drug release and absorption. The amount first released is enough to achieve a loading dose for the therapeutic response required and the maintenance dose is then released at a controlled rate over a set period of time [11].

According to Gronia and Heun [12], there are three major potential tasks in developing oral controlled drug delivery systems. These include:

1. The need to develop a practicable delivery system capable of conveying an API at a therapeutically effective rate to a needed site within a period required for peak treatment
2. The need to reduce drug elimination through hepatic first pass by providing measures either to bypass or minimize it to an insignificant level
3. The need to adjust the gastrointestinal transit time to enable transportation of the drug delivery system to a target or an absorption site that will remain there for an extended period of time thus maximizing dose supply

Advances in oral dosage form design that have been developed to address these concerns include:

1. Oral Extended Release Drug Delivery System (OERDDS)

Oral extended release drug delivery system (OERDDS) is one of the innovations of oral dosage forms developed to act as drug reservoirs from which the API can be released over a defined period of time at a predetermined and controlled rate [13]. They are particularly useful for APIs having biological half-life between 2 to 8 hours. If the half-life is less than 2 hours, there will be the need for large doses and higher rates of elimination from the blood circulation [14]. The drug should also be easily absorbed and stable in the gastrointestinal tract environment and have pronounced oral effectiveness [15]. Moreover, the preferable single dose of such drug moiety should be less than 500mg because increase in the bulk of the drug increases the volume of the product. In addition, the therapeutic range must be wide enough to prevent release variations that may exceed minimal levels of toxicity [16].

OERDDS avoids high blood concentrations while equally maintaining therapeutic concentrations over a prolonged period [17]. There is also improvement in treatment efficacy and reduced toxicity since drug absorption is slowed-down. The duration of activity of drugs with short half-life is increased and drug accumulation is reduced even with chronic dosing [16]. The short comings of this delivery system include the risk of dose dumping when fast initial release of drug occurs and the dose and dosage regimens cannot be easily adjusted [16]. Moreover, therapy cannot be urgently terminated even when acute toxicity occurs and the cost of preparation is also high. The rates of release are affected by food and OERDDS have large sizes which cause ingestion difficulties and hinder gut transit [18].

Table 1. Extended release dosage forms available in the market

Brand Name	Active Ingredient
Altiva – D Tab	Fexofenadine HCl and Pseudoephidrine sulphate
Augmentin – XR Tab	Amixicillin and Potassium Clavulanate
Betacap –TR Cap	Propranolol HCl
Carvidon – MR Tab	Trimetazidine HCl
Cefoclox – XL Tab	Cefpodoxime Dicloxacillin and Lactic acid bacillus
Dayo – OD Tab	Divolproex Sodium
Divaa – OD Tab	Divalproex Sodium
Embeta – XR Tab	Metoprolol Succinate
Epsolin ER Cap	Phenytoin Sodium
Etomax – ER Tab	Etodolac
Etura Tab	Etodolac
Exermet GM 502 Tab	Glimepiride and Metformin HCl
Fecontin – F Tab	Ferrous Glycine Sulphate and Folic acid
Gabaneuron – SR Tab	Gabapentin and Methylcobalamin
Glimestar PM Tab	Glimipride,Pioglitazone and metformin
Glizid – MR Tab	Gliclazide
Gluconorm – SR Tab	Metformin HCl
Gluconorm G Tab	Metformin HCl
Gluconorm PG Tab	Glimepiride, Pioglitazone and Metformin HCl
Glycomet – 1 GM Tab	Metformin HCl
Intalith CR	Lithium Carbonate
Licab – XL Tab	Lithium Carbonate
Lithosun SR Tab	Lithium Carbonate
Mahacef – XL Tab	Cefpodoxime Dicloxacillin and Lactic acid bacillus
Metapure-XL Tab	Metoprolol Succinate
Metaride Tab	Glimipiride and Metformin HCl
Metocontin Tab	Metoclopramide HCl
Metzok Tab	Metoprolol Succinate
Minipress –XL Tab	Parazocin HCl
Pari – SR Tab	Proxitine HCl
Perinorm – CD Cap	Sodium Valproate and Valproic Acid
Pomed – EX Tab	Pantaprozol and domperidone
Reolol – AM 25/5 Tab	Metoprolol Succinate
Revelol – XL Tab	Metoprolol Succinate
Riomet – Trio 2 Tab	Metformin HCl
Sentosa – ER Tab	Venlafaxine
Sporidex – AF Tab	Cefalaxin
Supermet – XL Tab	Metoprolol Succinate
Tegritol - CR Tab	Carbemezapine
Tolol AM Tab	Metoprolol Succinate
Unicontin – E Tab	Theophylline
Valprol – CR Tab	Metoprolol Succinate and Amlodipine
Vasovin- XL Tab	Nitroglycerin
Venlor – XR Tab	Venlafexine HCl
Wellbutrin - XL Tab	Buproprion HCl
Zanocin – OD Tab	Ofloxacin
Zen Retard Tab	Carbemezapine
Zetpol CR Tab	Carbemezapine

Extended release dosage form with prolonged residence time in the stomach are highly desirable for drugs that are locally active in the stomach, have an absorption window in the stomach or in the upper small intestine, unstable in the intestinal or colonic environment or have low solubility at high pH values [9, 19]. Some of the oral extended release drug delivery systems present in the international market are presented in Table 1 [20].

Mechanisms of Oral Extended Release System

Diffusion Controlled Drug Release

Diffusion-controlled drug release can occur in two different formulations i.e., the reservoir device and the matrix or monolithic device. In the reservoir devices, the drug reservoir is covered with a thin polymer layer which functions as a rate-controlling membrane. At the steady state, the drug release rate remains constant to result in a zero-order release. On the other hand, in the matrix (or monolithic) devices, a drug is usually dispersed inside the polymer matrix, and the drug is released into the environment without any rate-controlling barrier layer. The drug release rate decreases over time since the drug molecules away from the surface have to migrate longer distances resulting in non-zero-order release [21]. The matrix system may comprise of drugs dispersed in an insoluble matrix of rigid non-swellable hydrophobic materials like polyvinylchloride, beeswax and stearic acid.

Dissolution Controlled Drug Release

Dissolution/degradation-controlled drug release is based on dissolution or degradation of a polymer membrane encapsulating the drug reservoir or a drug-containing polymer matrix. The drug becomes available for dissolution when the polymeric coating or the polymer matrix dissolves [3]. In the coated formulations, variation of coat thickness and composition can be used to control the release rate of the drug. Water insoluble biodegradable polymers, such as poly(glycolic acid), poly(lactic acid), and poly(ε-caprolactone) have been used for controlled drug release because they degrade slowly by hydrolysis for weeks and months.

Osmotically Controlled Drug Release

The rate of release of drug in these formulations is controlled by the constant in- flow of water across a semi permeable membrane into a reservoir which contains an osmotic agent (osmogens). Generally, the release is not changed by the GI environment but depends entirely on the entry of water into the dosage form. A change in the pore size and type of osmogen can be used to modify the rate of release [22].

Swelling Controlled Drug Release System

Drug release from this system is controlled by the use of hydrophilic polymers which could be naturally occurring hydrophilic gums e.g., acacia, tragacanth, guar gum, alginates, albizia gum and khaya gum, or semi-synthetic polymers e.g., HPMC and xanthan [23, 24]. The drug and polymers are granulated together with a solvent such as alcohol or water, and compressed into tablets. The release of drug from initially dehydrated hydrogels involves adsorption of water and desorption of drug from a swelling controlled diffusion system. As the polymer swells the drug diffuses out [25].

Chemically Controlled Drug Release

Chemically controlled systems include all polymeric formulations which solute diffusion is controlled by chemical reaction such as dissolution of the polymer matrix or cleavage of the drug from a polymer backbone. Depending on the type of degradation reaction, the system may be classified as chemically degradable (e.g., hydrolysis) or biodegradable (e.g., by enzymatic reaction). It is important that the biodegradable system and their metabolites be eliminated from the body without permanent accumulation and they must be nontoxic, non carcinogenic and non teratogenic [26].

2. Mucoadhesive Drug Delivery Systems (MDDS)

Bioadhesion implies attachment of a drug carrier system to a specific biological location like epithelial tissue called mucoadhesion - if the adhesive is attached to a mucus membrane [27, 28]. The luminal surface of the GI tract is a richly glycosylated tissue that presents considerable advantages for formulations with mucoadhesive properties to adhere to the surface. The mucosal route has short residence time which is usually within minutes and mucoadhesive systems can be used to increase the residence time. The adhesive localizes the delivery system and elongates the contact time at the absorption location thus enhancing drug absorption in a site-specific manner [29, 30]. Mucoadhesive drug delivery systems have been utilized for the treatment of periodontal disease and the delivery of proteins and peptides [31]. Tablets have also been formulated as multilayered systems and matrix devices for mucoadhesive delivery. Such tablets are placed under the upper lip (e.g., prochlorperazine adhesive tablets) to avoid the clearance by salivary gland [32].

Mucoadhesive characteristics are affected by the properties of the bioadhesive polymer such as molecular weight, flexibility, hydrogen bonding capacity, cross-linking density, charge, concentration, and hydration (swelling) of the polymer [33] as well as the medium in which the polymer exists. The molecular weight of a polymer above 100,000 has been shown to have a direct relationship with its bioadhesive properties as well as the degree of flexibility for the bioadhesive to effectively entangle with the mucosal surface. Viscosity and diffusion coefficients also have a part to play in polymer mobility and flexibility since the mucosal network experiences higher diffusion when the polymer is more flexible [33].

Table 2. Some mucoadhesive dosage forms available in the market

Name and Form	*Active ingredient*	*Application Site*
Aftach tablet	*Triamcinolone acetonide*	*Oral cavity*
Susadrin tablet	*Nitroglycerin*	*Buccal*
Buccostem tablet	*Prochlorperazine maleate*	*Buccal*
Salcoat powder spray	*Beclomethasone dipropionate*	*Oral cavity*
Soloseryl paste	-	*Gingival*
Orabase gel	-	*Oral cavity*
Orahesive bandage	-	*Oral cavity*
Sucralfate	*Aluminum hydroxide*	*Gastrointestinal ulcers*

In addition, mucoadhesion can effectively take place with polymers that contain functional groups with ability to form hydrogen bonds. The charge on a polymer also affects its degree of mucoadhesion. For example, nonionic polymers have superior mucoadhesive properties when compared to anionic polymers. In the same vein, cationic polymers display higher levels of mucoadhesion when in a neutral or slightly alkaline medium [34]. The density of cross-linking affects diffusion of water into the polymer network and the higher the density, the lower the diffusion rate. This usually causes inadequate swelling of the polymer and a reduced inter-penetration rate between the polymer and mucin. Low concentrations of polymer gives a reduced number of penetrating polymer chains per unit volume of the mucus thus rendering the interaction between polymer and mucus unstable [35]. When the polymer concentration is high, a longer penetrating chain length and enhanced adhesion is obtained. Nevertheless, there exists a critical concentration above which the polymer develops a significantly coiled structure which reduces accessibility of solvent to the polymer and a reduced chain penetration occurs. Therefore, higher concentrations of polymers do not necessarily improve mucoadhesive properties and could sometimes reduce it [36]. Furthermore, hydration (swelling) helps to expand and create a proper macromolecular mesh of sufficient size and also induce mobility in the polymer chains. This is important for the interpenetration process between polymer and mucin [37]. The mucoadhesive properties of a polymer also depend on the surrounding influences next to the polymer such as pH, gastrointestinal movement during talking, eating or drinking and gastrointestinal content. Therefore, an optimum time period for the administration of the dosage form is necessary in order to avoid many of these interfering factors [33].

Polymers have played an important role in designing mucoadhesive drug delivery systems and they include natural polymers such as tragacanth, pectin, gelatin and sodium alginate and semi-synthetic polymers such as the cellulose derivatives [38, 39].

The advantages of MDDS include: rapid absorption due to enormous blood supply and appreciable rates of blood flow in the mucus membranes; the residence time of the dosage form at the site of absorption is prolonged hence increased therapeutic efficacy of the drug; the drug administration is easier thus encouraging patient compliance [40]. In addition, the onset of action is faster due to a high mucosal surface. Oral mucoadhesive drug delivery provides advantages of high accessibility and low enzymatic activity [40]. Some of the oral mucoadhesive drug delivery systems present in the international market are presented in Table 2 [41].

3. Oral Fast Disintegrating/Dissolving Tablets (ODT)

Oral disintegrating tablets are tablets that disintegrate and/or dissolve rapidly in the saliva remarkably fast (usually within a few seconds) without the need for water [42]. They often contain ingredients that enhance the rate of tablet disintegration in the oral cavity. Fast or ODT tablets have been formulated for pediatric, geriatric, and bedridden patients and for active patients who are busy or travelling and may not have access to water [43]. They combine the advantages of dry and liquid formulations. They are suitable for patients who have difficulties in taking conventional oral dosage forms because of hand tremors and dysphagia such as geriatric population, institutionalized patients, psychiatric patients and patients with nausea, vomiting, and motion sickness complications [44 - 47]. ODTs should have sufficient strength to withstand the rigors of the manufacturing process and post-manufacturing handling. They should have a pleasant mouth feel and should not be sensitive to environmental conditions such as humidity and temperature. In addition, they should be adaptable and amenable to existing processing and packaging machineries and cost-effective [48]. ODTs should have sufficient mechanical strength and good package design which is portable and without fragility concern [49].

ODTs should be pleasantly flavored with good taste to increase the acceptability of bitter drugs by various groups of population. Effective taste masking technologies should be adopted for bitter tasting drugs. Some novel ODT technology allow high drug loading, have an acceptable taste with a pleasant mouth feel, leaving minimal residue in the mouth after oral administration [46]. ODT have also been investigated for their potential in improving bioavailability of poorly soluble drugs through enhancing the dissolution profile of the drug and reducing the hepatic metabolism of the drugs. Freeze-drying technique has been used in order to improve the dissolution rate and oral bioavailability of drugs with poor solubility and high permeability [50].

Super disintegrants such as sodium starch glycolate and crospovidone are usually used to facilitate the fast disintegration of the tablets [51]. Despite their advantages, Oral fast disintegrating tablets are quite expensive and they can be fragile and highly friable making storage difficult [52].

Table 3. ODT products available in the international market

Oral tablet	Active ingredients	Manufacturer
Nimpain MD	Nimesulide	Prompt cure pharma
Imodium lingual	Imodium	R.P. Scherer Corp., U.S.A
Pepcidin Rapitab	Pepcid	Merck & Co., U.S.A
Calritin Reditabs	Calritin	Schering Plough, U.S.A
Nurofen Flashtab	Ibuprofen	Boot healthcare
Hyoscyamine sulfate ODT	Hyoscyamine sulfate	Ethex Corporation
Cibalginadue Fast	Ibuprofen	Novartis Consumer Health
Zyprexa	Olanzepine	Eli Lilly
Zofran ODT	Ondansetron	Glaxo Smithkline
Risperdal M Tab	Risperidone	Janssen
Imocdium Instant Melts	Lopermide HCl	Janssen
Propulsid Quick Sol	Cisapride monohydrate	Janssen
Zomig-ZMT and Rapimelt	Zolmitriptan	Astra Zeneca
Alavert	Loratadine	Wyeth Consumer Healthcare
NuLev	Hyoscyamine Sulfate	Schwarz Pharma
Kemstro	Baclofen	Schwarz Pharma
Benadryl Fast Melt	Diphenhydramine Citrate	Pfizer
Nasea OD	Ramosetoron HCl	Yamanouchi
Gaster D	Famotidine	Yamanouchi
Excedrin Quick Tabs	Acetaminophen	Bristol-Myers Squibb
Zolpidem ODT	Zolpidem tartrate	Biovail
Fluoxetine ODT	Fluoxetine	Biovail

Orally disintegrating tablets technologies which entered the market in the 1980s, have grown steadily in demand, and their product pipelines are rapidly expanding. A list of some of the ODTs in the international market is presented in Table 3. New ODT technologies address many pharmaceutical and patient needs, ranging from enhanced life-cycle management to convenient dosing for paediatric, geriatric, and psychiatric patients with dysphagia [46].

4. Oral Fast Disintegrating/Dissolving Films

Oral fast disintegrating/dissolving films (OFDF) consists of ultra-thin films which disintegrate/dissolve rapidly in seconds as it comes in contact with saliva and do not require water for swallowing. They were made to overcome the deficiencies of oral fast disintegrating tablets [53]. Oral films are unique formulation available in various sizes and shape with excellent mucoadhesion properties containing the active pharmaceutical ingredients (API) and excipients [54]. They are useful for patients having diarrhea, emesis, mental problems, incapacitated patients, cough and allergic attacks [55]. Dissolution of the API in the films occurs in the oral cavity and efficacy is improved. Oral films are useful for all categories of patients but more for paediatric and geriatrics both for local and systemic effects [56]. However, they are very sensitive to environmental moisture and the shelf life of most films depends on the API but is generally about two years [57].

The advantages of oral fast dissolving films include: delivery of accurate and precise doses; avoidance of the risk of choking; provision of good mouth feel for patients; rapid disintegration and dissolution in the large surface area of the oral cavity; enhanced bioavailability by pre-gastric absorption thus reducing the frequency of dosing with an overall improvement in patient compliance. Oral films avoids first pass metabolism due to direct absorption from the buccal mucosa into the systemic circulation, with consequent reduction of side effects [58, 59]. Despite these advantages, oral films are limited to drugs having low doses, packaging is expensive and high oral bioavailability is required [60].

Table 4. Marketed product of oral films in the market

Oral film	Active ingredients	Manufacturer	marketed Category
Klonopin® Wafers	Clonazepam	Solvay pharmaceuticals	Antianxiety
Listerine cool mint pocket paks ®	Cool Mint	Pfizer	Mouth freshener
Benadryl ®	Diphenhydramine HCl	Pfizer	Antiallergic
Listerine ®	cool mint	Pfizer	Mouth freshener
Chloraseptic®	Benzocaine/ Menthol	Prestige	Sore throat
Gas-X ®	Simethicone	Novartis	Anti Flatuating
Sudafed PE®	Phenylephrine	Wolters Kluwer Health Inc.	Releliving Congestion
SupressR ®	Menthol	InnoZenR, Inc	Cough suppressants
Triaminic ®	Diphenhydramine HCl	Novartis	Anti allergic
Theraflu ®	Dextromethorphan hydrobromide	Novartis	Cough suppressants

Oral fast dissolving films have been prepared by five methods namely solvent casting, semisolid casting, hot melt extrusion and solid dispersion extrusion [59 - 63].

Polymers such as gelatin, alginate, pectin, HPMC, hydroxypropylcellulose, carboxymethylcellulose, and polyvinylpyrrolidone are used in film formation and can be used alone or in combination [58, 64]. The strength and other properties of the film depend on the type and amount of polymer used in the formulation [65]. Often times, the polymers used are hydrophilic to enhance rapid dissolution when the film contacts the saliva in the buccal cavity [66]. It is also important that the polymers should be non-toxic, non-irritant, tasteless, readily available, have sufficient shelf-life, free from leachable impurities and have good spreading and wetting properties [67]. Some of the ODF in the market are listed in Table 4 [68].

5. Pulsatile Drug-delivery Systems

Pulsatile drug delivery systems are characterized by time period of no release (lag time) followed by a rapid and complete drug release i.e., programmed pattern at appropriate time and/or at appropriate site of action ([69, 70]. They are suitable for drugs with high first-pass effect or special chronopharmacological needs. Pulsatile drug-delivery systems can be classified into site-specific systems in which the drug is released at the desired site within the intestinal tract (e.g., the colon), or time-controlled devices in which the drug is released after a well-defined time period [71]. Site-controlled release is usually controlled by environmental factors, like the pH or enzymes present in the intestinal tract, whereas the drug release from time-controlled systems is controlled primarily by the delivery system and ideally, not by the environment [70, 72]. A delayed release delivery system (where time controls the release) would meet the needs of chronopathologies with symptoms mostly recurring at night time or in the early morning [73] whereas site-specific delivery into the colon district might enable an improvement in the treatment of inflammatory bowel disease and oral bioavailability of peptide drugs [74, 75]. Pulsatile delivery systems aim to deliver the drug at a rate similar to a biological requirement of a given disease therapy and thus manage the disease while minimizing the side effects [76].

In time controlled delivery systems, the release profile is determined by formulation parameters while in site specific controlled delivery systems the release profile is determined by parameters related to gastrointestinal environment. Time controlled systems are divided into those using barrier technologies around the active agent designed to degrade or dissolve after a certain time, and in those that the degradation of the polymer itself induces the release of the active agent [77]. High viscosity types of HPMC (e.g., Methocel® K4M) are often used to retard drug release *in vivo* by forming mechanically strong gel layers able to withstand extensive erosion [78]. For example a product that is already in the market (Chronotropic® or Time Clock® system) [79] consists of two coating layers a hydrophilic (HPMC) or lipophilic (carnauba or beeswax) coating layer and an enteric coating layer in order to prevent premature drug release from the drug containing core. On the other hand, examples of environmental stimuli used to induce release include tablet formulated with three or four different compressed compositions with different release rates mixed and granulated together [80], capsule capable of delivering therapeutic agents into the body in a time controlled or position-controlled pulsatile release fashion [81], capsule composed of one or more population of multicoated particulates such as beads, pellets, granules, etc [82], multi-particulate dosage form comprising of a mixture of two types of beads, immediate release beads and timed pulsatile release beads [83].

Diseases where in pulsatile drug delivery systems are promising include asthma, peptic ulcers, cardiovascular ailments, arthritis and attention deficit syndrome in children and hypercholesterolemia. Some of the marketed technologies of pulsatile drug delivery systems are presented in Table 5.

6. Floating Drug Delivery Systems

Floating drug delivery systems (FDDS) are hydrodynamically balanced systems that remain buoyant in the stomach by virtue of their floating properties without affecting the gastric emptying rate for a prolonged period of time [84]. While the system is floating on the gastric contents, the drug is released slowly from the system at a desired rate. This results in an increase in the gastroretentive time (GRT) due to the delayed gastric emptying which results in reduced fluctuations in the plasma levels of drugs. After the release of drug, the residual system is emptied from the stomach. In order for a dosage form to float in the stomach, the density of the dosage form should be less than the gastric contents i.e., density of less than 1.0 g/ml [85, 86].

Table 5. Marketed Pulsatile Delivery Technologies

Brand	Technology	Manufacturer
Diffucaps®	Multiparticulate system	Eurand
Orbexa®	Microbeads produced by granulation, spheronization and extrusion techniques	Eurand
OROS® Push Pull™	Osmotic controlled bilayer/trilayer tablet	Alza
CODAS™	Chronotherapeutic oral drug delivery system using microbeads	Elan
SODAS®	Spheroidal oral drug delivery system using microbeads	Elan
SyncroDose®	Tablets coated with TIMERx-based material	Penwest
Geoclock®	Chronotherapeutic coated tablets	SkeyPharma
Geomatrix™	Multilayered tablet	SkeyPharma
Pulsincap®	Plugged capsule	Scherer DDS, Ltd
Port®	Coated gelatin capsule with osmotic core	Port Systems, LLC
EGALET® Time release	Three compartments coated tablet	Egalet
OSDrC®	Multicoated tablet with a variety of pulsatile drug release profiles	OSDrC
PULSYS ™	Tablet containing multiple pellets with different release profiles	MiddleBrook Pharmaceuticals™
COLAL®	Coated pellets, tablets or capsules	Alizyme Therapeutics Limited

Factors that have been shown to affect the GRT include specific gravity and food. The effect of food on GRT dosage forms depend on its nature, caloric content and the frequency of intake [85 - 87]. Obviously, when the gastroretentive properties of a floating dosage form are independent of meal size, the dosage form can be suitable for patients with a wide range of eating habits [88]. In addition, buoyant delivery systems might provide a beneficial strategy for the treatment of gastric and duodenal cancers.

One of the disadvantages of floating systems is that they require a sufficiently high level of fluids in the stomach for the drug delivery to remain buoyant [89]. Thus, coating the dosage form with bioadhesive polymers which enables them to adhere to the mucous lining of the stomach wall may prove beneficial [90]. Alternatively, the dosage form may be administered with a glass full of water (200–250 ml). Floating systems are not suitable for drugs that are irritant to gastric mucosa and for those that have solubility or stability problems in gastric fluids. Drugs such as nifedipine, which is well absorbed along the entire GI tract and do not undergo significant first-pass metabolism, may not be desirable candidates for FDDS since the slow rate of gastric emptying may lead to reduced systemic bioavailability [91].

The currently available FDDS designed on the basis of delayed gastric emptying and buoyancy principles are the effervescent and non-effervescent delivery systems. The effervescent FDDS utilize matrices prepared with swellable polymers such as Methocel® or polysaccharides, e.g., chitosan, and effervescent components, e.g., sodium bicarbonate and citric or tartaric acid [92] or matrices containing chambers of liquid that gasify at body temperature [93 - 95]. The matrices are fabricated such that on arrival in the stomach, carbon dioxide is liberated by the acidity of the gastric contents and is entrapped in the jellified hydrocolloid. This produces an upward motion of the dosage form and maintains its buoyancy. A decrease in specific gravity causes the dosage form to float on the chime [92]. The carbon dioxide generating components may be intimately mixed within the tablet matrix, in which case a single-layered tablet is produced [96], or a bilayered tablet may be compressed which contains the gas generating mechanism in one hydrocolloid containing layer and the drug in the other layer formulated for a sustained release effect [97]. This concept has also been exploited for floating capsule systems which have been prepared by filling the capsule with a mixture of sodium alginate and sodium bicarbonate, and in vitro tests has shown that the generation of carbon dioxide that was trapped in the hydrating gel network on exposure to an acidic environment causes the capsule to float [98].

The preparation of non effervescent FDDS involves intimate mixing of drug with a gel-forming hydrocolloid, which swells in contact with gastric fluid after oral administration and maintains a relative integrity of shape and a bulk density of less than unity within the outer gelatinous barrier [99]. The air trapped by the swollen polymer confers buoyancy and the gel structure acts as a reservoir for sustained drug release since the drug is slowly released by a controlled diffusion through the gelatinous barrier [100]. As the exterior surface of the dosage form goes into solution, the gel layer is maintained by the immediate adjacent hydrocolloid layer becoming hydrated and the drug dissolves in and diffuses out with the diffusing solvent, creating a 'receding boundary' within the gel structure [100]. Polymers used for these delivery system are gel-forming or highly swellable cellulose type hydrocolloids, polysaccharides, and matrix forming polymers such as polycarbonate, polyacrylate, polymethacrylate and polystyrene. Some floating drug delivery systems available in the market are presented in Table 6 [101, 102].

Table 6. Floating drug delivery systems available in the market

Brand Name	Active Ingredient(s)
Cifran OD ®	Ciprofloxacin
Madopar ®	L-DOPA and Benserazide
Valrelease ®	Diazepam
Topalkan ®	Aluminum -magnesium antacid
Almagate FlatCoat ®	Aluminum -magnesium antacid
Liquid Gavison ®	Aluminium hydroxide
Conviron	Ferrous sulfate
Cytotec®	Misoprostal

Conclusion

Oral drug delivery systems will continue to be the most preferred form of drug delivery due to their ease of administration and high patient acceptance and compliance. There is an increasing number of dosage form designed to provide efficient delivery systems that will increase the bioavailability of drug, reduce the frequency of administration, reduce the fluctuation blood concentration and provide targeted drug delivery. It is believed that increasing number of more efficient systems would become commercially available in the years to come.

References

[1] S. J. Hwang, H. Park, K. Park, Gastric retentive drug-delivery systems, *Crit. Rev. Ther. Drug Carrier Syst.*, 5 (1998) 243–284.

[2] K. P. S Kumar, D. Bhowmik, Dutta, A. S. Paswan, L. Deb, Recent trends in scope and opportunities of control release oral drug delivery systems, *Crit. Rev. Pharm. Sci.*, 1 (2012) 20-40.

[3] G. M. Jantzen, J. R. Robinson, Sustained-controlled release drug delivery systems. In: Modern Pharmaceutic,. (eds) Banker, G. S., Rhodes, C. T. 4th edition. Marcel Dekker Inc., New York. pp. (2002) 503-530.

[4] H. G. Shivakumar, D. V. Gowda, T. M. P. Kumar, Floating controlled drug delivery systems for prolonged gastric residence: a review, *Ind. J. Pharm. Educ.*, 38 (2004) 172-78.

[5] S. Desai, S. A. Bolton, Floating controlled release system: In vitro – In-vivo evaluation. *Pharm. Res.*, 10 (1993) 1321-1325.

[6] S. Garg, S. Sharma, Gastroretentive drug delivery systems. *Business Briefing Pharmatech.* (2003) 160-164.

[7] S. Lindgren, L. Janzon. Dysphagia: prevalence of swallowing complaints and clinical findings. *Med. Clin. North Am.*, 77 (1993) 3–5.

[8] A. A. Deshpande, C. T. Rhodes, N. H. Shah, A.W. Malick, Controlled-release drug delivery systems for prolonged gastric residence: An overview, *Drug Dev. Ind. Pharm.*, 22 (1996) 531–539.

[9] K. B. Aher, G. B. Bhavar, H. P. Joshi, S. R. Chaudhari, Recent advances in compression-coated tablets as a controlled drug delivery system. *Saudi Pharm. J.*, 1 (2011) 1-14.

[10] S. M. A. El-halim, M. M. Amin, O. N. E. Gazayerly, N. A. A. E. Gawad, Salbutamol sulphate controlled release hydrophilic matrix tablets, RGUHS *J. Pharm. Sci.* 01, (2011) 194-200.

[11] M. G. Khan, Controlled release oral dosage forms: Some recent advances in matrix type drug delivery systems. *The Sciences*, 1 (2001) 350-354.

[12] R. Gronia, G. Heun, Oral dosage forms with controlled gastrointestinal transit, *Drug Dev. Ind. Pharm.*, 10 (1984) 527- 39.

[13] Y. W. Chein, Oral drug delivery and delivery systems, Marcel dekker Inc., New York, (1992) pp. 139-196.

[14] N. K. Jain, Controlled and novel drug delivery system, In: progress in controlled and novel drug delivery system, C B S publishers and distributors, New Delhi. (2004) pp. 419-435.

[15] M. Q. Ahsan, M. M. Rahman, M. K. Jha, I. Ahmed, M. M. R. Moghal, M. H. Rahman, Development and *in-vitro* evaluation of sustained release matrix tablets of salbutamol sulphate using methocel K100M CR polymer. *Int. J. Pharm. Sci. Res*. 02 (2011) 567-576.

[16] B. Jayanthi, P M. Manna, S. Madhusudhan, G. P. Mohanta, R. Manavalan, Per oral extended release products- A overview. *J. Appl. Pharm. Sci.*, 01 (2011) 50-55.

[17] M. Pogula, S. Nazeer, Extended release formulation. *Int. J. Pharm. Technol.*, 02 (2010) 625-84.

[18] P. M. Dandagi, V. S. Masthiholimath, M. B. Patil, F. V. Manvi, A. P. Gadad, R. Sharma, Development and evaluation of theophylline and salbutamol sulphate sustained release matrix tablets. *Indian Drugs*, 76 (2005) 598-602.

[19] B. N. Singh, H. K Kim, Floating drug delivery systems: an approach to oral controlled drug delivery via gastric retention, *J. Control. Rel.*, 63 (2000) 235-59.

[20] S. Kumar, A. Kumar, V. Gupta, K.. Malodia, P. Rakha, Oral extended release drug delivery system: A promising approach. *Asian J. Pharm. Tech.*, 2 (2012) 38-43.

[21] G. Acharya, K.. Park, Mechanisms of controlled drug release from drug-eluting stents, *Adv. Drug Del. Rev.*, 58 (2006) 387–401.

[22] F. Theeuwes, Elementary osmotic pump, *J. Pharm. Sci.*, 64 (1975) 1987-1991.

[23] O. A. Odeku, J. T. Fell, Evaluation of khaya gum as a directly compressible matrix system for controlled release, *J. Pharm. Pharmacol.*, 56 (2004) 1365-1370.

[24] O. A. Odeku, J. T. Fell, Effects of the method of preparation on the compression, mechanical and release properties of khaya gum matrices, *Pharm. Dev. Technol.*, 11 (2006) 435-441.

[25] C. Maderuelo, A. Zarzuelo, J. M. Lanao, Critical factors in the release of drugs from sustained release hydrophilic matrices, *J. Control. Rel.*, 154 (2011) 2-19.

[26] V. V. Renade, J. P. Cannon, Drug delivery systems. 3rd Edition. *CRC Press*, FL.(2011) pp. 79-124.

[27] K. P. R. Chowdary, L. Srinivas, Mucoadhesive drug delivery systems: A review of current status, *Indian Drugs,* 37 (2000) 400-406.

[28] M. Davidovich-Pinhas, H. Bianco-Peled, Alginate-PEGAc: a new mucoadhesive polymer. *Acta Biomater*., 7 (2011) 625-633.

[29] X. Yang, J. R. Robinson, Bioadhesion in mucosal drug delivery. In: Biorelated polymers and gels: controlled release and applications in biomedical engineering. Okano, T. (ed.) San Diego, CA: Academic Press; (1998) pp. 135–192.

[30] V. M. Patel, B. G. Prajapati, M. M. Patel, Formulation, evaluation and comparison of bilayered and multilayered mucoadhesive buccal devices of propranolol hydrochloride, *AAPS Pharm Sci. Tech*, 8 (2007) 22-28.

[31] S. S. Davis, J. G. Hardy, M. J. Taylor, A. Stockwell, D. R. Whalley, C. G. Wilson, The *in vivo* evaluation of an osmotic device using gamma scintography. *J. Pharm. Pharmacol.*, 36 (1984) 740-742.

[32] N. Nafee, F. Ismail, N. Boraie, L. Mortada, Mucoadhesive buccal patches of miconazole nitrate: in vitro/in vivo performance and effect of ageing, *Int. J. Pharm.*, 264 (2003) 1-14.

[33] S. S. Lahoti, S. G. Shep, R. V. Mayee, S. S. Toshniwal, Mucoadhesive drug delivery system: A review, *Indo-Global J. Pharm. Sci*., 1 (2011) 243-251.

[34] E. L. McConnell, H. M. Fadda, A. W. Basit, Gut instincts: explorations in intestinal physiology and drug delivery, *Int. J. Pharm.,* 364 (2008) 213-226.

[35] R. H. Muller, C. Jacobs, Buparvaquone mucoadhesive nanosuspension: preparation, optimisation and long-term stability, *Int. J. Pharm*., 237 (2002) 151-161.

[36] R. Shaikh, T. R. Raj Singh, M. J. Garland, A. D. Woolfson, R. F. Donnelly, Mucoadhesive drug delivery systems, *J. Pharm. Bio-allied Sci.,* 3 (2011) 89-100.

[37] P. Tangri, S. Khurana, N.V.S. Madhay, Mucoadhesive drug delivery: mechanism and methods of evaluation, *Int. J. Pharma Bio. Sci*., 2 (2011) 458-467.

[38] H. S. Ch'ng, H. Park, P. Kelly, J. R. Robinson, Bioadhesive polymers as platform for oral controlled drug delivery., II: Synthesis and evaluation of some swelling water insolublebioadhesive polymers. *J. Pharm. Sci*., 74 (1985) 399-405.

[39] D. Harris, J.R. Robinson, Drug delivery via the mucous membranes of the oral cavity, *J. Pharm. Sci*., 81 (1992) 1-10

[40] G. P. Andrew, T. P. Laverty, D. S. Jones, Mucoadhesive polymeric for controlled drug delivery, *Eur. J. Pharm. Biopharm*., 71 (2009) 505-518.

[41] *A. Ahuja, R. K. Khar, J. Ali, Mucoadhesive drug delivery systems, Drug Dev. Ind. Pharm., 23 (1997) 489-515.*

[42] K. B. Patel, S. N. Shete, V. S. Belgamwar, A. R. Tekade, Formulation design and optimization of taste-masked mouth-dissolving tablets of tramadolol hydrochloride, *Asian J. Pharm*., 4 (2010) 239-245.

[43] A. Arunachalam, M. Karthikeyan, S. A Kumar, K. Konam, P. H., Prasad, S. Sethuraman, S. Manidipa, Fast dissolving drug delivery system: A review, *J. Global Trends Pharm. Sci*., 1 (2010) 92-110.

[44] H. Seager, Drug-delivery products and the zydis fast-dissolving dosage form, *J. Pharm. Pharmacol.,* 50 (1998) 375-382.

[45] L. H. Reddy, B. Ghosh, Fast dissolving drug delivery systems: a review of the literature, *Indian J. Pharm. Sci*., 64 (2002) 331- 336.

[46] B. Shyamala, G. Y. Narmada, Rapid dissolving tablets: A novel dosage form, *The Indian Pharm.* 13 (2002) 09-12.

[47] A. Modi, P. Tayade, Enhancement of dissolution profile by solid dispersion (kneading) technique, *AAPS Pharm. Sci. Tech*., 7 (2006) 68-75.

[48] J. Hirani, D. Rathod, K. Vadalia, Orally disintegrating tablets: A review. *Trop. J. Pharm. Res*., 8 (2009) 161-172.

[49] S. Velmurugan, S. Vinushitha, Oral disintegrating tablets: an overview, *Int. J. Chem. Pharm. Sci*., 1 (2010) 1-12.

[50] M. Kumar, K. R. Sethipooja, G. K. Saraogi, A. K. Singhai, Orally disintegrating tablets: A review, *Int. Res. J. Pharm*., 2 (2011) 16-22.

[51] N. G. Swamy, N. Sachin, Z Abbas, Design and characterization of oral dispersible tablets of enalapril maleate using a co-processed excipient, *J. App. Pharm. Sci*., 2 (2012) 040-049.

[52] V. K.. Mudgal, P. R. Sethi, R. Kheri, G. K.. Saraogi, A. K. Singhai, Orally disintegrating tablets: a review, *Int. Res. J. Pharm*., 2 (2011) 16-22.

[53] S. Kalyan, M. Bansal, Recent trends in the development of oral dissolving films, *Int. J. Pharm. Tech. Res*., 4 (2012) 725-735.

[54] A. Arya, A. Chandra, V Sharma, K.. Pathak, Fast Dissolving oral films: An innovative drug delivery system and dosage form, *Int. J. Chem. Tech Res*., 2 (2010) 576-583.

[55] M. Malke, Shidhaye, V. J. Kadam, Formulation and evaluation of oxacarbazine fast dissolving tablets, *Indian J. Pharm. Sci*., 69 (2007) 211-214.

[56] D. Meenu, S. S. Shahiwala, F. Aliasgar, A review on mouth dissolving films, *Curr. Drug Del.*, 6 (2009) 469-476.

[57] R. Saurabh, R. Malviya, P. K Sharma, Trends in buccal film: Formulation characteristics. Recent studies and Patents. *Eur. J. Appl. Sci*., 3 (2011) 93-101.

[58] S. L. Patil, P. R. Mahaparale, M. A. Shivnikar, S. S. Tiwari, K. V. Pawar, and P. N. Sane, Fast dissolving oral films: an innovative drug delivery syste,. *Int. J. Res. Rev. Pharm. Appl. Sci.*, 2 (2010) 482-496.

[59] R. Bradoo, Fast dissolving drug delivery systems. *JAMA India*. 4 (2001) 27-31.

[60] B. Bhyan, S. Jangra, M. Kaur, H. P. Singh, Orally fast dissolving films: innovation in formulation and technology, *Int. J. Pharm. Sci. Rev. Res*., 9 (2011) 50-57.

[61] B. R. Yasmeen, S. Firoz, Y. Chandra, A. Vikram, A. Mahitha, U. Aruna, Preparation and evaluation of oral fast dissolving films of citalopram hydrobromide, *Int. J. Biopharm*., 3 (2012) 103-106.

[62] R. Kaur, R. Bala, Formulation and evaluation of Ivabradine hydrochloride fast dissolving film, *J. Pharm. Res*., 5 (2012) 3327-3330.

[63] M. Nishigakia, K. Kawaharab, M. Nawac, M. Futamurac, M. Nishimurad, K.. Matsuuraa, K.. Kitaichi, Y. Kawaguchic, T. Tsukiokad, K.. Yoshidac, Y. Itoha, Development of fast dissolving oral film containing dexamethasone as an antiemetic medication: Clinical usefulness, *Int. J. Pharm*., 424 (2012) 12– 17.

[64] A. S. Kulkarni, H. A. Deokule, M. S. Mane, D. M Ghadge, Exploration of different polymers for use in the formulation of oral fast dissolving strips, *J. Curr. Pharm. Res.*, 2 (2010) 33-35

[65] A. Fini, V. Bergamante, G.C. Ceschel, C. Ronchi, C.A. Fonseca de Moraes, Fast dispersible/slow releasing ibuprofen tablets, *Eur. J. Pharm. Biopharm.*, 69 (2008) 335–341.

[66] Y. D. Priyanka, Y. A. Chaudhary, T. E. G Murthy, B. Seshagiri, Approaches for taste masking of bitter drugs: a review, *J. Adv. Drug Res.*, 2 (2011) 58-67.

[67] R. P. Dixit, S. P. Puthli, Oral strip technology: Overview and future potential, *J. Control. Rel.*, 139 (2009) 94–107.

[68] P. Saini, A. Kumar, P. Sharma, S. Visht, Fast disintegrating oral films: a recent trend of drug delivery, *Int. J. Drug Dev. Res.*, 4 (2012) 80-94.

[69] L. E. Kalantzi, Karavas E, E. X. Koutris, D. N. Bikiaris, Recent advances in oral pulsatile drug delivery, *Rec. Pat. Drug Del. Form*, 3 (2009) 49-63.

[70] T. Bussemer, I. Otto, R. Bodmeier, Pulsatile drug-delivery systems, *Crit. Rev. Ther. Drug Car. Sys.*, 18 (2001) 433-458.

[71] B. G. Stubbe, S. C. De Smedt, J. Demeester, Programmed polymeric devices for pulsed drug delivery, *Pharm Res.*, 21 (2004) 1732-1740.

[72] A. Kikuchi, T. Okano, Pulsatile drug release control using hydrogels, *Adv. Drug Del. Rev.*, 54 (2002) 53-77.

[73] N. A. Peppas, W. Leobandung, Stimuli-sensitive hydrogels: ideal carriers for chronobiology and chronotherapy, *J. Biomat. Sci. Polym. Ed.*, 15 (2004) 125-144.

[74] A. Gazzaniga, A. Maroni, M.E Sangalli, L. Zema, Time-controlled oral delivery systems for colon targeting. *Expt. Opin. Drug Del.*, 3 (2006) 583-597.

[75] A. Gazzaniga, L. Palugan, A Foppoli, M.E Sangalli, Oral pulsatile delivery systems based on swellable hydrophilic polymers, *Eur. J. Pharm. Biopharm.*, 68 (2008) 11-18.

[76] R. Yoshida, K. Sakai, T.Okano, Y. Sakurai, Pulsatile drug delivery systems using hydrogels, *Adv. Drug Del. Rev.*, 11 (1993) 85-108.

[77] J. B Kohn, D. M. Schachter, US20037326425 (2003).

[78] M. E. Sangalli, A., Maroni, A. Foppoli, L. Zemaa, F. Giordano, A. Gazzaniga, Different HPMC viscosity grades as coating agents for an oral time and/or site-controlled delivery system: A study on process parameters and *in vitro* performances, *Eur. J. Pharm. Sci.*, 22 (2004) 469-476.

[79] A. Maroni, L. Zema, M. Cerea, M. E. Sangalli, Oral pulstile drug delivery systems, *Expert Opin. Drug Del.*, 2 (2005) 855-871.

[80] M. Dittgen, S. Fricke, C. Timpe, H. Gerecke, A. Eichardt. US20006117450 (2000).

[81] P. J. Percel, G. M. Venkatesh, K. S. Vishnupad, KWO58433. (2001).

[82] G. P Venkatesh. US2006246134. (2006).

[83] P. J. Percel, N. H. Vyas, K. S. Vishnupad, G. M. Venkatesh. US2005025824. (2005).

[84] N. Brahma, S. Kwon, H. Kim, Floating drug delivery systems - an approach to oral controlled drug delivery via gastric retention, *Journal of Controlled Release*, 63 (2000) 235-259.

[85] P. Mojaverian, R. K. Ferguson, P. H. Vlasses, M. L. Rocci, A. Oren, J. A. Fix, L. J. Caldwell, C. Gardner. Estimation of gastric residence time of the Heidelberg capsule in humans: effect of varying food composition. *Gastroenter.*, 89 (1985) 392–397.

[86] M. Oth, M. Franz, J. Timmermans, A. Möes, The bilayer floating capsule: a stomach-directed drug delivery system for misoprostol. *Pharm. Res.*, 9 (1992) 298–302.

[87] J. G. Moore, P. E Christian, J. A. Brown, C. Brophy, F. Datz, A. Taylor, N. Alazraki. Influence of meal weight and caloric content on gastric emptying of meals in man. *Dig. Dis. Sci.* 29 (1984) 513–519.

[88] L. Whitehead, J. T. Fell, J. H. Collett, H. L. Sharma, A. M. Smith, Floating dosage forms: an in vivo study demonstrating prolonged gastric retention, *J. Control. Release*, 55 (1998) 3–12.

[89] J. Timmermans, A. J. Moes, Factors controlling the buoyancy and gastric retention capabilities of floating matrix capsules: New data for reconsidering the controversy, *J. Pharm. Sci.*, 83 (1994) 18-24.

[90] V. S Chitnis, V. S. Malshe, J. K. Lalla, Bioadhesive polymers-synthesis, evaluation and application in controlled release tablets, *Drug Dev. Ind. Pharm.*, 17 (1991) 879–892.

[91] N. Rouge, P. Buri, E. Doelker, Drug absorption sites in the gastrointestinal tract and dosage forms for site-specific delivery. *Int. J. Pharm.*, 136 (1996) 117–139.

[92] A. Rubinstein, D. R. Friend, Specific delivery to the gastrointestinal tract. In: Polymeric site-specific pharmacotherapy, A. J. Domb (Ed.), Wiley, Chichester (1994) pp. 282–283.

[93] A. S. Michaels, Drug delivery device with self actuated mechanism for retaining device in selected area. US Patent 3, 786, 813 (1974).

[94] A. S. Michaels, J. D. Bashwa, A. Zaffaroni, Integrated device for administering beneficial drug at programmed rate. US Patent 3, 901, 232 (1975).

[95] W. A. Ritschel, Targeting in the gastrointestinal tract: new approaches, *Methods Find. Exp. Clin. Pharmacol.*, 13 (1991) 313–336.

[96] H. Hashim, A. Li Wan Po, Improving the release characteristics of water-soluble drugs from hydrophilic sustained release matrices by in situ gas-generation, *Int. J. Pharm*, 35 (1987) 201–209.

[97] H. M. Ingani, J. Timmermans, A. J. Möes, Conception and *in vivo* investigation of peroral sustained release floating dosage forms with enhanced gastrointestinal transit, *Int. J. Pharm.*, 35 (1987) 157–164.

[98] A. F. Stockwell, S. S. Davis, S. E. Walker, *In vitro* evaluation of alginate gel systems as sustained release drug delivery systems, *J. Control. Rel.*, 3 (1986) 167–175.

[99] A. K. Hilton, P. B. Deasy, *In vitro* and *in vivo* evaluation of an oral sustained-release floating dosage form of amoxycillin trihydrate, *Int. J. Pharm.*, 86 (1992) 79–88.

[100] P. R. Sheth, J. Tossounian, The hydrodynamically balanced system (HBS™): a novel drug delivery system for oral use. *Drug Dev. Ind. Pharm.* 10 (1984) 313–339.

[101] G. Chawla, P. Gupta, A. K. Bansal, Gastroretentive drug delivery systems. In: Progress in controlled and novel drug delivery systems. Jain, N. K. (ed.) CBS Publishers and Distributors. New Delhi. (2004) pp. 76-97.

[102] S. P. Vyas, R. K. Khar, Gastroretentive systems. In: Controlled drug delivery. Vallabh Prakashan, Delhi, India. (2006) pp. 197-217.

In: Recent Advances in Drug Delivery Research
Editor: Valerio Voliani
ISBN: 978-1-62948-228-6

Chapter 3

Recent Progress in pH-Sensitive Nanocarriers for an Efficient Delivery of Biomolecules to Specific Targets

Daniele R. Nogueira, Montserrat Mitjans and M. Pilar Vinardell*
Departament de Fisiologia, Facultat de Farmacia, Universitat de Barcelona,
Av. Joan XXIII s/n, Barcelona, Spain

Abstract

The pH variations in the body are particularly important in the development of nanocarriers that have the ability to promote a triggered release of active biomolecules in a pH-dependent fashion. These kind of specific devices have been studied as drug delivery systems of anti-cancer drugs to tumour cells, peptides and proteins to the gastrointestinal tract, anti-inflammatory drugs to inflamed tissues, proteins and growth factors to ischemia tissues, and drugs and genes to the intracellular compartments. Different approaches have been taken to develop pH-sensitive delivery devices, including the incorporation of pH-responsive polymers, peptides, surfactants and fusogenic lipids. pH induced decomposition or changes in the conformation and permeability of the nanocarriers form the basis for the pH-sensitive behaviour of these delivery systems. The pH targeting approach is regarded as a promising strategy that can sharply increase the therapeutic efficacy of various treatment protocols and, in specific cases, overcome the multidrug resistance of many bacterial and tumour cells. This chapter focuses on the advances in the development of pH-sensitive nanocarriers and their performance as nano-scale strategies for the efficient drug and gene delivery to the intracellular compartments and specific tissues with an acidic environment.

Keywords: Nanotechnology, nanocarriers, drug delivery, pH-sensitive activity, acidic environment

---

* E-mail: mpvinardellmh@ub.edu.

Introduction

Nanocarriers offers a suitable means as drug delivery systems with promising application for delivering diagnostic and imaging agents, and therapeutic compounds such as drugs and genes [1-3]. These nanodevices have the ability to improve the existing treatments through their altered pharmacokinetics and biodistribution profiles. Furthermore, they have the capacity to protect the active molecule from undesirable interactions with biological milieu components, to improve the solubility of hydrophobic compounds and to provide controlled release of the contents [4].

In addition, significant advances made in nanoscience and nanotechnology over the last decade have led to the development of new platforms with the aim to further improve on the nanocarriers therapeutic efficacy. Researchers have explored the use of nanodevices that have the ability to produce physicochemical changes in their structure when exposed to some external stimuli. These stimuli favor drug release at the target site and can include (a) physical signals such as temperature, electric field, magnetic field, and ultrasound; and (b) chemical signals such as pH, ionic strength, redox potential, and enzymatic activities [5, 6]. In stimuli-sensitive drug delivery, required amounts of the active biomolecule can be released at the site of action in response to one or more of these stimuli.

Among the environmental stimuli mentioned above, the pH targeting approach is regarded as a promising strategy that can sharply increase the therapeutic efficacy of various treatment protocols and, thus, has developed rapidly and has been widely used to design novel drug delivery devices [7-10]. This kind of nanocarriers can be divided into two types: one induces drug release at higher pH, which is usually used for oral drug delivery; and other that release its content under acidic conditions and, thus, can be used to target tumor, inflamed and ischemia tissues, as well as endosomal or lysosomal compartments, where the pH is relatively low.

This chapter focuses on the recent progress in pH-sensitive nanocarriers that can efficiently delivery anti-cancer drugs to tumor cells, peptides and proteins to the gastrointestinal tract, anti-inflammatory drugs to inflammatory disorders, proteins and growth factors in ischemia conditions, or drugs and genes to the intracellular compartments. In particular, the design of pH-responsive nanodevices for selective drug delivery comprises targeting the variations of pH at the level of organs, tissues or cell organelles. At the cellular level, especially at the intracellular compartments, pH-sensitive nanocarriers have been designed to escape the acidic environment of the endosomes for cytoplasmic drug release [9, 11]. At the tissue level, the pH-responsive formulations have been exploit to target solid tumors [12, 13], inflamed [14, 15] and ischemia [16, 17] tissues, which have a characteristic acidic extracellular environment different from healthy tissues. Finally, at the organ level, pH-responsive nanodevices have been formulated for oral delivery and differential drug uptake along the gastrointestinal (GI) tract that is characterized by a pH gradient [18, 19].

Design of pH-Sensitive Nanocarriers

The ability of a nanocarrier to selectively reach and delivery its content in the site of action determines its utility and potential biomedical applications. In this line, a brief and efficient approach on pH-tunable nanomaterials is a promising strategy to target a specific pathological area. The therapeutic efficacy of biomolecules encapsulated in pH-responsive drug delivery systems depends on the specificity of the selected nanodevice for the acidic environment of target organs, tissues or cell organelles. This specific release activity allow the bioactive compound to reach potential target sites including tumor interstitium; inflammatory and ischemia tissues; GI tract (especially the small intestine); and intracellular compartments such as the cytosol (RNAi, drugs targeting cytosolic proteins) [20, 21], nucleus (DNA-active drugs, DNA gene vectors) [22, 23], and other cellular compartments including Golgi apparatus, endoplasmic reticulum and mitochondria [24, 25] (Figure 1).

The knowledge about the physiological pH in organs, tissues and cellular compartments determines the use of the pH targeting approach for the development of novel drug delivery systems. The pH variation along the GI tract is well known and should be taken into consideration when developing oral administrations. The stomach has a strongly acidic pH of ~1.5, while the pH in the small intestine and colon is almost neutral. Therefore, pH-sensitive nanodevices that are stable in the acidic environment of GI tract might be useful to deliver acid-sensitive drugs such as peptides and proteins through the oral route [18, 26]. The solid tumors, in part due to the high glycolysis, usually show extracellular pH slightly deviates to the acidic region from pH 7.4, by which pH-sensitive delivery of anti-cancer drugs may be developed [27]. The pH value in tumor matrix is affected by tumor histology, tumor volume and the location within a tumor, and can be as low as 5.7 [28, 29]. The inflammatory tissues are also known to be acidic, reaching values of pH as low as 5.0 [14].

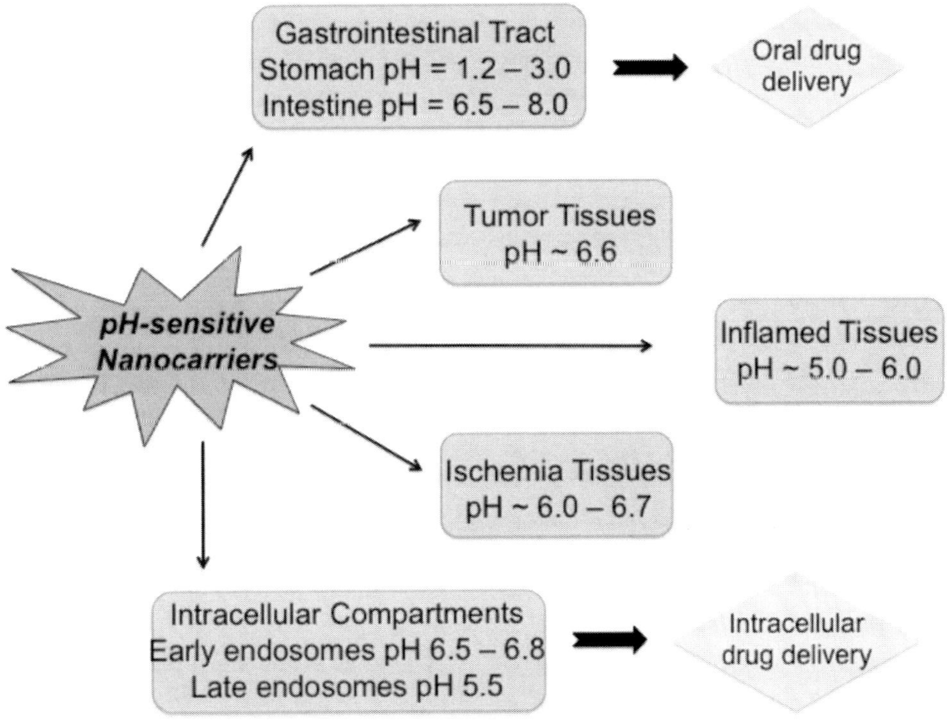

Figure 1. Different targets that can be reached by pH-sensitive nanocarriers.

In this same line, the ischemia tissues have an acidic environment, which can reach pH of about 6.0 or even lower values under severe conditions [30]. Finally, the pH variation in different cellular compartments is the basis for the pH-sensitive intracellular delivery of drugs. Early endosomal compartments have a pH from 6.5 to 6.8, while the lumen of late endosomes has a lower pH, of about 5.5 [31, 32]. The lysosomes have a pH as low as 4.6 to 5.0 [33] and contain degradative enzymes, which may destroy the nanocarriers that are unable to escape from endosomes [34]. Thus, considering the different pH range along the intracellular compartments, the design of pH-triggered drug delivery systems is a promising approach for a specific release of bioactive molecules.

During the design and development of a new formulation with pH-responsive activity, the researchers concern about the selection of a bioactive compound that has the ability to change its conformity and lytic properties as a function of the pH variations. Different approaches have been taken to develop pH-sensitive delivery devices, including the incorporation of pH-responsive polymers, peptides, surfactants and fusogenic lipids. In the next sections of the present chapter, it is presented a description of the recent trends and innovative applications of these classes of bioactive compounds for a pH-triggered delivery of drugs and genes.

pH-Responsive Activity: Tumor Targeting

Compared with traditionally used drug carriers, nanoparticulated drug delivery systems possess unique abilities to pass through the smallest capillary vessels, with prolonged duration in blood stream, and to penetrate cells and tissue gap to arrive at target organs. However, the delivery of nanocarriers to a solid tumor is especially determined by physiological factors including tumor interstitial fluid pressure, lymphatic drainage and tumor blood vasculature [4]. There are several major differences between the blood and lymph vasculatures in tumor and normal tissues, which may favor the preferential extravasion and retention of nanocarriers in these pathological tissues [35]. The defective lymphatic drainage that decreases the clearance mechanisms, together with leaky tumor blood vessels, result in accumulation and retention of high molecular weight compounds in solid tumors, a phenomenon recognized as the enhanced permeability and retention (EPR) effect [36]. Considering these particular characteristics of the tumor tissues, colloidal drug delivery systems have been used extensively to improve the specificity, safety and efficacy of chemotherapeutic treatment for solid tumors. The pathophysiological EPR effect is considered as the driving force for their tumor tropic distribution patterns. On the other hand, the physicochemical properties of the nanocarrier such as surface charge, hydrophobicity and particle size also affect its fate after the systemic administration and should be considered during the design of novel nanomedicines.

The human solid tumors have been shown to exhibit acidic extracellular pH environments (pH_e) of about 6.6; however, can usually vary from 5.7 to 7.8 [28], being this disparity dependent upon tumor histology, tumor volume, and location inside a tumor. This acidity is caused in part by lactic acid accumulation in rapidly growing tumor cells owing to their elevated rates of glucose uptake but reduced rates of oxidative phosphorylation [37].

Therefore, considering this particular environment, researchers have increasingly exploit the acidic environment of the tumors to develop pH-sensitive nanocarriers that can target solid tumors, achieve high local drug concentration and also minimize overall systemic exposure, which avoid many adverse effects characteristic of the chemotherapeutic agents [38]. Noteworthy is that the majority of research in the cancer area is focused on targeting the membrane proteins enriched in tumor cells [4]; however, the pH targeting approach is regarded as a promising strategy that can sharply increase the therapeutic efficacy of various treatment protocols and, in specific cases, overcome the multidrug resistance of many tumour cells.

Nanoparticles have been formulated for pH-dependent tumor-specific drug release by using especially polymers that have the ability to change their physicochemical properties, such as the swelling capacity and the increased solubility as a function of local pH levels. pH-sensitive polymeric nanocarriers are generally negatively charged and stable at pH 7.4 but become neutralized and leaky at acidic pH, which prompted their potential application to target the tumor extracellular matrix [38].

A multifunctional targeting strategy was proposed by Shen et al. [12], in which a novel pH-sensitive polymethacrylate (PMA)-grafted poly(amidoamine) (PAMAM) nanodelivery system was designed to be responsive to the acidic tumor microenvironment, and thereby trigger drug release in the intratumoral space. The folate-PEGylation of these nanoparticles enhanced tumor drug accumulation, and the combination of this surface property with the pH-responsive behavior led to a strong inhibition of tumor growth in tumor-bearing mice.

More recently, a functionalized PAMAM nanocarrier conjugated poly(2-(N,N-diethylamino)ethyl methacrylate) (pDEA) and methoxy-poly(ethylene glycol) 2000 was designed to deliver anticancer drugs [13]. pDEA has pH-sensitive properties, showing hydrophobicity in neutral environments and hydrophilicity in weakly acidic environments because of the presence of tertiary amines, and was therefore considered a functional layer coating the antitumor drug 5-fluorouracil in neutral environments and releasing it in the acidic environment of tumors, which led to greater anticancer effects. In other study, Zheng et al. [39] proposed a pH-sensitive poly(glutamic acid) grafted mesoporous silica nanoplatform, that might allow rapid release of doxorubicin specifically in cancerous tissues.

Chitosan-based nanoplatforms have also been explored for tumor targeting. Nanoparticles created with poly(lactic-co-glycolic acid) (PLGA) and low molecular-weight chitosan (LMWC) were formulated by Amoozgar et al. [40] as a novel nanocarrier for a specific drug release and greater cytotoxicity in the weakly acidic microenvironment of tumors. The hydrophilic LMWC layer reduced opsonization and phagocytic uptake after systemic applications.

Recently, it was also explored the ability of chitosan nanoparticles incorporating a biocompatible pH-sensitive surfactant derived from the amino acid lysine to promote an increased release of methotrexate in the tumor acidic environment [8]. It was shown a triggered release of payload under acidic conditions that might be due to the pH-dependent activity of the surfactant incorporated. This specific activity also prompted an enhanced cytotoxicity in tumor cell lines (Figure 2), which may be attributable to the combined effect of increased protonation of surfactant and chitosan chemical groups on the nanoparticle surface at tumor pH. The greater protonation increases binding to the cell membrane, leading to higher cytotoxic effects.

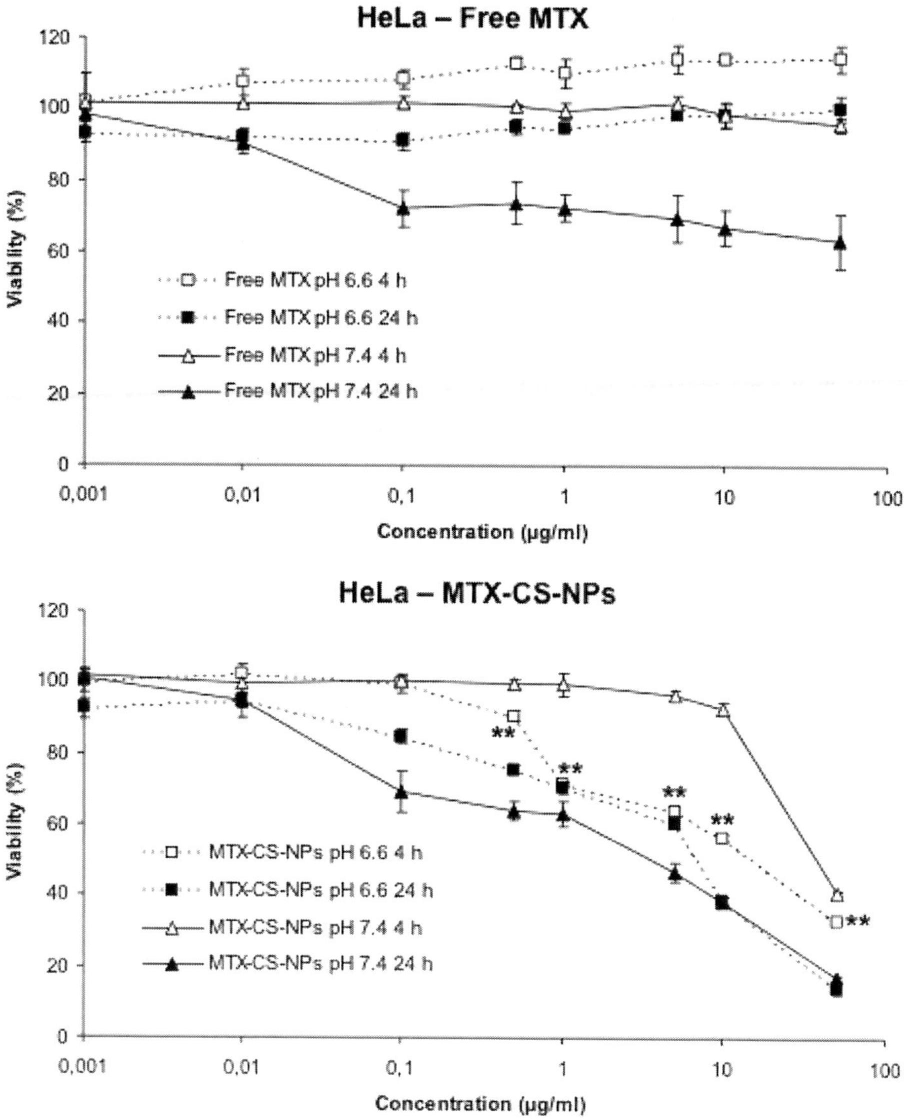

Figure 2. pH-dependent cytotoxicity of free methotrexate and chitosan nanoparticles encapsulating methotrexate against HeLa tumor cells after 4 and 24 h incubation, as determined by a MTT assay. The cytotoxicity assays were performed at physiological conditions (pH 7.4) and at pH 6.6, characteristic of the tumors microenvironment. $^{**}p < 0.005$ denote significant differences from the cytotoxic effects at pH 7.4. The data are reprinted and adapted from Nogueira et al. [8], with permission from Elsevier.

Polymeric micelles are another approach that has been widely used to improve the efficacy of cancer therapy due to their high drug loading capacity and well-controlled sizes. Micellar structures formulated with pH-responsive block copolymers displayed a specific doxorubicin release at tumor environment, while a stable structure was maintained at blood pH [41]. The acidic pH of tumors prompted a phase transition, which allowed the drug release and a more potent anti-cancer activity than free doxorubicin. In this same context, multi-arm star triblock copolymers were used to prepare pH-sensitive micelles for controlled delivery of doxorubicin [42]. Due to the swelling of the micelles at lower pH values, the drug release was significantly accelerated, which provided enhanced anticancer activity and bioavailability of doxorubicin. Another innovative nanocarrier based on self-assembling co-polymer stearoyl-PEG-poly-sulfadimethoxine methacrylate was prepared by Ravazzolo et al. [43] to obtain micelles with responsive behavior in the physiopathologic pH range of tumors. The colloidal formulations were stable at pH 7.4 for several hours, while at pH 6.5, they rapidly rearranged and aggregated, which led to the increased paclitaxel antitumor activity. In another study, Wu et al. [44] formulated pH-responsive micelles using PEG-poly(β-amino ester) polymers that present hydrophobic-to-hydrophilic transitions dependent on the pH. At pH 6.4-6.8, characteristic of the tumor tissues, amine protonation increased polymer solubility and induced a sharp micellization-demicellization transition for drug release.

Biodegradable strontium carbonate nanoparticles with pH-sensitive properties were also developed as new anticancer vehicles [45]. A faster release of the antitumor drug took place in the acidic microenvironment of tumors, which might be due to the acid-degradable nature of these nanoparticles. Furthermore, Mok et al. [46] designed a small interfering RNA nanovector, composed of an iron oxide magnetic nanoparticle, for targeted treatment of cancer. The nanoparticles were coated with polyethyleneimine (PEI), which have its primary amine group blocked with citraconic anhydride and, thus, have an increase biocompatibility at physiological conditions. When this blockage agent was removed at acidic conditions, the nanovector elicited a pH-sensitive cytotoxic effect in the acidic tumor tissue.

On the other hand, Huang et al. [22] developed an innovative nanoparticle system modified with activable cell-penetrating peptides that respond to the lowered tumor extracellular pH_e. These nanocarriers with pH-triggered activity allow the exposure of the peptide in the tumor environment, which also drive the nanoparticles' internalization into the intratumoral cells for an effective delivery of their contents. In another innovative study, He et al. [47] proposed a new generation of pH-responsive nanoplatforms engineered with acetylated α-cyclodextrin materials. These nanocarriers showed pH-modulated hydrolysis and pH-triggered paclitaxel delivery capability, which led to an improved cytotoxic activity against various tumor cells.

Liposomes have been also created for the specific tumor targeting. Jiang et al. [48] developed dual-functional liposomes with pH-responsive cell-penetrating peptide and active targeting hyaluronic acid for tumor-target drug delivery. When paclitaxel was loaded into these liposomes, it was demonstrated a remarkably stronger cytotoxicity toward hepatic cancer cells at pH 6.4 relative to at pH 7.4.

It is worthy mentioning that most of the previously mentioned pH-sensitive drug delivery nanodevices designed for tumor targeting also have the ability to specifically target the pH of the endosomal compartments to promote an efficient intracellular drug delivery [7, 8, 22, 43, 48]. The development of this kind of nanocarriers comprises the recent efforts that focused on the specific drug delivery to the cytosol and nucleous. In this line, a more detailed discussion of this class of nanocarriers is present in the next section of this chapter.

pH-Responsive Activity: Intracellular Delivery

Many therapeutic agents, such as proteins, peptides, DNA and some drugs, act at intracellular sites, and thus their therapeutic efficacy depends on efficient intracellular trafficking pathways [49]. The nanocarriers usually cannot directly cross the plasma membrane and their uptake into cells is mediated by endocytosis that confines the internalized active compounds to endosomes. It is know that following endocytosis, rapid endosomal acidification occurs due to a vacuolar proton ATPase-mediated proton influx, which justify the design of drug carriers that have the ability to change their conformation under an acidic environment. Therefore, one of the challenges for the efficient intracellular delivery of therapeutic compounds is to facilitate their release into the cytosol by destabilizing endosomal membranes under mildly acidic conditions, which circumvent the non-productive trafficking to lysosomes, where degradation may occur [32, 50].

The process of cell internalization is mediated especially by phagocytic and pinocytic endocytosis [51]. Phagocytosis occurs in specialized cells, while pinocytosis is used by all cells and can be divided in three types: fluid-phase, absorptive, and receptor-mediated endocytosis (e.g., clathrin- or caveolae-mediated endocytosis) [52]. In contrast, the non-endocytic processes are less prominent compared to endocytosis. This kind of process can occur through fusing of the vehicle, especially the lipid-based vehicles, with the plasma membrane, resulting in concomitant release of its contents into the cytosol [4].

Successful endosomal escape enables the nanocarrier to target the cytosol, the nucleus or other subcellular organelles, which are the site of action of multiple genes and drugs. Considering that generally the nanocarrier cannot directly cross the endosomal membrane, many strategies, based especially in the use of bioactive agents, are applied to induce the fusion of the nanocarrier with the membrane, in order to disrupt the endosome and promote the release of its contents to the cytoplasm. Among the agents used to promote nanocarrier escape/release from endosomes, the polymers have been the mostly explored. Polymers with buffering capability at pH 5.0 – 6.0, generally induce a mechanism hypothesized proton sponge effect. The unsaturated amino groups in the polymers structure absorb and sequester protons at endosomal pH, which cause the influx of chloride ions and water molecules, leading to an increase in osmotic pressure inside the endosomal compartment, followed by plasma membrane disruption and nanocarrier release into the cytoplasm [4].

Copolymers such as poly(styrene-*co*-maleic acid) were applied to confer pH-responsive properties to liposomes [10]. This copolymer exhibits conformational transition from a charged extended structure to an uncharged globule at acidic pH encountered inside cellular endosomes, resulting in destabilization of liposomes due to vesicle fusion and/or channel formation within the membrane bilayer, and ultimately in the release of the encapsulated cargo. In another recent study, Cajot et al. [53] proposed pH-responsive hybrid micelles based mainly on an ABC miktoarm star copolymer in association with a target star or linear copolymer. The protonation of the external poly(2-vinyl-pyridine) (P2VP) segments locates positive charges to the micelles that triggered their cell internalization. Once inside the cell, the lower pH of the endosomes induces further protonation of the P2VP block of the whole micelle, which led to the rupture of the endosomes, possibly thanks to proton sponge effect. In this same context, core-cross linked pH-sensitive degradable micelles were developed based on diblock copolymers that contain acid-labile acetyl and photo-cross linkable acryloyl groups [54]. The micelles displayed high stability at pH 7.4 and suffered rapid hydrolysis at mildly acidic pH, which allowed the rapid intracellular release of the loaded drugs. Finally, polymersomes with pH-tuning on-off membrane were prepared by the self-assembly of poly(β-amino ester)-based amphiphilic copolymers [55]. Below a pH of 7.0, and especially at pH 5.5, the membrane of this pH-sensitive polymer-some-like vesicle structure forms tunnels through which the drug cargo can be rapidly released.

To increase the selectivity, an innovative nanocarrier is formulated using a hollow gold nanosphere equipped with a biomarker-specific aptamer [56], which allowed an internalization process exclusively into the targeted tumor cells. Furthermore, this carrier has the advantage to be stable under normal biological conditions, whereas appears ultrasensitive to pH change at the endo-lysosomal compartments.

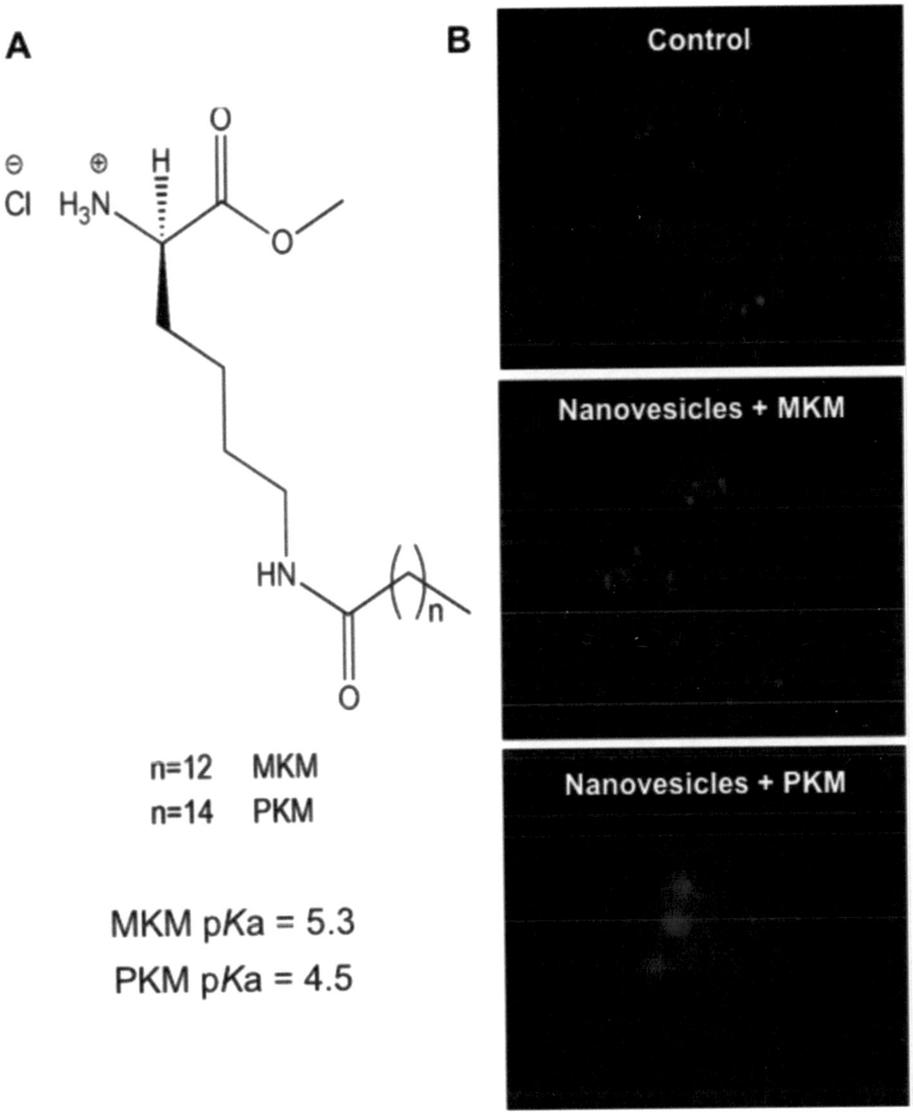

Figure 3. (A) Chemical structure of the cationic pH-sensitive lysine-based surfactants (MKM and PKM) included in the nanovesicle formulations. (B) Fluorescence microscopy images of HeLa cells showing the subcellular distribution of calcein fluorescence. The cells were treated with calcein (control), and both calcein and pH-sensitive nanovesicles. Images were acquired at 3 h after 1 h of uptake. Calcein is a tracer molecule, which is internalised by the cell through endocytosis and is used to monitor the stability of endosomes following nanocarrier uptake. The diffuse fluorescence in the cell cytosol indicates disruption of the endosomal membrane.

Another approach that has been used to target the intracellular compartments is the PEG-sheddable nanocarriers, in which PEG is grafted via pH-labile cross-linkers [57]. An example is the development of pH-responsive assemblies with the helper lipid dioleoylphosphatidylethanolamine (DOPE) (PEG-lipid:DOPE liposomes) containing tunable and bifunctional phenyl-substituted vinyl ether (PIVE) cross-linkers [23]. The PIVE linkage was designed to hydrolyze under acidic conditions, and the acid-catalyzed hydrolysis of PIVE leads to destabilization of the acid labile PEG-PIVE-lipid:DOPE liposomes via dePEGylation, thereby triggering a pH-dependent content release that allowed a higher DNA transfection efficiency.

Bioactive surfactants, such as cationic lysine-based surfactants, have also been used to develop pH-sensitive nanovesicles with potential application for the intracellular delivery of drugs and genes [9].

The pH-responsive lytic activity of the endosomal membrane by the nanovesicles with the bioactive surfactants might be explained by a modification in their hydrophobic/hydrophilic balance in the pH range of the endosomes. The surfactants become more protonated at acidic pH, which might induced they interaction with negatively-charged endosomal membranes, leading to influx of water and ions, and eventually bring about endosome destabilization (Figure 3).

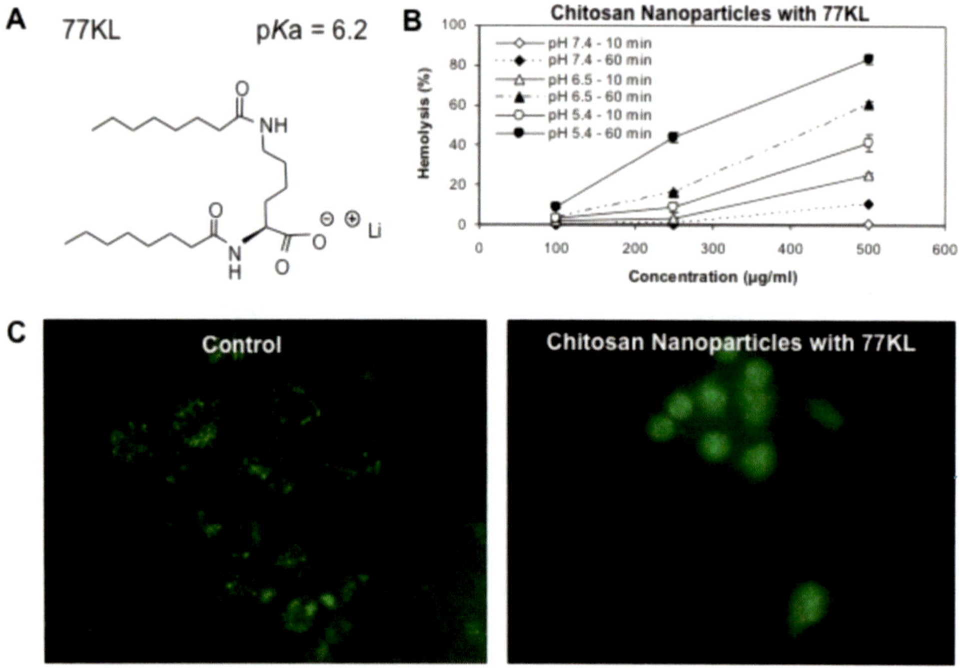

Figure 4. (A) Chemical structure of the anionic pH-sensitive lysine-based surfactant (77KL). (B) pH-sensitive membrane-lytic activity of chitosan nanoparticles containing 77KL. Nanopartilce-induced hemoglobin release from rat erythrocytes was expressed as a function of pH, concentration and incubation time. (C) Fluorescence microscopy images of HeLa cells showing the subcellular distribution of calcein fluorescence. The cells were treated with calcein (control), and both calcein and pH-sensitive nanoparticles. Images were acquired at 3 h after 1 h of uptake. The data are reprinted and adapted from Nogueira et al. [8], with permission from Elsevier.

As an example of drug nanocarriers with the ability to target the acidic environment of both the tumor tissues and the endosomal compartments, it can be mentioned the chitosan nanoparticles modified with a bioactive anionic lysine-based surfactant with pH-responsive properties [8]. The membrane-lytic activity of the nanoparticles in the pH range of the endosomes might be due to the increasing protonation state of the carboxylic group of the surfactant in this condition (Figure 4). It was stated that the protonation of the surfactant molecule makes it non-ionic and enhances its hydrophobicity, which would increase binding to the endosomal membrane and, thus, its lysis.

pH-sensitive liposomes based on zwitterionic oligopeptide lipids, with multistage pH-response to tumor microenvironmental pH and endosomal/lysosomal pH successively, have been also recently reported [7]. These nanocarriers were negative at physiological pH, positive at pH 6.5 and more positive at lower pH, which allowed higher tumor cellular uptake due to electrostatic absorptive endocytosis at pH_e and proton sponge effect for endo-lysosomal escape.

Novel nanostructure lipid carriers containing L-arginine lauryl ester were proposed by Li et al. [58] as pH-sensitive membranolytic and lysosomolytic nanocarriers. The better tumor targeting and *in vivo* anticancer activity proved the potential applicability of these nanocarriers. On the other hand, Paliwal et al. [59] proposed estrogen-anchored pH-sensitive liposomes that showed fusogenic potential at acidic pH (5.5), which allowed intracellular delivery and further nuclear localization of the encapsulated drug.

Besides the polymers and surfactants, peptides with amphiphilic structure and pH-sensitive properties have also been used for drug and gene delivery to the intracellular compartments. An example is the peptide GALA, which suffer a change in its structure from a random coli to an amphipathic α-helix when the endosomal pH decrease from 6.0 to 5.0, and thereby promotes the peptide binding to endosomal membranes and results in membrane lysis [60]. In a recent report, GALA was used to modify lipid envelope-type nanoparticles, which displayed high transfection efficiency when loaded with condensed complexes of pH-responsive polycation stearylated-octahistidine (STR-H8) and siRNA [61]. The use of the pH-sensitive fusogenic GALA peptide was also reported in combination with cell penetrating peptides and cleavable PEG-lipids to make liposomes for delivering siRNA to the cytosol [62, 63].

pH-Responsive Activity: Oral Drug Delivery

Oral administration is the most desirable way among all the drug delivery routes due to its high convenient and comfortable means of administering drugs to patients, and may also solve the current noncompliance-related problems associated with injections of peptide and protein drugs [64]. As it is well known, each segment of GI tract maintains its own characteristic pH level, from highly acidic in the stomach lumen (pH 1.2–3.0), to slightly basic in the intestine (pH 6.5– 8.0). Such pH variations and also the high number of digestive enzymes present in the GI tract can induced denaturation and/or degradation of highly sensible proteins and peptides, leading to loss of their activity [18, 65]. Therefore, it has proven to be a challenge to achieve an effective and consistent bioavailability levels for orally administered drugs [66].

Nanosized drug delivery devices have showed outstanding advantages in promoting drug absorption of oral biomacromolecules: (a) protect the bioactive macromolecules from pH and enzyme degradation, (b) offer bioadhesion properties that might increase the interaction between the nanocarrier and the mucosa, and (c) provide a huge surface area that might achieve greater dispersion of the drug molecules [67].

The use of the nanotechnology to develop vehicles that promote enhancing absorption of biomacromolecules in the small intestine, have been considered by many researchers during the design of novel formulations for oral administration of various peptides and proteins [64]. More recently, new technologies have prompted the inclusion of pH-responsive mechanisms in the design of nanocarriers for improving systemic exposure of drugs after oral administration. This greater exposure, achieved by using pH-sensitive vehicles, is described to be via higher gastric retention, transepithelial transport, and cellular targeting with surface-functionalized ligands [68, 69].

Different from the pH-sensitive vehicles that trigger acidic conditions, the nanocarriers design for oral administration induces drug release at higher pH environments of the GI tract. This specific activity can be achieved due to the presence of e.g., ionizable functional groups on the backbone or side chain of the polymer used to prepare pH-sensible nanoparticles [69]. Nanocarriers with pH-tunable properties have been currently used for oral drug delivery, where a physiological pH shift in GI tract facilitates the swelling or dissolution of the carriers.

Poly(methacrylic acid-co-ethylacrylate) copolymers (trade name: Eudragits) are commonly used for preparation of controlled release formulations. For example, Eudragit L100 dissolves at pH > 6, while Eudragit S100 dissolves at pH > 7. Similarly, Eudragit L100-55 contains an anionic copolymer based on methacrylic acid and ethyl acrylate, which dissolves when the pH is higher than 5.5. Following the pH-responsive properties of this class of polymers, researchers have designed pH-sensitive nanoparticles based on Eudragit L100 as an oral insulin delivery system [19] and on Eudragits L100, S100 and L100-55 to improve the oral bioavailability of cyclosporine A [70]. It is demonstrated that this kind of nanocarriers are a promising novel tool to improve the absorption of proteins, peptides and low water-soluble drugs in the intestinal tract.

Hydroxypropyl methylcellulose phthalate (HPMCP), especially the types HP50 and HP55, which dissolve at pH 5.0 and 5.5, respectively, are usually used to prepare pH-sensitive nanoparticles. HP55 nanoparticles containing also the polymer PLGA was developed as drug carriers for orally insulin delivery by a modified emulsion solvent diffusion method [71]. The release studies of insulin from the nanoparticles in simulated gastric fluid showing the pH-dependent character of these formulations. Wu et al. [11] have developed HP55-coated pH-sensitive capsule containing PLGA/Eudragit RS nanoparticles also for the oral delivery of insulin. The results obtained indicated that the integration of pH-responsive HP55-coated capsule with cationic nanoparticles may be a promising platform for oral delivery of proteins with high bioavailability, which could be attributed to the selectively drug release from nanoparticles in the intestinal tract, instead of stomach.

Other currently strategy applied to prepare pH-sensitive nanoparticles for oral drug delivery is the use of the cationic polymer chitosan. pH-responsive nanoparticle carrier system self-assembled by hydrophilic chitosan and poly-γ-glutamic acid (γ-PGA) [72], and by N-trimethyl chitosan (TMC) and γ-PGA [26], were created and proposed as a platform technology for oral delivery of hydrophilic macromolecules via the paracellular pathway. The application of the former nanoparticles for the oral administration of insulin resulted in a significant hypoglycemic action in diabetic rats, whereas the last carriers showed the ability to open the tight junctions of Caco-2 cells to allow the transport of insulin.

As a next step of the previous studies, Sung et al. [18] focuses on the premise that pH-responsive nanoparticles shelled with chitosan can adhere to and infiltrate the mucus layer in the small intestine. The experimental results led to the proposal of a mechanism of action: the infiltrated nanoparticles transiently open the tight junctions and, due to their pH-sensitivity, become less stable and disintegrate, releasing the load insulin, which thus permeates through the opened paracellular pathway and moves into the systemic circulation.

In another research, chitosan in combination with γ-PGA was also used for the development of pH-responsive multi-ion-cross linked nanoparticles [73]. The polymeric components of the nanoparticles were blended with tripolyphosphate (TPP) and $MgSO_4$, and the experimental results demonstrated that these carriers are significantly more effective to transport insulin and to improve its transmucosal delivery in the small intestine. Insulin was encapsulated at pH < 6 and released at higher pH by chitosan deprotonation and destabilization.

In addition, researchers have designed pH-responsive heparin-chitosan nanoparticles to treat *Helicobacter pylori* infections [74]. These carriers were stable in the gastric lumen due to electrostatic interactions within the structures and, upon contact with an *H. pylori* infection along the gastric epithelium (pH ~ 7.4), the deprotonation of chitosan occurs, which weakened electrostatic interactions and led to nanoparticle collapse and drug release.

Finally, and also in the context of the development of enhanced treatments for the diabetes mellitus, pH-sensitive silica-based nanomatrix encapsulating glucagon-like peptide-1 (GLP-1) was designed and prepared by Qu et al. [67]. The results indicated that these nanocarriers have a greater intestinal mucosa permeability and significantly higher proteolytic stability compared to the native GLP-1.

pH-Responsive Activity: Inflamed Tissues Targeting

An important pathophysiological change caused by inflammation is acidosis. Based on this altered environment, the developed of pH-responsive drug delivery systems is an interesting strategy to achieve a greater therapeutic efficacy. The local acidosis-triggered drug release might provide superior therapeutic efficacy and potentially reduced side effects [75].

A strategy to achieve a higher efficacy in the treatment of arthritis was proposed by Wang et al. [76], which was based on the development of pH-sensitive conjugates of dexamethasone and *N*-(2- hydroxypropyl)methacrylamide copolymer. The results obtained have shown that the delivery system specifically accumulates in inflamed tissues in an animal model of arthritis, and the pH-sensitive drug release (extracellular and intracellular) in arthritic joints provides a unique method for selective targeting of glucocorticoids to inflamed joints, which may potentially reduce systemic side effects.

Recently, a novel pH-sensitive drug delivery system based on functionalized silica nanotubes was developed for the incorporation of non-steroidal anti-inflammatory drugs (NSAIDs), aimed at a tailored drug release in acidic conditions characteristic of inflamed tissues [14]. The electrostatic interaction between the carboxylic group of the anti-inflammatory drug with the polycationic nanotube surface may lead to ideal drug delivery systems because this linkage ensures effective release of the drug in the slightly acidic inflamed tissues, while maintaining the conjugates stable in the bloodstream (pH 7.4). The authors highlight that these optimized silica nanotubes are an attractive pH-sensitive delivery system for inflammatory diseases that can largely diminish the adverse side effects associated with continuous use of the NSAIDs.

Some research was also directed to the development of pH-sensitive Eudragit P-4135F nanoparticles for the local treatment of inflamed bowel tissue [77]. In this case, the therapeutic principle is based on the selective drug release triggered by luminal pH, and not by the pH of the inflamed tissue. However, this can prevent premature drug absorption during passage through the small intestine until the lower ileal tissue is reached, which allow increased efficiency and tolerability through the selective drug delivery to the site of inflammation.

On the other hand, pH-sensitive liposomes radiolabelled with 99mTc have also been used to identify inflammatory regions in a rat focal inflammation model [15]. The results obtained indicated that these pH-responsive nanocarriers presents a high tropism for inflammatory regions and may be useful as a radiopharmaceutical to identify inflamed tissues.

pH-Responsive Activity: Ischemia Tissues Targeting

Myocardial extracellular pH drops from 7.4 to less than 6.7 during severe cardiac ischemia [78]. Brain tissue pH typically falls to 6.0-6.5 during ischemia under normoglycemic conditions and can fall below 6.0 during severe ischemia or under hyperglycemic conditions [30]. Therefore, this knowledge prompted the development of pH-sensitive nanocarriers for the specific and effective drug delivery in ischemia tissues.

A nano-sized pH-sensitive positively charged polymeric micelle was prepared by self-assembling human serum albumin as a model protein and degradable block copolymer methoxy poly(ethylene glycol)-poly(b-amino ester) containing piperidine and imidazole rings [16]. The authors demonstrated that when the pH is lower than pH 7.0, the polymeric micelles bear a gradually increasing net positive charge due to the ionized amino groups in the copolymer chain. By these results, the authors stated that this polymeric nanocarrier could be used as a pH-triggered targeting agent and an effective drug delivery system in cerebral ischemia models.

pH-responsive heparin-functionalized chitosan/poly(g-glutamic acid) nanoparticles were proposed as effective drug delivery devices for multi-functional release of basic fibroblast growth factor (bFGF) and heparin in ischemia tissues [17]. The pH-tunable properties of these polymeric nanoparticles could sustain bFGF release at pH 6.7 (simulate the pH of ischemia tissue) and allow rapid disintegration at pH 7.4 (simulate the pH of repaired tissue) to continuously release heparin. These features make these nanoparticles a potential therapeutic method for enhancing ischemic tissue regeneration and preventing harmful clots formation.

Conclusion

Nanotechnology tools have become important approaches for the design and development of novel therapeutics and diagnostics agents. In this context, pH-tunable nanocarriers have received growing attention due to their efficiency to enhance targeting to specific pathological areas with an acidic environment (e.g., tumor, inflamed and ischemic tissues), as well as to endosomal compartments (aiming to achieve an efficient intracellular drug delivery), and to GI tract (intending to promote an enhancing absorption of biomacromolecules in the intestine).

Important considerations for a pharmaceutical or scientist in developing innovative approaches to treat a variety of diseases depend especially on the specificity of the formulation to the target organ, tissue or cell. As discussed in the course of this chapter, the use of the pH variations in the body is a great strategy to be considered during the design and development of specific nanocarriers.

Therefore, here it was presented the recent progress that has been reached in this research field, highlighting the wide range of pH-sensitive bioactive compounds used, the novel production technologies and especially the potential outcomes that might lead to a greater therapeutic efficacy during clinical applications.

Based on sustained effort in using innovative nanotechnology for pharmaceutical purposes, the environmentally sensitive nanomedicines, especially the pH-responsive nanocarriers, are expected to result in the next-generation of therapeutical approaches with extensive and efficient medical applications.

Abbreviations

2,5-diphenyl-3,-(4,5-dimethyl-2-thiazolyl) tetrazolium bromide (MTT); basic fibroblast growth factor (bFGF); dioleoylphosphatidylethanolamine (DOPE); enhanced permeability and retention (EPR); gastrointestinal (GI); glucagon-like peptide-1 (GLP-1); hydroxypropyl methylcellulose phthalate (HPMCP); low molecular-weight chitosan (LMWC); N^{ε}-myristoyl lysine methyl ester (MKM); N^{α},N^{ε}- dioctanoyl lysine with a lithium counterion (77KL); non-steroidal anti-inflammatory drugs (NSAIDs); N^{ε}-palmitoyl lysine methyl ester (PKM); N-trimethyl chitosan (TMC); phenyl-substituted vinyl ether (PIVE); poly(2-(N,N-diethylamino)ethyl methacrylate) (pDEA); poly(2-vinyl-pyridine) (P2VP); polyethyleneimine (PEI); poly-γ-glutamic acid (γ-PGA); poly(lactic-co-glycolic acid) (PLGA); polymethacrylate (PMA); polymethacrylate-grafted poly(amidoamine) (PAMAM); stearylated-octahistidine (STR-H8); tripolyphosphate (TPP)

Acknowledgment

The authors acknowledge the financial support of the project MAT2012-38047-C02-01 of the *Ministerio de Economía y Competitividad* (Spain).

References

[1] R. Liu, B. He, D. Li, Y. Lai, J. Chang, J.Z. Tang, Z. Gu, Effects of pH-sensitive chain length on release of doxorubicin from mPEG-b-PH-b-PLLA nanoparticles, *Int. J. Nanomedicine*, 7 (2012) 4433-46.

[2] Y. Sato, H. Hatakeyama, Y. Sakurai, M. Hyodo, H. Akita, H. Harashima, A pH-sensitive cationic lipid facilitates the delivery of liposomal siRNA and gene silencing activity in vitro and in vivo, *J. Control. Release*, 163 (2012) 267-76.

[3] G. Ting, C.H. Chang, H.E. Wang, Cancer nanotargeted radiopharmaceuticals for tumor imaging and theraphy, *Anticancer Res.*, 29 (2009) 4107-18.

[4] Y. Li, J. Wang, M.G. Wientjes, J.L.-S. Au, Delivery of nanomedicines to extracellular and intracellular compartments of a solid tumor, *Adv. Drug Deliv. Rev.*, 64 (2012) 29-39.

[5] M.S. Muthu, C.V. Rajesh, A. Mishra, S. Singh, Stimulus-responsive targeted nanomicelles for effective cancer therapy, *Nanomedicine*, 4 (2009) 657–67.

[6] M.A.C. Stuart, W.T.S. Huck, J. Genzer, M. Muller, C. Ober, M. Stamm, G.B. Sukhorukov, I. Szleifer, V.V. Tsukruk, M. Urban, F. Winnik, S. Zauscher, I. Luzinov, S. Minko, Emerging applications of stimuli-responsive polymer materials, *Nat. Mater.*, 9 (2010) 101–13.

[7] R. Mo, Q. Sun, N. Li, C. Zhang, Intracellular delivery and antitumor effects of pH-sensitive liposomes based on zwitterionic oligopeptide lipids, *Biomaterials*, 34 (2013) 2773-86.

[8] D.R. Nogueira, L. Tavano, M. Mitjans, L. Pérez, M.R. Infante, M.P. Vinardell, In vitro antitumor activity of methotrexate via pH-sensitive chitosan nanoparticles, *Biomaterials*, 34 (2013) 2758-72.

[9] D.R. Nogueira, M.C. Morán, M. Mitjans, L. Pérez, D. Ramos, J. de Lapuente, M.P. Vinardell, Lysine-based surfactnats in nanovesicle formulations: the role of cationic charge position and hydrophobicity in in vitro cytotoxicity and intracellular delivery, *Nanotoxicology*, (2013). doi:10.3109/17435390.2013.793779.

[10] S. Banerjee, K. Sen, T.K. Pal, S.k. Guha, Poly(styrene-co-maleic acid)-based pH-sensitive liposomes mediate cytosolic delivery of drugs for enhanced cancer chemotherapy, *Int. J. Pharm.*, 436 (2012) 786-97.

[11] Z.M. Wu, L. Zhou, X.D. Guo, W. Jiang, L. Ling, Y. Qian, K.Q. Luo, L.J. Zhang, HP55-coated capsule containing PLGA/RS nanoparticles for oral delivery of insulin, *Int. J. Pharm.*, 425 (2012) 1-8.

[12] M. Shen, Y. Huang, L. Han, J. Qin, X. Fang, J. Wang, V.C. Yang, Multifunctional drug delivery system for targeting tumor and its acidic microenvironment, *J. Control. Release*, 161 (2012) 884-92.

[13] L. Du, Y. Jin, J. Yang, S. Wang, X. Wang, A functionalized poly(amidoamine) nanocarrier-loading 5-fluorouracil: pH-responsive drug release and enhanced anticancer effect, *Anticancer Drugs*, 24 (2013) 172-80.

[14] C.T. Sousa, C. Nunes, M.P. Proença, D.C. Leitão, J.L.F.C. Lima, S. Reis, J.P. Araújo, M. Lúcio, pH sensitive silica nanotubes as rationally designed vehicles for NSAIDs delivery, *Colloids Surf. B Biointerfaces*, 94 (2012) 288-95.

[15] V.A. Carmo, C.S. Ferrari, E.C. Reis, G.A. Ramaldes, M.A. Pereira, M.C. de Oliveira, V.N. Cardoso, Biodistribution study and identification of inflammation sites using 99mTc-labelled stealth pH-sensitive liposomes, *Nucl. Med. Commun.*, 29 (2008) 33-8.
[16] G.H. Gao, M.J. Park, Y. Li, G.H. Im, J.H. Kim, H.N. Kim, J.W. Lee, P. Jeon, O.Y. Bang, J.H. Lee, D.S. Lee, The use of pH-sensitive positively charged polymeric micelles for protein delivery, *Biomaterials*, 33 (2012) 9157-64.
[17] D.W. Tang, S.H. Yu, Y.C. Ho, F.L. Mi, P.L. Kuo, H.W. Sung, Heparinized chitosan/poly(γ-glutamic acid) nanoparticles for multi-functional delivery of fibroblast growth factor and heparin, *Biomaterials*, 31 (2010) 9320-32.
[18] H.-W. Sung, K. Sonaje, Z.-X. Liao, L.-W. Hsu, E.-Y. Chuang, pH-responsive nanoparticles shelled with chitosan for oral delivery of insulin: From mechanism to therapeutic applications, *Acc. Chem. Res.*, 45 (2012) 619–29.
[19] Y. Zhang, X. Wu, L. Meng, Y. Zhang, R. Ai, N. Qi, H. He, H. Xu, X. Tang, Thiolated Eudragit nanoparticles for oral insulin delivery: preparation, characterization and in vivo evaluation, *Int. J. Pharm.*, 436 (2012) 341-50.
[20] Y. Obata, S. Tajima, S. Takeoka, Evaluation of pH-responsive liposomes containing amino acid-based zwitterionic lipids for improving intracellular drug delivery in vitro and in vivo, *J. Control. Release*, 142 (2010) 267-76.
[21] S. Kobayashi, I. Nakase, N. Kawabata, H.H. Yu, S. Pujals, M. Imanishi, E. Giralt, S. Futaki, Cytosolic targeting of macromolecules using a pH-dependent fusogenic peptide in combination with cationic liposomes, *Bioconjugate Chem.*, 20 (2009) 953-9.
[22] S. Huang, K. Shao, Y. Kuang, Y. Liu, J. Li, S. An, Y. Guo, H. Ma, X. He, C. Jiang, Tumor targeting and microenvironment-responsive nanoparticles for gene delivery, *Biomaterials*, 34 (2013) 5294-302.
[23] H.K. Kim, D.H. Thompson, H.S. Jang, Y.J. Chung, J. van den Bossche, pH-responsive biodegradable assemblies containing tunable phenyl-substituted vinyl ethers for use as efficient gene delivery vehicles, *ACS Appl. Mater. Interfaces*, 5 (2013) 648-58.
[24] Y. Yamada, H. Harashima, Mitochondrial drug delivery systems for macromolecule and their therapeutic application to mitochondrial diseases, *Adv. Drug Deliv. Rev.*, 60 (2008) 1439-62.
[25] M.T. Tarrago-Trani, B. Storrie, Alternate routes for drug delivery to the cell interior: pathways to the Golgi apparatus and endoplasmic reticulum, *Adv. Drug Deliv. Rev.*, 59 (2007) 782-97.
[26] F.-L. Mi, Y.-Y. Wu, Y.-H. Lin, K. Sonaje, Y.-C. Ho, C.-T. Chen, J.-H. Juang, H.-W. Sung, Oral delivery of peptide drugs using nanoparticles self-assembled by poly(γ-glutamic acid) and a chitosan derivative functionalized by trimethylation, *Bioconjugate Chem.*, 19 (2008) 1248-55.
[27] I.F. Tannock, D. Rotin, Acid pH in tumors and its potential for therapeutic exploitation, *Cancer Res.*, 49 (1989) 4373-84.
[28] R. van Sluis, Z.M. Bhujwalla, N. Raghunand, P. Ballesteros, J. Alvarez, S. Cerdan, J.P. Galons, R.J. Gillies, In vivo imaging of extracellular pH using 1 H MRSI, *Magn. Reson. Med.,* 41 (1999) 743-50.
[29] K. Engin, D.B. Leeper, J.R. Cater, A.J. Thistlethwaite, L. Tupchong, J.D. Mcfarlane, Extracellular pH distribution in human tumors, *Int. J. Hyperthermia*, 11 (1995) 211-6.

[30] Z.G. Xiong, X.M. Zhu, X.P. Chu, M. Minami, J. Hey, W.L. Wei, J.F. MacDonald, J.A. Wemmie, M.P. Price, M.J. Welsh, R.P. Simon, Neuroprotection in ischemia: blocking calcium-permeable acid-sensing ion channels, *Cell*, 118 (2004) 687-98.

[31] N.M. Moore, C.L. Sheppard, T.R. Barbour, S.E. Sakiyama-Elbert, The effect of endosomal escape peptides on in vitro gene delivery of polyethylene glycol-based vehicles, *J. Gene Med.*, 10 (2008) 1134-49.

[32] P.S. Stayton, A.S. Hoffman, N. Murthy, C. Lackey, C. Cheung, P. Tan, L.A. Klumb, A. Chilkoti, F.S. Wilbur, O.W. Press, Molecular engineering of proteins and polymers for targeting and intracellular delivery of therapeutics, *J. Control. Release*, 65 (2000) 203-20.

[33] I. Mellman, Endocytosis and molecular sorting, *Annu. Rev. Cell Dev. Biol.*, 12 (1996) 575-625.

[34] M. Dominska, D.M. Dykxhoorn, Breaking down the barriers: siRNA delivery and endosome escape, *J. Cell Sci.*, 123 (2010) 1183-9.

[35] F. Yuan, M. Dellian, D. Fukumura, M. Leunig, D.A. Berck, V.P. Torchilin, R.K. Jain, Vascular-permeability in a human tumor xenograft-molecular-size dependence and cutoff size, *Cancer Res.*, 55 (1995) 3752-6.

[36] A.K. Iyer, G. Khaled, J. Fang, H. Maeda, Exploiting the enhanced permeability and retention effect for tumor targeting, *Drug Discov. Today*, 11 (2006) 812-8.

[37] J. Kim, C.V. Dang, Cancer's molecular sweet tooth and the warburg effect, *Cancer Res.*, 66 (2006) 8927–30.

[38] E.S. Lee, Z. Gao, Y.H. Bae, Recent progress in tumor pH targeting nanotechnology, *J. Control. Release*, 132 (2008) 164-70.

[39] J. Zheng, X. Tian, Y. Sun, D. Lu, W. Yang, pH-sensitive poly(glutamic acid) grafted mesoporous silica nanoparticles for drug delivery, *Int. J. Pharm.*, 450 (2013) 296-303.

[40] Z. Amoozgar, J. Park, Q. Lin, Y. Yeo, Low molecular-weight chitosan as a pH-sensitive stealth coating for tumor-specific drug delivery, *Mol. Pharm.*, 9 (2012) 1262-70.

[41] C.-Y. Chen, T.H. Kim, W.-C. Wu, C.-M. Huang, H. Wei, C.W. Mount, Y. Tian, S.-H. Jang, S.H. Pun, A.K.-Y. Jen, pH-dependent, thermosensitive polymeric nanocariers for drug delivery to solid tumors, *Biomaterials*, 34 (2013) 4501-9.

[42] Y.Q. Yang, B. Zhao, Z.D. Li, W.J. Lin, C.Y. Zhang, X.D. Guo, J.F. Wang, L.J. Zhang, pH-sensitive micelles self-assembled from multi-arm star triblock co-polymers poly(ε-caprolactone)-b-poly(2-(diethylamino)ethyl methacrylate)-b-poly(poly(ethylene glycol) methyl ether methacrylate) for controlled anticancer drug delivery, *Acta Biomater.*, 9 (2013) 7679-90.

[43] E. Ravazzolo, S. Salmaso, F. Mastrotto, S. Bersani, E. Gallon, P. Caliceti, pH-responsive lipid core micelles for tumour targeting, *Eur. J. Pharm. Biopharm.*, 83 (2013) 346-57.

[44] X.L. Wu, J.H. Kim, H. Koo, S.M. Bae, H. Shin, M.S. Kim, B. Lee, R. Park, I. Kim, K. Choi, I.C. Kwon, K. Kim, D.S. Lee, Tumor-targeting peptide conjugated pH-responsive micelles as a potential drug carrier for cancer therapy, *Bioconjugate Chem.*, 21 (2010) 208–13.

[45] W.-Y. Qian, D.-M. Sun, R.-R. Zhu, X.-L. Du, H. Liu, S.-L. Wang, pH-sensitive strontium carbonate nanoparticles as new anticancer vehicles for controlled etoposide release, *Int. J. Nanomedicine*, 7 (2012) 5781-92.

[46] H. Mok, O. Veiseh, C. Fang, F.M. Kievit, F.Y. Wang, J.O. Park, M. Zhang, pH-sensitive siRNA nanovector for target gene silencing and cytotoxic effect in cancer cells, *Mol. Pharm.,* 7 (2010) 1930-9.

[47] H. He, S. Chen, J. Zhou, Y. Dou, L. Song, L. Che, X. Zhou, X. Chen, Y. Jia, J. Zhang, S. Li, X. Li, Cyclodextrin-derived pH-responsive nanoparticles for delivery of paclitaxel, *Biomaterials*, 34 (2013) 5344-58.

[48] T. Jiang, Z. Zhang, Y. Zhang, H. Lv, J. Zhou, C. Li, L. Hou, Q. Zhang, Dual-functional liposomes based on pH-responsive cell-penetrating peptide and hyaluronic acid for tumor-target anticancer drug delivery, *Biomaterials*, 33 (2012) 9246-58.

[49] C. Plank, W. Zauner, E. Wagner, Application of membrane-active peptides for drug and gene delivery across cellular membranes, *Adv. Drug Deliv. Rev.*, 34 (1998) 21-35.

[50] R. Chen, S. Khormaee, M.E. Eccleston, N.K.H. Slater, The role of hydrophobic amino acid grafts in the enhancement of membrane-disruptive activity of pH-responsive pseudo-peptides, *Biomaterials*, 30 (2009) 1954-61.

[51] T. Soldati, M. Schliwa, Powering membrane traffic in endocytosis and recycling, *Nature Rev. Mol. Cell Biol.*, 7 (2006) 897-908.

[52] I.A. Khalil, K. Kogure, H. Akita, H. Harashima, Uptake pathways and subsequent intracellular trafficking in nonviral gene delivery, *Pharmacol. Rev.*, 58 (2006) 32-45.

[53] S. Cajot, K.V. Butsele, A. Paillard, C. Passirani, E. Garcion, J.P. Benoit, S.K. Varshney, C. Jérôme, Smart nanocarriers for pH-triggered targeting and release of hydrophobic drugs, *Acta Biomater.*, 8 (2012) 4215-23.

[54] Y. Wu, W. Chen, F. Meng, Z. Wang, R. Cheng, C. Deng, H. Liu, Z. Zhong, Core-crosslinked pH-sensitive degradable micelles: a promising approach to resolve the extracellular stability versus intracellular drug release dilemma, *J. Control. Release*, 164 (2012) 338-45.

[55] I.K. Jeong, G.H. Gao, Y. Li, S.W. Kang, D.S. Lee, A biodegradable polymersome with pH-tuning on-off membrane based on poly(β-amino ester) for drug delivery, *Macromol. Biosci*, (2013). doi: 10.1002/mabi.201200468.

[56] N. Zhao, J. You, Z. Zeng, C. Li, Y. Zu, An ultra pH-sensitive and aptamer-equipped nanoscale drug-delivery system for selective killing of tumor cells, *Small*, (2013). doi: 10.1002/smll.201202694.

[57] B. Romberg, W.E. Hennink, G. Storm, Sheddable coatings for long-circulating nanoparticles, *Pharm. Res.*, 25 (2008) 55–71.

[58] S. Li, Z. Su, M. Sun, Y. Xiao, F. Cao, A. Huang, H. Li, Q. Ping, C. Zhang, An arginine derivative contained nanostructure lipid carriers with pH-sensitive membranolytic capability for lysosomolytic anti-cancer drug delivery, *Int. J. Pharm.*, 436 (2012) 248-57.

[59] S.R. Paliwal, R. Paliwal, H.C. Pal, A.K. Saxena, P.R. Sharma, P.N. Gupta, G.P. Agrawal, S.P. Vyas, Estrogen-anchored pH-sensitive liposomes as nanomodule designed for site-specific delivery of doxorubicin in breast cancer therapy, *Mol. Pharm.*, 9 (2012) 176-86.

[60] W.J. Li, F. Nicol, F.C. Szoka, GALA: a designed synthetic pH-responsive amphipathic peptide with applications in drug and gene delivery, *Adv. Drug. Deliv. Rev.*, 56 (2004) 967-85.

[61] N. Toriyabe, Y. Hayashi, H. Harashima, The transfection activity of R8-modified nanoparticles and siRNA condensation using pH sensitive stearylated-octahistidine, *Biomaterials*, 34 (2013) 1337-43.
[62] H. Hatakeyama, E. Ito, H. Akita, M. Oishi, Y. Nagasaki, S. Futaki, H. Harashima, A pH-sensitive fusogenic peptide facilitates endosomal escape and greatly enhances the gene silencing of siRNA-containing nanoparticles in vitro and in vivo, *J. Control. Release*, 139 (2009) 127-32.
[63] Y. Sakurai, H. Hatakeyama, H. Akita, M. Oishi, Y. Nagasaki, S. Futaki, H. Harashima, Efficient short interference RNA delivery to tumor cells using a combination of octaarginine, GALA and tumor-specific, cleavable polyethylene glycol system, *Biol. Pharm. Bull.*, 32 (2009) 928-32.
[64] X.-Q. Wang, Q. Zhang, pH-sensitive polymeric nanoparticles to improve oral bioavailability of peptide/protein drugs and poorly water-soluble drugs, *Eur. J. Pharm. Biopharm.*, 82 (2012) 219-29.
[65] M. Goldberg, I. Gomez-Orellana, Challenges for the oral delivery of macromolecules, *Nat. Rev. Drug Discovery*, 2 (2003) 289–95.
[66] Y.J. Yamanaka, K.W. Leong, Engineering strategies to enhance nanoparticle-mediated oral delivery, *J. Biomater. Sci. Polym.* Ed., 19 (2008) 1549–70.
[67] W. Qu, Y. Li, L. Hovgaard, S. Li, W. Dai, J. Wang, X. Zhang, Q. Zhang, A silica-based pH-sensitive nanomatrix system improves the oral absorption and efficacy of incretin hormone glucagon-like peptide-1, *Int. J. Nanomedicine,* 7 (2012) 4983-94.
[68] E. Roger, F. Lagarce, E. Garcion, J. Benoit, Biopharmaceutical parameters to consider in order to alter the fate of nanocarriers after oral delivery, *Nanomedicine*, 5 (2010) 287–306.
[69] P. Colombo, F. Sonvico, G. Colombo, R. Bettini, Novel platforms for oral drug delivery, *Pharm. Res.*, 26 (2009) 601–11.
[70] J. Dai, T. Nagai, X. Wang, T. Zhang, M. Meng, Q. Zhang, pH-Sensitive Nanoparticles for Improving the Oral Bioavailability of Cyclosporine A, *Int. J. Pharm.*, 280 (2004) 229–40.
[71] F.D. Cui, A.J. Tao, D.M. Cun, L.Q. Zhang, K. Shi, Preparation of insulin loaded PLGA-Hp55 nanoparticles for oral delivery, *J. Pharm. Sci.,* 96 (2007) 421–7.
[72] K. Sonaje, K.J. Lin, J.J. Wang, F.L. Mi, C.T. Chen, J.H. Juang, H.W. Sung, Self-assembled pH-sensitive nanoparticles: A platform for oral delivery of protein drugs, *Adv. Funct. Mater.*, 20 (2010) 3695–700.
[73] Y.-H. Lin, K. Sonaje, K.M. Lin, J.-H. Juang, F.-L. Mi, H.-W. Yang, H.W. Sung, Multi-ion-crosslinked nanoparticles with pH-responsive characteristics for oral delivery of protein drugs, *J. Control. Release,* 132 (2008) 141-9.
[74] Y. Lin, C. Chang, Y. Wu, Y. Hsu, S. Chiou, Y. Chen, Development of pH-responsive chitosan/heparin nanoparticles for stomach-specific anti-Helicobacter pylori therapy, *Biomaterials*, 30 (2009) 3332–42.
[75] S. Mitragotri1, J.-W. Yoo, Designing micro- and nanoparticles for treating rheumatoid arthritis, *Arch. Pharm. Res.,* 34 (2011) 1887-97.
[76] D. Wang, S.C. Miller, X.-M. Liu, B. Anderson, X.S. Wang, S.R. Goldring, Novel dexamethasone-HPMA copolymer conjugate and its potential application in treatment of rheumatoid arthritis, *Arthritis Res. Ther.*, 9 (2007) R2.

[77] Y. Meissner, Y. Pellequer, A. Lamprecht, Nanoparticles in inflammatory bowel disease: Particle targeting versus pH-sensitive delivery, *Int. J. Pharm.*, 316 (2006) 138–43.

[78] S.P. Sutherland, C.J. Benson, J.P. Adelman, E.W. McCleskey, From the cover: acid-sensing ion channel 3 matches the acid-gated current in cardiac ischemia-sensing neurons, *PNAS*, 98 (2001) 711-6.

In: Recent Advances in Drug Delivery Research
Editor: Valerio Voliani
ISBN: 978-1-62948-228-6

Chapter 4

Bio-Inspired Chimeric Drug Delivery Nanosystems (chi-DDnSs): Their Fractal Morphology and Regulatory Aspects

Natassa Pippa[1,2], *Stergios Pispas*[2,*] *and Costas Demetzos*[1]
[1]Department of Pharmaceutical Technology, Faculty of Pharmacy, Panepistimioupolis Zografou, National and Kapodistrian University of Athens, Athens, Greece
[2]Theoretical and Physical Chemistry Institute, National Hellenic Research Foundation, Athens, Greece

Abstract

Pharmaceutical Nanotechnology can provide challenges for producing innovative drugs based on bioinspired nanostructures that can be used as advanced Drug Delivery nanosystems (aDDnSs). These systems could be correlated to the living organisms due to their self-assembly properties, their hierarchical structural organization, as well as to their biocompatibility and biodegradability characteristics. aDDnSs can be considered as new therapeutic outcomes in nanomedicine, that could be able to deliver pharmacomolecules to specific tissues and can improve their PK/PD (pharmacokinetics/pharmacodynamics) behavior and affect their total bioavailability. Drug delivery is a scientific sector that promotes the innovation by design and such formulation approaches that can produce aDDnSs. It has been accepted that the living organisms, composed of different biomaterials, achieve their higher functionality due to the cooperative nature of the system's elements. This observation give raise to the production of bio-inspired nano Drug Delivery Systems that offer the possibility of increasing the therapeutic index of the encapsulated pharmacomolecules by improving their effectiveness and efficacy, diminishing their toxicity against physiological tissues and achieving controlled functionality of the delivery system. The proper choice of a drug delivery system can alter the solubility and ameliorate the stability of candidate drugs, improving their overall absorption, distribution, metabolism and excretion (ADME) profile. Drug nanocarriers produced by the combination of bionanomaterials, such as liposomes, polymers and

* E-mail: pispas@eie.gr.

dendrimers, are considered as new classes of complex self-assembled soft nanostructures. These nanosystems can be characterized as *chimeric* aDDnSs due to the combination of different in nature bionanomaterials and are used for delivery of pharmacomolecules. The major advantage of such bio-inspired delivery systems lies in the ability to control the size, the structure and the morphology of the nano-assembly, due to the cooperativity of the components. The morphology of nanoparticles has been recently described via fractal analysis. The experimentally determined fractal dimension could be a useful tool for the development and characterization of innovative nanocarriers for pharmacomolecules with complete knowledge of their structural characteristics. This approach can disclose the pharmacokinetic reality of behavior of the candidate drugs, and can improve their therapeutic value by highlighting the interdependence of particle morphology and biological and pharmacokinetic processes. Additionally, there is growing effort to refine methodologies for preparation and physicochemical characterization, in order these new technologies to have the potential to meet regulatory requirements.

Keywords*:* Pharmaceutical Nanotechnology, advanced Drug Delivery nanosystems, bio-inspired nanoparticles, chimeric liposomes, copolymers, fractal morphology

Introduction

Pharmaceutical Nanotechnology, Drug Delivery Systems, Soft Matter Self-assembly and Fractals

Nanoscience and nanotechnology can offer advantages in the development process of new drugs and they represent a new approach to research in this field. These areas offer benefits for the development of innovative products and promote new properties of the materials used, which could be essential in the effectiveness of the final product. Scientists in this field work at the atomic, molecular and supramolecular levels, and can manufacture new nanodevices and nanosystems with new properties and functions.

Nanotechnology is the *art* of producing little devices and machines at the microscopic and molecular scale. Pharmaceutical Nanotechnology and nanomedicine have branched out in different directions, each of them embodying the key insight that the ability to structure materials, devices and systems at the molecular or supramolecular scale can bring enormous immediate benefits in the research of drug delivery systems and diagnostic methods. According to the European Medicines Agency: "Nanotechnology is defined as the production and application of structures, devices and systems by controlling the shape and size of materials at nanometer scale". The nanometer scale ranges from the atomic level at around 0.2 nm (2 Å) up to around 100 nm" while: "Nanomedicine is defined as the application of nanotechnology in view of making a medical diagnosis or treating or preventing diseases. It exploits the improved and often novel physical, chemical and biological properties of materials at nanometer scale".[1]

Over the last decades, biology has made significant advances in providing a rational understanding of the molecular mechanisms governing life's processes. New

[1] European Medicines Agency (2006). CHMP Reflection paper on nanotechnology-based medicinal products for human use. http://www.ema.europa.eu/docs/en_GB/document_library/Regulatory_and_procedural_guideline/2010/01/WC500069728.pdf

bionanomaterials have emerged from biological systems, which chemists and physicists have then promptly fabricated, manipulated and addressed at the molecular scale. The emblematic example is DNA technology, which affords the elaboration of programmable chemical synthesis routes to build complex architectures and functions with molecular precision, and sheds light on a new generation of robust tools [1, 2].

A fundamental connection between systems biology and nanotechnology is the ultimate goal besides their differences. Systems biology aims to uncover the fundamental operation of the cell in an effort to predict the exact response to specific stimuli and genetic variations [2, 3]. Nanotechnology does not aspire to be so precise nor is it required; nanotechnology is chiefly concerned with useful design. Systems biology is a scientific discovery problem whereas nanotechnology is an engineering design problem [2, 3].

Inspired by nature, scientists in the field of nanotechnology have been endeavored to explore supramolecular self-assembly to reveal the mechanism for the biological self-assembly and understand the way in which biological objects and structures are organized; mimic the complicated but efficient self-assembly process in nature to design hierarchical structures possessing biological activities and create innovative structures at nanoscale capable of novel biological functions [2]. Soft Nanotechnology is a relatively young scientific and technological discipline [4-6]. Self-assembly of soft materials, which is a minimalistic route to the fabrication of nanomaterials, can be exploited to create a panoply of nanostructures for a wide variety of applications [1].

Additionally, nanotechnology driven technologies, closing the gap between medicines, medical devices and advanced therapeutics, will allow new clinical technologies to facilitate healthcare in infectious and chronic progressive disorders. Pharmaceutical nanotechnology presents potential opportunities to create more effective and safe drugs by using advanced Drug Delivery nanoSystems (aDDnSs) [7-10].

According to Rowland and his colleagues [11], a drug delivery system (DDS) is defined as a technological formulation or a device that enables the introduction of a therapeutic substance in the body and improves its efficacy and safety by controlling the rate, time, and place of release of drugs in the body. The pharmacological properties of conventional drugs can be improved through better drug delivery systems (DDS), which include carriers and their associated therapeutics. In the last three decades, the development of supramolecular self-assembly has offered new choices for versatile nanocarriers used in drug delivery. The drug carriers can be nanoparticles like liposomes, micelles, dendrimers, polymersomes and nanotubes.

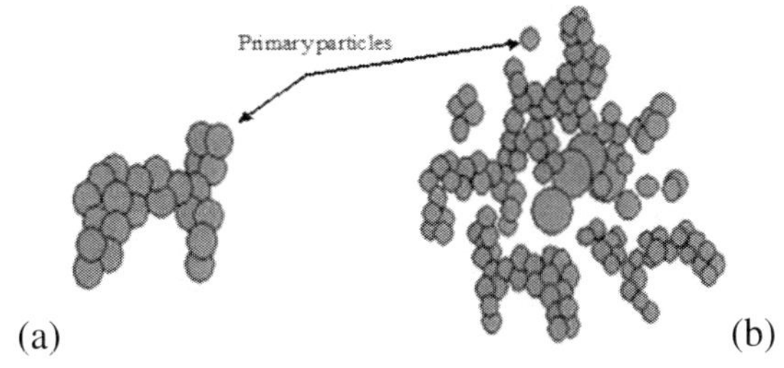

Figure 1. The structure of a. an aggregate and b. an agglomerate.

According to Commission Recommendation of 18 October 2011 on the definition of nanomaterial (2011/969/EU) particle means a minute piece of matter with defined physical boundaries, while agglomerate means a collections of weakly bound particles or aggregates where the resulting external surface area is similar to the sum of the surface areas of the individual components and aggregate means a particle comprising of strangle bound and fused particles (Figure 1).

As mentioned above, Pharmaceutical Nanotechnology is oriented in the area of targeted drug delivery, especially in colloidal nanocarriers [12]. Nanocarriers have the possibility of providing endless opportunities in the area of drug delivery and higher ratio of surface area to volume. For this reason, they improve the solubility of hydrophobic compounds and increase the stability of wide variety of therapeutic agents and biomolecules like peptides. They also have improved pharmacokinetic characteristics; minimize the toxicity and the risk-to-benefit ratio. Colloidal nanocarriers like liposomes, polymeric nanoparticles, etc., can be classified in a more general category of "soft matter", which includes a wide range of materials, that cannot classified as solid or liquid and that can deform easily because their molecules simply rearrange. These materials are characterized by softness (can be considered synonymous with deformability) because for these materials, the entropy changes related to the bond energy variations are dominated by the modification due to molecules or biomolecules configuration and structural changes [12].

Another important feature is particle shape, which is related to the specific surface and determines the presence of attractive or repulsive forces within dispersed and dispersive phases, which are present in a colloidal dispersion [13]. The interactions which play a key role in particle shape include ionic interactions, dipole-dipole interactions, steric interactions and hydrogen bonding [12, 13]. The structural interactions are related to the physical laws of quantum mechanics, which are responsible for space filling and local order. In life sciences, knowledge of the interaction mechanism at short distances between the biomolecules immersed in an electrolyte solution is very important to elucidate the essential biological processes involved in many cellular phenomena like membrane fusion. Furthermore, self-assembly is one of the most interesting properties that arise in nanoscale or microscopic level. Molecular self-assembly is a nano-manufacturing strategy that implies molecular and over-molecular design, in a way that complementarity brings to aggregation in the desired structure [6, 12, 13]. Figure 2 (a., b. and c.) presents several self-assembled nanocarriers which are used as drug delivery systems. The self-assembly driven building mechanism brings different advantages: it realizes the most difficult steps in nano manufacturing, that is, the ones involving atomic-level matter modifications, in a clean way, and it tends to produce stable and relatively perfect structures, since it requires the output structures to be the most thermodynamically stable. Materials have uniquely functional properties at nanometer-scale dimensions that, if harnessed effectively, could lead to novel engineered systems with highly useful characteristics. On the other hand, biomaterials are highly organized from the molecular to the nano- and macroscales, often in a hierarchical manner, with intricate nano-architectures that ultimately make up a myriad of different functional soft and hard tissues [4, 5, 6, 12]. Most of the natural objects and systems encountered in the real word are built in a completely irreversible and disordered fashion [13]. In irreversible processes the details of growth mechanism seem to play a key role in determining the resulting shapes of the objects [14, 15, 16, 17].

Mandelbrot was the first to model this irregularity mathematically [18]. According to Mandelbrot: "clouds are not spheres, mountains are not cones, coastlines are not circles, and dark is not smooth, nor does lightning travel in a straight line" and coined the world fractal for structures in space and processes in time that cannot be characterized by a single spatial or temporal scale.

In fact, the fractal objects, systems and processes in time have multiscale properties and self-similar patterns are frequently observed in Nature, especially in nanoscale. The physiological implications of the fractal concepts are serious since fractal structures, systems and processes are ubiquitous in living things, e.g., the lung, the neural networks, ion channel kinetics, the convoluted surface of the brain, and the distribution of blood flow through the blood vessels [19].

Besides, many applications of fractals exist for the morphology of surfaces, e.g., the surface area of a drug particle and surface reactions on proteins [20-22]. Additionally, Fractal Geometry is the tool to describe systems and devices in the nanoworld and the kinetics of physical phenomena like aggregation and membrane fusion in this scale [14 - 17, 23].

Recent Advances in Drug Delivery Systems Based on Bio-Inspired Material Chemistry

Fabricated nano-sized devices or drug carriers, often called nanocarriers or nanovehicles, provide various advantages for effective drug delivery. Nanocarriers can carry poorly soluble, unstable, or systemically toxic drugs with extended blood half-lives and reduced side effects [24].

The proper choice of delivery system can overcome problems related to hydrophobicity and especially to solubility, can regulate bioavailability and can therefore improve the ADME profile (*A*bsorption, bio*D*istribution, *M*etabolism and *E*xcertion) of the bioactive molecule or of the candidate drug.

In addition, intravenously injected nanovehicles travel along the blood stream without blocking vessels. Floating nanoparticles are accumulated at the inflamed site having leaky blood vessels by the enhanced permeability and retention (EPR) effect [11, 24]. The presence of targeting molecules at the surface of nanocarriers increases the targeting ability, resulting in higher accumulation at the target site. Below, we summarize the main conventional drug delivery systems used in the Pharmaceutical Nanotechnology.

Amphiphilic Block Copolymer Micelles

Amphiphilic block copolymers consisting of two blocks of different solubility behavior in water, i.e., a hydrophobic and a hydrophilic one are a widely studied case of soft matter. Asymmetric amphiphilic block copolymers self-assemble in aqueous media, to form core-shell micellar structures and morphologies, with a mesoscopic or nanoscopic narrow size range (Figure 2c.) (in the order of 10-100 nanometers) [25, 26].

The core forms the inside of the particle and is created by the aggregation of the insoluble (minority) blocks and the corona, which is exposed to aqueous medium, is made by the soluble blocks. Several different aggregate morphologies have been also observed depending on copolymer composition and physicochemical parameters of the dispersion.

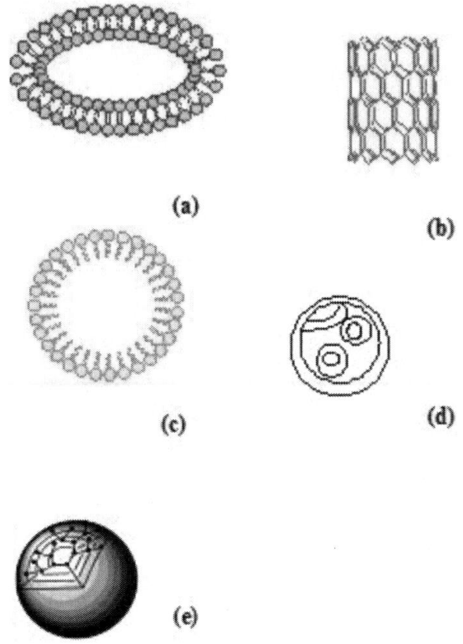

Figure 2. Examples of conventional Drug Delivery nanosystems (cDDnSs): a. Liposomes b. Nanotubes and c. Micelles and of advanced Drug Delivery nanosystems (aDDnSs): d. Liposomes in Liposomes (LiLs) and e. Liposomal "locked in" dendrimers, chi-aDDnSs.

The aforementioned applications of block copolymers in nanomedicine and pharmaceutics lead to the pursue for a deeper understanding of their self-organizing properties, which in a significant way define their application potential [25, 26]. For example, the nanoscale property of the self-assembled structure allows easy cellular uptake, while the detailed chemical structure of the copolymer and the morphology of the nanoassemblies formed in solution defines the drug loading ability and capacity of polymeric nanostructures.

Liposomes

Liposomes (Figure 2a.) are spherical, self-closed nanostructures composed of curved lipid bilayers which entrap some part of the solvent into their interior and their sizes are in the range of 20nm to micrometers [27, 28]. Liposomes are spherical structures composed of single or multiple concentric bilayers resulting from the self-assembly of amphiphilic molecules, such as phospholipids, in an aqueous medium. The polar head groups are located at the surface of the membranes, in contact with the medium, whereas the fatty acid chains form the hydrophobic core of the membranes, shielded from the water. These vesicles entrap in their interior volume part of the water phase and, consequently can capture and segregate polar molecules; moreover, because of the physicochemical properties of their constituents, they can also dissolve hydrophobic molecules in their bilayers. Conventional liposomes are in general thermodynamically unstable in biological media. The size or radius of curvature of liposomes is an important parameter that determines their physical properties.

Polymersomes

Polymersomes are artificial vesicles, formed by amphiphilic block copolymers, which contain an aqueous solution in the core surrounded by a bilayer membrane [29] where block copolymer chains reside. The bi-layer membrane is composed of hydrated hydrophilic coronas (e.g., made up of biocompatible poly(ethylene glycol (PEG) chains) both at the inside and outside of hydrophobic middle part of the membrane (made up of the hydrophobic block of the copolymer). The aqueous core can be utilized for the encapsulation of therapeutic hydrophilic molecules and the membrane can integrate hydrophobic drugs within its hydrophobic part [30-32]. Due to the relatively thick membranes, polymersomes can be rather stable. The presence of a hydrophilic PEG brush on the surface will reduce the protein adsorption onto the polymersomes during the blood circulation. Permeability, rate of degradation and stimuli-sensitivity of the membranes can be varied by using various biodegradable and/or stimuli-responsive block copolymers to modulate the release of the encapsulated drugs [29, 33].

Dendrimers

The history of dendrimers started about 30 years ago, and today there are many kinds that all share a similar structure. Dendrimers are quite different from traditional linear polymers [34]. Generally, their constructions consist of branched branches emanating from a core, along with a well-defined number of active groups on their surface area. Their unique structural features hold out promise of many applications in the fields of nanoelectronics and sensors, or they can be used as carriers of active substances, drugs, anti-prion agents, insulating materials, and transfecting agents [35-39]. Dendrimers, a 4th architectural class of polymers, represent a new category of drug delivery systems. The dendritic macromolecular structure consists of a central core, branching units and terminal functional groups which can be modified [34]. Due to their precise architecture, dendrimers possess an advantage over other generally polydisperse nanoparticles and this allows for greater control over their pharmacodynamic profile, while as vehicles for drug delivery they can be used either for encapsulation of bioactive compounds or for their covalent or non-covalent attachment at the periphery. They also offer other potential advantages such as prolongation of drug circulation time, protection of a drug from its surroundings, increase in drug stability (and possibly effectiveness) and the ability to target diseased tissues. There are two well-known strategies for the dendrimers' synthesis; the divergent strategy introduced by Vogtle, Tomalia and Newkome and the convergent synthetic path introduced by Hawker and Frechet [40].

Chimeric Advanced Drug Delivery Nanosystems Based on Biologically Inspired Nanotechnology

The first attempt for the creation of a mixed nanocarrier consisting of liposomes and dendrimers was the work performed by Khopade et al. [41]. Cationic polyamidoamine (PAMAM) dendrimers were incorporated in the aqueous interior of liposomes in order to increase the encapsulation efficiency of the acidic anticancer drug methotrexate [41]. The loading of the drug was indeed increased proportionally to dendrimer generation while the leakage of the drug from the system decreased. It has been demonstrated that, differently to what had been suggested in the first article concerning aDDnSs, pH and solubility gradient is presumably not the basis of the drug release modulation [41]. The amelioration of the release profile is not caused, mainly, by the forces developed between dendrimer and drug but by the induction of a more "stable" and, probably, less permeable lipid membrane due to the existence of the dendrimer-drug complex in the interior of the vesicle [41]. A further study of such systems was made by Papagiannaros and his collogues [42] in which a PAMAM G4-doxorubicin complex was formed prior to encapsulation in liposomes. From the results obtained this system seems to be quite promising in terms of drug release and cytotoxic activity against cancer cell lines. Recently other polymeric materials with dendritic architecture known as hyperbranched polymers (HBPs) have been used for the preparation of aDDnSs [43].

By combining liposomes with amphiphilic (block) copolymers, more stable systems could be obtained, usually known as Stealth or Sterically Stabilized liposomes. Stealth liposomes are defined as "second-generation liposomes" and are characterized by enhanced colloidal properties, including high stability [44, 45]. Stealth liposomal technology was achieved by modifying the surface of liposomal membrane by engineering hydrophilic polymer conjugates, such as polyethylene glycol (PEG), which is the most widely used polymer conjugate, while reducing mononuclear phagocyte system uptake because the circulation time increases with increasing PEGylated lipid concentration [46]. Such liposomes are called sterically stabilized liposomes and can be produced in two different ways, by grafting or by absorption of the polymer to the liposomal surface. The penetration of phospholipid bilayers by water-soluble surface-active block copolymers is an interesting approach for the design and the development of targeted and controlled drug delivery systems.

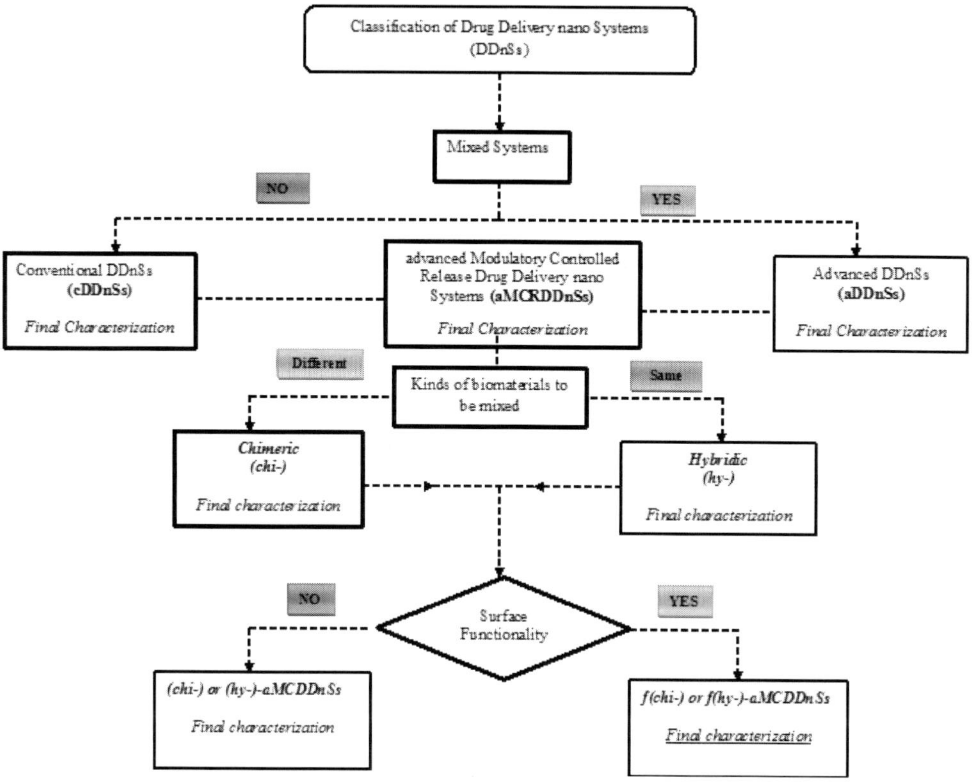

Scheme 1. The classification of Drug Delivery nanosystems.

The nontoxicity, high biocompatibility, low immunogenicity and antigenicity of stealth nanovectors are of interest for their clinical applications [47, 48]. Polymer-stabilized liposomes are often used in drug delivery applications to prolong the circulation time in the bloodstream, too.

It is generally assumed that the macrophage-resistant property of sterically protected nanocontainers is due to suppression in surface opsonization and protein adsorption. The large group of triblock copolymers with a hydrophilic middle block (poly-(propylene oxide); PPO) and hydrophilic end blocks (poly-(ethylene oxide); PEO) are an interesting alternative to PEGylated lipids for steric stabilization and because of their commercial availability and low cost [49].

Advanced Drug Delivery nanosystems (aDDnSs) can be characterized as mixed nanosystems due to the combination of different in nature bionanomaterials and are used for biomimetic delivery [50]. Recently, the Modulatory Controlled Release nanosystems were classified in *hybrid* and *chimeric* (Scheme 1) [51-59]. *In vitro* studies have shown that aDDnSs can interfere with the release profile of the incorporated bioactive molecules [54, 55, 57- 62]. The interest in such nanosystems stems from the possibilities for basic understanding of biological behavioral motifs, since biological systems extensively uses mixed materials to create multi-functional self-assembled nanostructures, too [63-66]. Additionally, the application of polymers in medicine as components of drug nanocarriers are considered essential for producing and developing new formulations against several human diseases. Amphiphilic block copolymers and vesicle forming surfactants have attracted major scientific interest in recent years due to their intriguing self-assembly behavior in aqueous media, which results in a plethora of nanoassemblies and their potential applications in drug delivery [63-65]. Lipopolymers self-assembled into biocompatible nanostructured multifunctional biomaterials offer many potential and attractive applications in drug, protein and nucleotide delivery, nanomedicine and diagnostics, too [67-69].

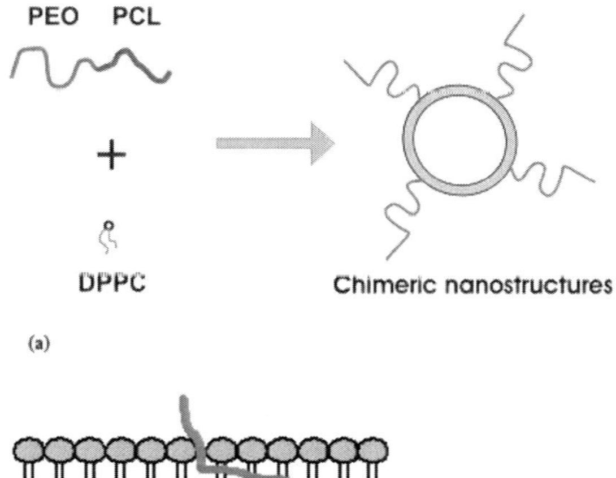

Figure 3. a. Structure of novel self-assembled chimeric nanostructures constructed from biocompatible PEO-b-PCL copolymer and lipids and b. the biomolecular sculpture of the DPPC/PEO-b-PCL mixed membrane. (Pippa, N., Kaditi, E., Pispas, S., Demetzos, C., (2013a). PEO-b-PCL/DPPC chimeric nanocarriers: self-assembly aspects in aqueous and biological media and drug incorporation. *Soft Matter*. 9, 4073-4082., Reproduced by permission of The Royal Society of Chemistry).

Amphiphilic block copolymers are able to form a range of different nanoparticulate morphologies for pharmaceutical applications [70]. A large number of studies indicate that it is possible to achieve absorption or penetration of block copolymers onto preformed liposomes or self-assembled superstructures in aqueous media [71-73]. The interactions and the insertion mechanism between lipids and block copolymers are of paramount importance due to their pharmaceutical applications [72-78]. Chimeric nanocarriers consisting of DPPC lipids and [(poly(ethylene oxide)-b-poly(ε-caprolactone) (PEO-b-PCL) block copolymers and poly(2-methyl-2-oxazoline)-grad-poly(2-phenyl-2-oxazoline) (MPOx)] gradient block copolymers were successfully prepared in aqueous media and in biological milieu (Figures 3 and 4) [57-59]. The gradient copolymer chain is expected to have several entry and exit points in the lipid membrane, in contrast to lipid-hydrophilic polymer conjugates and amphiphilic diblock copolymers, where the hydrophobic part is incorporated into the lipid membrane and the hydrophilic polymer chain is anchored on the membrane (Figure 4). This gradient copolymer chain arrangement may have several consequences in the structure and properties of the membrane itself and the chimeric nanostructure as a whole, as the current results indicate. In Figure 4, the MPOx macromolecules are shown anchored on the outer surface of chimeric nanovectors. It is most probable that the polymeric molecules can also anchor on the inner surface. In our opinion, the MPOx molecules, which are anchored on the outer surface of nanocarriers, are responsible for steric stabilization of the produced nanovectors and for their interactions with the environment. The physicochemical behavior of the chimeric nanoassemblies was found to depend on the molar ratio between the components, the temperature and the dispersion medium. It was concluded that the incorporation of block copolymers into liposomal bilayer increases the stability of the initial liposomal vesicles. On the other hand, the incorporation of block copolymers leads to liposomes of smaller size in PBS at the higher concentration of polymeric component. The morphology of chimeric liposomal nanovectors in HPLC-grade water and in PBS present statistically significant difference as the ratio of polymeric component increased. The fractal dimension values increased during the heating process only for chimeric nanocarriers while R_h decreased for chimeric liposomes in PBS in the process of heating up to 50°C. Incorporation of indomethacin was achieved in these chimeric nanocarriers to an extend depending on lipid/gradient copolymer ratio and dispersion medium. The present studies show that there are a significant number of parameters that can be used in order to alter the morphology of chimeric aDDnSs (chi-aDDnSs) and this is advantageous to the design and the development of "smart" nanocarriers for drug delivery. The results presented highlight the existing potential for controlling the colloidal behavior and the morphology of chimeric nanosystems in different media and conditions.

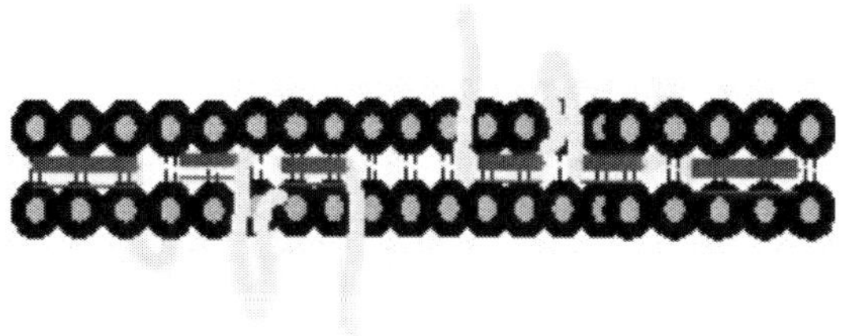

Figure 4. The biomolecular sculpture of the DPPC/MPOx chimeric membrane. The MPOx gradient copolymer structure results in a different incorporation of the polymer chain in the bilayer.

Physicochemical Characterization of aDDnSs

Controlling the morphology of nanoparticles is of key importance for exploiting their functionality and their properties in several emerging technologies [79]. The morphology of nanoparticles is critical to their biological interactions, like protein binding. For example, the factors influencing plasma protein-liposome interactions are surface coatings, surface charge and lipid dose, which affect the nanocarriers' morphology and surface structure [80]. Polymers induce significant morphological perturbations when included in lipid mixtures used for preparation of liposomal bilayers. According to the recent literature, the demixing of lipid-rich and polymer-rich membrane domains within the same vesicle bilayer was demonstrated and these morphological and structural differences were discussed as the possible resultant interdomain interactions within the mixed liposomal membrane [73]. The morphology and the shape of these systems are directly related to their colloidal behavior. Validated assays are important for detecting and quantifying nanopharmaceuticals, drug delivery systems or biologically active drug products, and how biophysical characteristics and structure may impact product quality in clinical use [80].

The studies of colloidal properties using liposomal and polymeric nanoparticles have already been evaluated, including the fractal approach and the biophysical formalism of the extended Derjaguin-Landau-Verwey-Overbeek (DLVO) theory [14-17, 23 81- 90].

Light scattering techniques are the primary tools used in order to elucidate the morphology and the physicochemical parameters of the conventional and chimeric liposomal carriers in different media and their ageing characteristics, as well as the aggregation kinetics. Table 1 presents fractal dimensions of liposomal nanoparticles as well as their aggregation kinetics equations. Fractal analysis is also used in molecular biology [91, 92] and applied chemistry [93-95].

Our previous works were related to the physicochemical characterization (size, polydispersity, ζ-potential) of liposomes composed of Dipalmitoylphosphatidylcholine (DPPC), DPPC: cholesterol (chol) (9:1 molar ratio) liposomes, DPPC:DPPG (9:1 molar ratio) and DPPC:DODAP (9:1 molar ratio) liposomes and the determination of their fractal dimension (mass fractal (d_f) and surface fractal (d_s)), in an aqueous (HPLC grade water) and in a biological (Fetal Bovine Serum-FBS) medium have been recently published [88, 89, 96].

Table 1. The aggregation kinetics and the fractal dimension of liposomal aggregates

Liposomal Composition	Dispersion medium	Aggregation kinetics	Fractal Dimension
DPPC	HPLC grade water	$R_h(t)=101.7t+55.196$ ($r^2=0.7415$)	2.50
DPPC	FBS	$R_h(t)=1.9193t+71.434$ ($r^2=0.8061$)	1.80
DPPC: cholesterol (9:1 molar ratio)	FBS	$R_h(t)=4.362t+135.96$ ($r^2=0.6617$)	2.40
DPPC:DODAP (9:1 molar ration)	PBS	$R_h(t)=1.9942t+39.653$ ($r^2=0.7381$)	1.80
DPPC:DPPG (9:1 molar ratio)	FBS	$R_h(t)=3.37t + 43.69$ ($r^2=0.967$)	1.4

Dynamic and static light scattering techniques were used to elucidate the structure and physicochemical parameters of liposomes in an ageing study in two different media, as well as their structural response in changes in concentration and temperature [88, 89]. Aggregation of DPPC liposomes in aqueous medium was observed, while d_f remained unchanged. The existence of Lateral Cluster-Cluster Aggregation could be a possible explanation to the observed behavior [97].

Physicochemical stability was observed for the DPPC:clolesterol (9:1) liposomes in the two dispersion media. The structural properties of DPPC liposomes in aqueous medium are quite different from those in FBS, as demonstrated from fractal analysis, especially for liposomes without cholesterol. The physical theories, which were developed for aggregation phenomena, include the fractal formalism for elucidating the shape of the resulting liposomal aggregates and structures, as mentioned above.

The fractal dimensionality of DPPC liposomes was decreased, while for DPPC: cholesterol (9:1) it remained unaffected in the two dispersion media. The structure of the liposomal systems, the process kinetics, and the fractal dimension are consistent with the Diffusion-Limited Cluster Aggregation (DLCA) and Reaction-Limited Cluster Aggregation (RLCA) models. DPPC:DPPG (9:1) and DPPC:DODAP (9:1) liposomes in HPLC-grade water were found to retain their original physicochemical characteristics at least for the time period that they were studied.

The liposomal stability indicates that electrostatic repulsion should be responsible for keeping the liposomes far enough to avoid aggregation or fusion. The fractal dimension, d_f, was found equal to 1.8 for reconstituted DPPC:DPPG (9:1) and DPPC:DODAP (9:1) liposomes in aqueous media. Aggregation of reconstituted DPPC:DPPG (9:1) and DPPC:DODAP (9:1) liposomes in FBS was observed. Their fractal dimensions were 1.46 and 2.45, respectively. The aggregation kinetics of unstable liposomal dispersions is presented in Table 1. Additionally, aggregation was observed for DPPC:DPPG (9:1) liposomes reconstituted in FBS. The first order kinetics describes the protein induced aggregation of cationic liposomes with serum components (Table 1).

According to the literature, shape is crucial to the nanoparticle's mechanism of cell internalization and the release rate and release profile of the therapeutic cargo [98-101]. On the contrary, shape effects on biological processes and mechanisms are still not fully understood, particularly at the nanoscale, primarily due to past limitations in the control of nanoparticle fabrication [100]. It should be note that certain shape specific delivery systems have demonstrated advantages over spherical nanosystems [102]. Furthermore, filamentous nanoparticles can help evade macrophage uptake, and shape-specific microparticles and/or nanoparticles can enhance vascular adhesion.

Drug Release from Chimeric aDDnSs

Manipulation of the biophysical properties of aDDnSs, especially for chimeric systems, provides improved control over the pharmacokinetics (PK) and pharmacodynamics (PD) of the encapsulated drugs relative to free drugs [46, 103]. The concept of fractal geometry can be applied to describe the complexity of the heterogeneous nature of drug processes in the human body and the dissolution of bioactive compounds [104 -107].

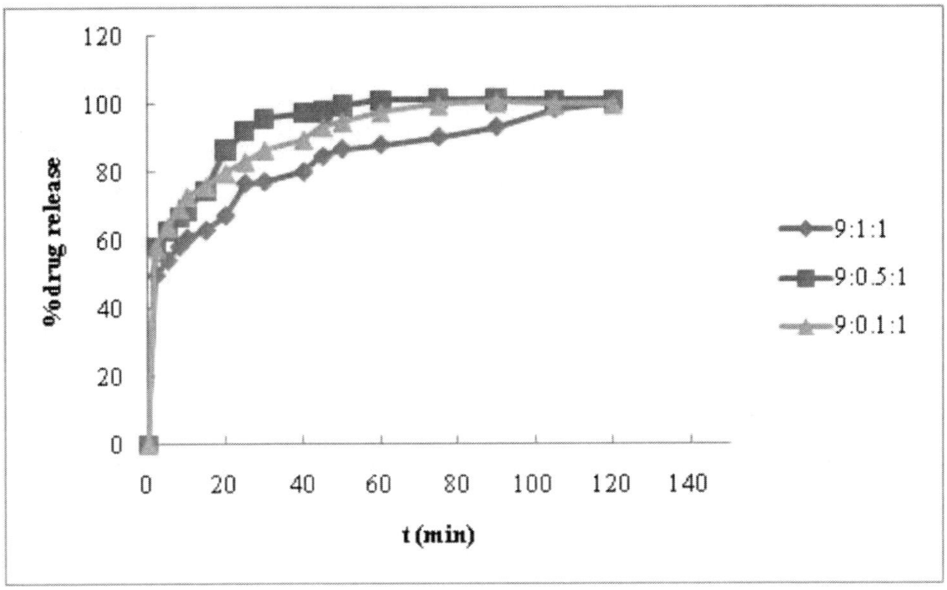

Figure 5. Cumulative drug release from DPPC:PEO-b-PCL: IND 9:0.1:1, 9:0.5:1 and 9:1:1 molar ratio (each value represents the mean ± S.D. of n = 3 independent experiments).

The *in vitro* release of the IND from the DPPC:PEO-b-PCL chimeric nanovectors is presented in Figure 5. It is observed that the *in vitro* release of the drug from the prepared chimeric nanostructures is quite fast especially for the mixed nanovectors prepared with the lower ratio of block copolymer. This phenomenology could serve as a control factor for the preparation and development of chimeric formulations with the desired release profile, modulating the release rate of the IND via the ratio of the components, improving its therapeutic index and finally decreasing any unwanted side effects. The combination of block copolymers with liposomes for the development of a novel chimeric nanovector appears very promising, mostly due to the fact that the PEO-b-PCL acts as a modulator for the release rate of the IND. Although the exact mechanism of release modulation is still under investigation, the initial results presented here show promise for developing advanced chimeric nanocarrier systems based on amphiphilic block copolymers and lipids.

It should be pointed out that drug release from the polymersomes is governed by the diffusion of the drug through the membrane [29, 108]. The driving force for the drug release is a concentration gradient of the drug between polymersomes and surrounding medium [29]. According to the literature, when the drug is diffusing from the core of the polymersomes to the surrounding medium the release rate is a function of the square root of time and for the polymersomes in polymersomes the release data can be fitted by the experimental law established by Peppas and Ritger and the size distribution of the polymersomes will also play a role in the overall release rate [29, 108, 109].

The *in vitro* release of the IND from the chimeric nanovectors and polymersomes at three different temperatures (25°C, 37°C and 45°C) is presented in Figure 6. It is observed that the *in vitro* release of the drug from the prepared chimeric nanostructures is quite fast only for the mixed nanovectors prepared with the lowest ratio of gradient block copolymer (DPPC:MPOx:IND 9:1:1) (Figure 6) at 25°C and at 37°C.

The combination of gradient block copolymers with phospholipids for the development of a novel chimeric nanovector appears very promising, mostly due to the fact that the MPOx acts as a modulator for the release rate of the IND. This phenomenology could serve as a control factor for the preparation and development of chimeric formulations with the desired release profile, modulating the release rate of the IND, improving its therapeutic index and finally decreasing any unwanted side effects.

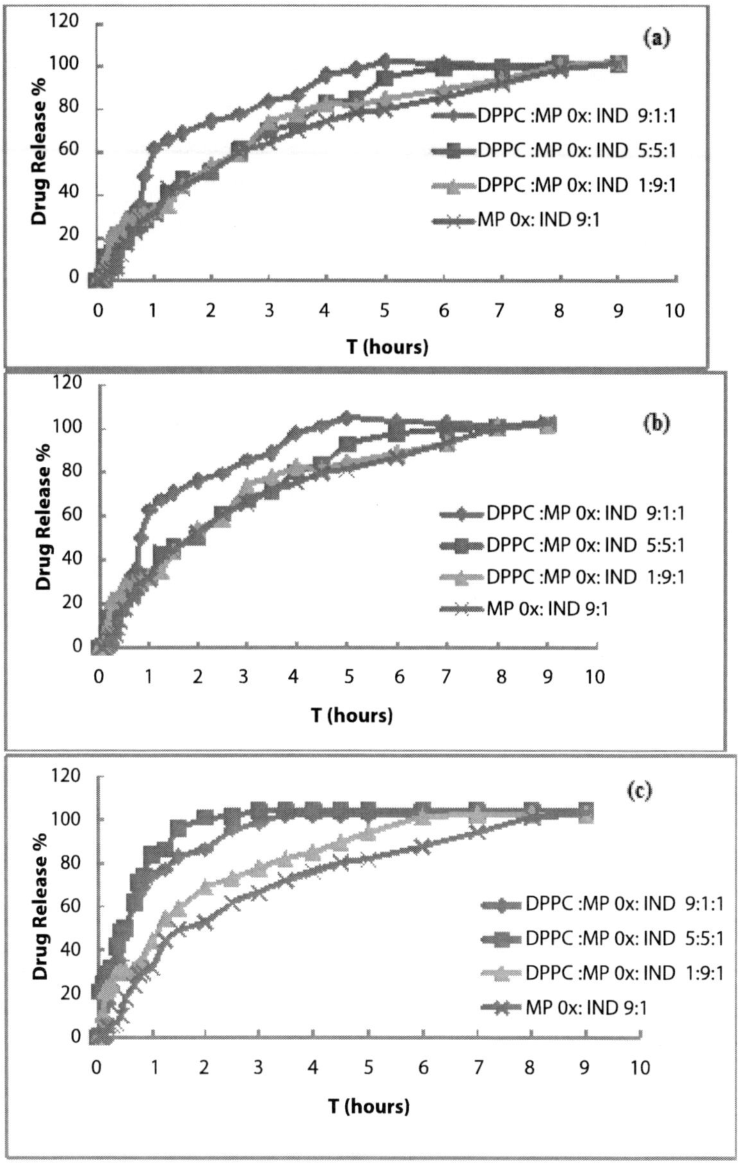

Figure 6. Cumulative drug release from DPPC:MPOx: IND 9:1:1, 5:5:1, 1:9:1 and MPOx:IND 9:1 molar ratio at (a) 25°C, (b) 37°C and (c) 45°C. Mean of three independent experiments run in triplicate, SD<10%. (Reprinted from Publication 450(1-2), Pippa, N., Merkouraki, M., Pispas, S., Demetzos, C., (2013b). DPPC:MPOx chimeric advanced Drug Delivery nanosystems (chi-aDDnSs): physicochemical and structural characterization, stability and drug release studies. 41-10. Int. J. Pharm. with permission from Elsevier).

On the other hand, polymersomes can be easily loaded with hydrophilic molecules in the internal cavity, as well as hydrophobic ones in the membrane, allowing for dual functioning therapy. They present low passive permeability to low-molecular-weight solutes, allowing a controlled release by external triggers such as temperature, pH and light.

It is observed that the *in vitro* release of the drug from the prepared polymersomes MPOx:IND (9:1 molar ratio) is quite slow in comparison with the chimeric nanocontainers (Figure 6). This kinetic behavior has been validated in simulation studies of drug release in fractal polymeric matrices.

In our opinion, it seems likely that the spatiotemporal variation in membrane permeability of the dynamically swelling MPOx polymer is close enough to the percolation threshold for non-classical diffusion effects to impinge on release kinetics [104-107]. The design of a Modulatory Controlled Release System at the nano scale level (MCRnS) is an issue that needs biomaterials which can modulate the release of the drug in a zero-kinetic order.

However, innovative therapies require innovative delivery systems by controlling the physicochemical properties of the biomaterials utilized, as well as their interactions between them and with the encapsulated drug [51-53, 109].

Furthermore, the *in vitro* release of the drug from the prepared chimeric nanostructures is faster only for all the chimeric nanovectors prepared at 45°C, temperature higher than T_m (=41°C) of DPPC lipids (Figure 6 (c)) in comparison to the other two lower temperatures (Figure (a) and (b)). In other words, for the chimeric nanovectors, the drug release rate increased with increasing temperature.

According to the literature, a conformational change of C-C single bonds in the alkyl chains of the DPPC lipids leads to an increase in the total volume occupied by the hydrocarbon chains in the membrane, and therefore increases the permeability of the mixed bilayer membrane. At T_m (41°C for DPPC lipids) permeability is additionally increased as result of the coexistence of membrane areas in both liquid crystalline phases [110-112]. The increase of the membrane permeability is most probably the reason for the increased release rates for chimeric liposomes at 45°C.

However, the presence of MPOx chains modulates the behavior since the chimeric nanovectors show different temperature dependent release rate, influences by the DPPC/MPOx ratio. On the other hand, the IND release rate for MPOx polymersomes remained unaffected by the increase of temperature (Figure 6) [108].

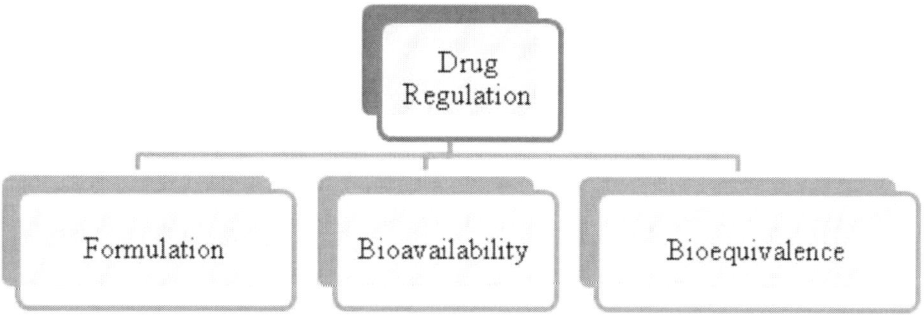

Figure 7. The trends in Drug Regulation.

From Bio-Inspired aDDnSs to Regulatory Aspects

According to the recent literature, so far there is no specific regulation framework in European Union which corresponds to the use of nanoscale products [113]. The development process seems to be conventional in terms of the properties of nanoparticles which are required to pass the regulatory criteria before approved for the market. The biocompatibility, the biodegradability and the nontoxic profile of newly prepared aDDnSs towards healthy tissues, should be taken into account in order to be acceptable for biomedical and pharmaceutical applications [11]. In these research orientations, focus is placed on new approaches for preparing advanced Drug Delivery nanoSystems (aDDnSs) with a Modulatory Controlled Release profile. Such complex and advanced nanosystems can alter the pharmacokinetic properties of the encapsulated drug and consequently its effectiveness. However, it is obvious that the regulatory framework in the European Union is considered to be extremely complicated and needs specific regulations to assure that the final product meets with the requirements concerning the pharmacokinetic parameters (active substance release, biodistribution, tissue accumulation, biodegradability, and clearance (Figure 7) [113]. The subject of the requirements concerning the pharmacokinetic and pharmacodynamic properties of the nanoscaled products still remains under discussion [3, 24]. It is obvious that the manufacturing process of using nanomaterials to produce nanoproducts is a difficult task and E.M.A. asked the participants in the workshop to debate and to propose non-clinical tools for regulating the developing process. The size distribution of nanoparticles, the physicochemical characterization, their stability in diverse media including biological, cell distribution, immune system effects, genotoxicity etc. are considered to be crucial for proposing the regulatory framework for nanoproducts [24]. Scientific challenges arise from the limitations of current testing methods and the unknown reliability of novel ones, because of the nanosize and the unique behavior of such nanosystems in biological structures. Further scientific research will be needed in order to provide a sound scientific basis for an adequate evaluation of the quality, safety and efficacy of emerging nanomedicines. The precise role of nanoparticles morphology and shape in drug delivery has not been fully elucidated, most likely due to the lack of easy-to-use methods and techniques available to control nanoparticles shape [24, 98, 100, 101]. Systems Pharmacology is a new scientific filed in these orientations and is an emerging discipline, which connects systems biology (i.e., genomics, proteomics, and metabolomics) to quantitative pharmacology (i.e., mechanism-based pharmacokinetic – pharmacodynamic modeling) to obtain fundamental insights in the relationships between drugs and diseases. Interest in this field has been increased substantially, recently. It is seen as a novel scientific approach to the design of (complex) therapeutic interventions to modify disease therapeutic processes. Such complex therapeutic interventions are referred to as systems therapeutics and include: personalized treatments, rational drug combinations and pre-emptive and preventive treatments [3].

Conclusion

Drug delivery has matured from its original goal of prolonging the duration of drug release; it now involves customized systems that are designed to achieve specific spatial and temporal control. Future generations of drug-delivery systems will incorporate "smart" biosensing functionalities that will enable unaided *in vivo* feedback control. In conclusion, bio-inspired delivery systems, especially chimeric aDDnSs, which are complex self-assembled soft nanostructures, act as facilitators for the development of innovative therapeutic devices, with added value and respond to the requirements of modern trends in the therapeutics, as indicated by systems pharmacology.

Abbreviations

DPPC, Dipalmitoylphosphatidylcholine; d_f, mass fractal; MPOx, poly(2-methyl-2-oxazoline)-grad-poly(2-phenyl-2-oxazoline); PBS, Phosphate Buffer Saline; aDDnSs, advanced Drug Delivery nanosystems; FBS, fetal bovine serum; DPPG, 1,2-dipalmitoyl-*sn*-glycero-3-phospho-(1'-*rac*-glycerol); DODAP, 1,2-dioleoyl-3-dimethylammonium-propane

References

[1] M. Lazzari, C. Ridríguez-Abreu, J. Rivas, M.A. Lópes-Quintela, Self-assembly: a minimalist route to the fabrication of nanomaterials, *J. Nanosci. Nanotechnol*, 6 (2006) 829-905.

[2] Y. Lin, C. Mao, C., Bio-inspired supramolecular self-assembly towards soft nanomaterials, *Front Mater. Sci.* 5 (2011) 247-265.

[3] R. Gaspar, B. Aksu, A. Cuine, M. Danhof, M.J. Takac, H.H. Linden, A. Link, A., E.M. Muchitsch, C.G. Wilson, P. Ohrngren, L. Dencker, L., Towards a European strategy for medicines research (2014-2020): The EUFEPS position paper on Horizon 2020, Eur *J. Pharm. Sci,* 47 (2012) 979-987.

[4] I.W. Hamley, Nanotechnology with soft materials. *Angew. Chem. Int.* Ed 42 (2003) 1692-1712.

[5] S. Nayak, L.A. Lyon, Soft nanotechnology with soft nanoparticles, *Angew. Chem. Int.* Ed Engl, 44(2005), 7686-7708.

[6] G.M. Whitesides, D.J. Lipomi, Soft nanotechnology: structure vs. function, *Faraday Discuss*, 143 (2009) 373-384.

[7] G.A. Hughes, G.A., Nanostructure-mediated drug delivery, *Nanomedicine* 1(2005) 22-30.

[8] R. Ravichandron, (2009). Nanotechnology – based drug delivery systems, *Nanobiotechnol*, 5(2009) 17-33.

[9] B. Mishra, B. Bhavesh, S. Patel, S. Tiwari, Colloidal nanocarriers: a review on formulation technology, types and applications toward targeted drug delivery, *Nanomedecine*, 6 (2010) 9-24.

[10] G.R. Souza, F.I. Staquicini, D.R. Christianson, M.G. Ozawa, J. Houston Miller, R. Pasqualini, W. Arap, Combinatorial targeting and nanotechnology applications. *Biomed. Microdevices*, 12 (2010) 597-606.

[11] M. Rowland, C.R. Noe, D.A. Smith, G.T. Tucker, D.J. Crommelin, D.J., C.C. Peck, M.L. Jr Rocci, L. Basançon, V.P. Shah, Impact of the pharmaceutical sciences on health care: a reflection over the past 50 years, *J. Pharm. Sci.* 101 (2012), 4075-4099.

[12] G. Bonacucina, M. Cespi, M. Misici-Falzi, G.F. Palmieri, Colloidal soft matter as drug delivery system, *J. Pharm. Sci.* 98(2009) 1-42.

[13] Y. Liu, J. Tan, A. Thomas, D. Ou-Yang, D., V.R. Muzykantov, The shape of things to come: importance of design in nanotechnology for drug delivery, *Ther. Deliv.* 3(2012),181-194.

[14] J. Sabín, G. Prieto, J.M. Ruso, F. Sarmiento, Fractal aggregates induced by liposome-liposome interaction in the presence of Ca^{2+}, *Eur. Phys. J. E.* 24 (2007) 201–210

[15] J. Sabín, G. Prieto, J.M. Ruso, P.V. Messina, F. Sarmiento, Aggregation of liposomes in presence of La^{3+}: a study of the fractal dimension, *Phys. Rev. E* 76 (2007) 011408 1-7

[16] S. Roldán-Vargas, R. Barnabas-Rodrígez, A. Martín-Molina, M. Quesada-Pérez, J. Estelrich, J. Callejas-Fernández, Growth of lipid vesicle structures: from surface fractals to mass fractals. *Physical Review E* 78 (2008) 010902(R) 1-4.

[17] S. Roldán-Vargas, R. Barnabas-Rodrígez, M. Quesada-Pérez, J. Estelrich, J. Callejas-Fernández, Surface fractals in liposome aggregation, The American physical society, *Phys. Rev.* 79(2009) 1-14.

[18] B.B. Mandelbrot, The Fractal Geometry of Nature, San Francisco: Freeman & Co. (1982).

[19] H.P. Koch, The concept of fractals in the pharmaceutical sciences, *Pharmazie*, 48 (1993) 643-659.

[20] A. Tromelin, J.C. Gnanou, C. Andrès, Y. Pourcelot, B. Chaillot, Study of morphology of reactive dissolution interface using fractal geometry, *J. Pharm. Sci.* 85(1996) 924-928.

[21] A. Tromelin, G. Hautbout, Y. Pourcelot, Application of fractal geometry to dissolution kinetic study of a sweetener excipients, *Int. J. Pharm.* 224 (2001) 131-140.

[22] P.A. Moreno, P.E. Vélez, E. Martínez, L.E., Garreta, N. Díaz, S. Amador, I. Tischer, J.M. Gutiérrez, A.K. Naik, F. García, The human genome: a multifractal analysis, *BMC Genomics*, 12 (2011) 506-523.

[23] N. Pippa, C. Demetzos, E. Danezis, The formalism of fractal aggregation phenomena of colloidal drug delivery systems, *J. Liposome Res*, 22 (2010) 55-61.

[24] D.J. Crommelin, A.T. Florence, Towards more effective advanced drug delivery systems, *Int. J. Pharm.* (2013) In press.

[25] V.P. Torchilin, Targeted polymeric micelles for delivery of poorly soluble drugs, *Cell Mol. Life Sci*, 61 (2004) 2549-2559.

[26] V.P. Torchilin, Micellar Nanocarriers: Pharmaceutical perspectives, *Pharm. Res*, 21 (2007) 1-15.

[27] A.D. Bangham, M.M. Standish, J.C. Watkins, Diffusion of univalent ions across the lamellae of swollen phospholipids, *J. Mol. Biol*, 13 (1965) 238–252.

[28] G. Gregoriadis, E.J. Wills, C.P. Swain, A.S. Tavill, Drug-carrier potential of liposomes in cancer chemotherapy, *Lancet* 1 (1974) 1313–1316.

[29] J.S. Lee, J. Feijen, Polymersomes for drug delivery: design, formation and characterization, *J. Control Release* 161(2012) 473-83.

[30] D.E. Discher, A. Eisenberg, Polymer vesicles, *Science* 297(2002) 967-973.

[31] F. Meng, Z. Zhong, Z., Polymersomes spanning from nano- to microscales: advanced vehicles for controlled drug delivery and robust vesicles for virus and cell mimicking, *J. Phys. Chem. Lett.* 2 (2011) 1533–1539.
[32] K.L. Thompson, P. Chambon, R. Versber, S.P. Armes, Can polymersomes form colloidosomes? *J. Am. Chem. Soc.* 134(2012) 12450-12453.
[33] J.F. Le Meins, O. Sandre, S. Lecommandoux, Recent trends in the tuning of polymersomes membrane properties, *Eur. Phys. J. E. Soft Matter*, 34(2011)1-16.
[34] D.A. Tomalia, In quest of a systematic framework for unifying and definig nanoscience, *J. Nanopart Res.* 11 (2006) 1251-1310.
[35] M. Cloninger, Biological applications of dendrimers, *Curr. Opin. Chem. Biol.* 6 (2002) 742-748.
[36] B. Klajernt, J. Janiszewska, Z. Urbancyz-Lipkowska, M. Bryszwska, D. Shcharbin, M. Labienniec, Biological propertiesof low molecular mass peptide dendrimers, *Int. J. Pharm*, 309 (2006) 208-217.
[37] B. Klajernt, M. Cortijo-Arellano, M. Bryszwska, J. Cladera, Influence of heparin and dendrimers on the aggregation of two amyloid peptides related to Alzheimer's and prion diseases, *Biochem. Biophys. Res. Commun*, 339 (2006) 577-582.
[38] J. Woo-Dong, K.M. Kamruzzaman Selimb, L. Chi-Hwa, I.K. Kang, Bioinspired application of dendrimers: from bio-mimicry to biomedical applications, *Prog. Polym. Sci*, 34 (2009) 1-23.
[39] S. Svenson, Dendrimers as versatile platform in drug delivery applications, *Eur. J. Pharm. Biopharm*, 71(2009) 445-462.
[40] C. Villalonga-Barber, M. Skretta-Micha, B.R. Steele, A. Georgopoulos, C. Demetzos, Dendrimers as biopharmaceuticsals: synthesis and properties, *Curr. Top Med. Chem.* 8 (2008) 1294-1309.
[41] A. J. Khopade, F.Caruso, P. Tripathi, S. Nagaich, N. K. Jain, Effect of dendrimer on entrapment and release of bioactive from liposomes, *Int. J. Pharm.* 232 (2002) 157-162.
[42] A. Papagiannaros, K. Dimas, G.T. Papaioannou, C. Demetzos, Doxorubicin-PAMAM dendrimer complex attached to liposomes: Cytotoxic studies against human cancer cell lines, *Int. J. Pharm*, 302 (2005) 29-38.
[43] E. A.Mourelatou, D. Libster, I. Nir, S. Hatziantoniou, A. Aserin, N. Garti, C. Demetzos, Type and Location of Interaction between Hyperbranched Polymers and Liposomes. Relevance to Design of a Potentially Advanced Drug Delivery Nanosystem (aDDnS), *J. Phys. Chem. B* 115(2011) 3400-8.
[44] L. Cattel, M. Ceruti, F. Dosio, From conventional to stealth liposomes: a new frontier in cancer chemotherapy, *J. Chemother*, 4 (2004) 94-97.
[45] M.L. Immordino, F. Dosio, L. Cattel, Stealth liposomes: review of the basic science, rationale, and clinical applications, existing and potential, *Int. J. Nanomedicine*, 1(2006),297-315.
[46] S.M. Moghimi, J. Szebeni, Stealth liposomes and long-circulating nanoparticles: critical issues in pharmacokinetics, opsonization and protein-binding properties, *Prog. Lipid Res.* 42 (2003) 463-478.
[47] A. Samad, Y. Sultana, M., Agil, Liposomal drug delivery systems: an update review, *Curr. Drug Deliv.* 4(2007) 297-305.

[48] M.S. Mufamadi, V. Pillay, Y.E. Choonara, L.C. Du Toit, G. GirishModi, G. Naidoo, V.M.K. Ndesendo, A review on composite liposomal technologies for specialized drug delivery, *J. Drug Delivery*, 2011 (2011) 939851-70.
[49] N. Bergstrand, K. Edwards, Effects of poly(ethylene oxide) – poly(propylene oxide) – poly(ethylene oxide) triblock copolymers on structure and stability of liposomal dioleoylphosphatidylethanolamine, *J. Colloid Interface Sci,* 276(2004) 400-407.
[50] S.C. Balmert, S.R. Little, Biomimetic delivery with micro- and nanoparticles, *Adv. Mater* 24 (2012) 3757-3778.
[51] C. Demetzos, Drug delivery nanosystems and their classification based on their dynamic variability. In: 2nd International Symposium on Biological Applications of Dendrimers, June 23–26, Porquerolles islands, France. (2010).
[52] C. Demetzos, Advances in drug delivery systems (DDSs). In: International Congress on *New Delivery Systems, Biosimilars, Bioequivalence-Biowaivers- Biotechnology Products*, July 2–3, Athens, Greece (2010).
[53] C. Demetzos, Drug Delivery nanosystems (DDnSs) and advances on their physical stability. In: Dendrimers as Composites of Advanced Drug Delivery nano-Systems (aDDnSs). Biomedical Applications, October 3-7, Athens, Greece (2011).
[54] K. Gardikis, C. Tsimplouli, K. Dimas, M. Micha-Skretta M., C. Demetzos, New chimeric advanced drug delivery nanosystems (Chi-aDDnSs) as doxorubicin carriers, *Int. J. Pharm.* 402(2010) 231-237.
[55] K.Gardikis, S. Hatziantoniou, M. Signorelli, M. Pusceddu, M. Micha-Scretta, A. Schiraldi, C. Demetzos, D. Fessas, Thermodynamics and structural characterization of liposomal locked-in dendrimers as drug carriers, *Colloids and Surfaces B: Biointerfaces*, 81 (2010) 11-19.
[56] K. Gardikis, D. Fessas, M. Signorelli, K. Dimas, C. Tsimplouli, M. Ionov, C. Demetzos, A new chimeric drug delivery nano system (chi-aDDnS) composed of PAMAM G 3.5 dendrimer and liposomes as doxorubicin's carrier. In vitro pharmacological studies, *J. Nanosci. Nanotechnol.* 5 (2011) 3764-72.
[57] N. Pippa, E. Kaditi, S. Pispas, C. Demetzos, PEO-b-PCL/DPPC chimeric nanocarriers: self-assembly aspects in aqueous and biological media and drug incorporation, *Soft Matter*, 9 (2013) 4073-4082.
[58] N. Pippa, M. Merkouraki, S., Pispas, C. Demetzos, DPPC:MPOx chimeric advanced Drug Delivery nanosystems (chi-aDDnSs): physicochemical and structural characterization, stability and drug release studies, *Int. J. Pharm.* 450 (2013) 1-10.
[59] N. Pippa, E. Kaditi, S. Pispas, C. Demetzos, DPPC/poly(2-methyl-2-oxazoline)-grad-poly(2-phenyl-2-oxazoline) chimeric nanostructures as potential drug nanocarriers, *J. Nanopart Res.* 15 (2013) 1685.
[60] K. Gardikis, K. Dimas, A. Georgopoulos, S. Pispas, E. Kaditi, C., Demetzos, β-lactam functionalized poly(isoprene –b-ethylene oxide) amphiphilic block copolymer micelles as a new nanocarrier system for curcumin, *Current Nanoscience* 6 (2010) 277-284.
[61] K. Gardikis, S. Hatziantoniou, M. Bucos, D. Fessas, M. Signorelli, T. Felekis, M. Zervou, C. Screttas, C., B. Steele, M. Ionov, M. Micha- Scretta, B. Klajnert, M. Bryszewska, C. Demetzos, New drug delivery nanosystem combining liposomal and dendrimeric technology (liposomal locked-in dendrimers) for cancer therapy, *J. Pharm. Sci.* 99 (2010) 3561-3571.

[62] K.N. Kontogiannopoulos, A.N. Assimopoulou, S. Hantziantoniou, K. Karatassos, C. Demetzos, V.P. Papageorgiou, Chimeric advanced drug delivery nanosystems (chi-aDDnSs) for shikonin combining dendritic and liposomal technology, *Int. J. Pharm.* 422 (2012) 381-389.
[63] S, Pispas, E. Sarantopoulou, Self-assembly in mixed aqueous solutions of amphiphilic block copolymers and vesicle-forming surfactant, *Langmuir* 23 (2007) 7484 -7490.
[64] S. Pispas, Self-assembled nanostructures in mixed anionic-neutral double hydrophilic block copolymer/cationic vesicle –forming surfactant solutions, *Soft Matter* 7 (2011) 474-482.
[65] S. Pispas, Vesicular structures in mixed block copolymer/surfactant solutions, *Soft Matter* 7 (2011) 8697-8701.
[66] E. Kaditi, G. Mountrichas, S. Pispas, C. Demetzos, Block copolymers for drug delivery nanosystems (DDnSs), *Curr. Med. Chem*, 19 (2012) 5088-100.
[67] Y. Liu, H. Miyoshi, M. Nakamura, Nanomedicine for drug delivery and imaging: A promising avenue for cancer therapy and diagnosis using targeted functional nanoparticles, *Int. J. Cancer*, 120 (2007) 2527-2537.
[68] J. Shi, A.R. Vortruba, O. Farokhzad, R. Langer, Nanotechnology in drug delivery and tissue engineering: from discovery to applications, *Nano Lett*, 10 (2010) 3223-3230.
[69] A. Angelova, B. Angelov, R. Mutafchieva, S. Lesieur, P. Counreur, Self-assembled multicompartmet liquid crystalline lipid carriers for protein, peptide, and nucleic acid drug delivery, *Acc Chem. Res*, 44 (2011) 2147-156.
[70] K. Letchford, H. Burt, A review of the formation and classification of amphiphilic block copolymer nanoparticulate structures: micelles, nanospheres, nanocapsules and polymersomes, *Eur. J. Pharm. Biopharm*, 65 (2007),259-269.
[71] R. Stoenescu, A. Graff, W. Meier, Asymmetric ABC-triblock copolymer membranes induce a directed insertion of membrane proteins, *Macromol Biosci*, 4 (2004) 930-935.
[72] D.L. Leiske, B. Meckes, C.E. Miller, C. Wu, T.W. Walker, B. Lin, M. Meron, H.A. Ketelson, M.F. Toney, G.G. Fuller, Insertion mechanism of a poly(ethylene oxide)-poly(butylenes oxide) block copolymer into DPPC monolayer, *Langmuir*, 27 (2011) 11444-11450.
[73] J. Nam, P.A. Beales, T.K. Vanderlick, Giant phospholipid/block copolymer hydrid vesicles: mixing behavior and domain formation, *Langmuir* 27(2011) 1-6.
[74] M.A. Firestone, S. Seifert, Interaction of nonionic PEO-PPO dublock copolymers with lipid bilayers, *Biomacromolecules* 6 (2005) 2678-2687.
[75] T. Ruysschaert, A.F.P. Sonnen, T. Haefele, W. Meier, M. Winterhalter, D. Fournier, Hydrid nanocapsules: interactions of ABA block copolymers with liposomes, *J. Am. Chem. Soc.* 127 (2005)6242-6247.
[76] E. Amado, A. Blume, J. Kressler, Novel non-ionic block copolymers tailored for interactions with phospholipids, *React. Funct. Polym*, 69 (2009) 450-456.
[77] F.E. Antunes, E.F. Marques, M.G. Miguel, B. Lindman, Polymer-vesicle association, *Adv. Colloid Interface Sci*, 147-148 (2009) 18-35.
[78] K. Kita-Tokarczyk, F. Itel, M. Grzelakwski, S. Egli, P. Rossbach, W. Meier, Monolayer interactions between lipids and amphiphilic block copolymers, *Langmuir*, 25(2009), 9847-9856.
[79] C.R. Henry, Morphology of supported nanoparticles, *Prog. Surf. Sci.* 80 (2005) 92-116.

[80] M.L. Chen, Lipid excipients and delivery systems for pharmaceutical development: A regulatory perspective, *Adv. Drug Deliv. Rev.* 60(2008),768-777.

[81] B.V. Derjaguin, L.D. Landau, Theory of the stability of stronglycharged lyophobic sols and of adhesion of strongly charged particles in solution of electrolytes *Acta Physicochim URRS,* 14 (1941) 633-62.

[82] E.J.B. Verwey, J.Th.G. Overbeek, Theory of the stability of lyophobic Colloids. Elsevier, Amsterdan (1948).

[83] M. Lattuada, H. Wu, M. Morbidelli, Estimation of fractal dimension of colloidal gels in the presence of multiple scattering, *Physical Review E* 64, 061404 (2001) 1-7.

[84] M. Lattuada, H. Wu, M. Morbidelli, A simple model for the structure of fractal aggregates, *J. Colloid Interface Sci*, 268 (2003)106-20.

[85] M. Lattuada, P. Sandkühler, H. Wu, J. Sefcik, M. Morbidelli, Aggregation kinetics of polymer colloids in reaction limited regime: experiments and simulations, *Adv. Colloid Interface Sci*, 103 (2003) 33-56.

[86] J. Sabín, G. Prieto, P.V. Messina, J.M. Ruso, R. Hidalgo-Álvarez, F. Sarmiento, On the effect of Ca^{2+} and La^{3+} on the colloidal stability of liposomes, *Langmuir* 21 (2005) 10968-10975.

[87] J. Sabín, G. Prieto, J.M. Ruso, R. Hidalgo-Álvarez, F. Sarmiento, Size and stability of liposomes: a possible role of hydration and osmotic forces, *Eur. Phys. J.*E 20 (2006) 401-408.

[88] N. Pippa, S. Pispas, C. Demetzos, The fractal hologram and elucidation of the structure of liposomal carriers in aqueous and biological media, *Int. J. Pharm*, 430 (2013) 65-73.

[89] N. Pippa, S. Pispas, C. Demetzos, The delineation of the morphology of charged liposomal vectors via a fractal analysis in aqueous and biological media: physicochemical and self-assembly studies, *Int. J. Pharm.* 437 (2012) 264-274.

[90] M. Hadjidemetriou, N. Pippa, S. Pispas, C. Demetzos, Incorporation of dimethoxycurcumin into charged liposomes and the formation kinetics of fractal aggregates of uncharged vectors, *J. Liposome Res*, 23(2013) 92-100.

[91] L.A. Mirny, The fractal globule as a model of chromatin architecture in the cell, *Chromosome Res* 19 (2011) 37-51.

[92] A. Bancaud, C. Lavelle, S. Huet, J. Ellenberd, A fractal model for nuclear organization: current evidence and biological implications, *Nucleic Acids Res*, 40 (2012) 8783-8792.

[93] Y.M Harshe, L. Ehrl, M. Lattuada, Hydrodynamic properties of rigid fractal aggregates of arbitrary morphology, *J. Colloid Interface Sci*, 352 (2010) 87-98.

[94] Y.M. Harshe, M. Lattuada, Viscosity contribution of an arbitraty shape rigid aggregate to a dilute suspension, *J. Colloid Interface Sci*, 367 (2012) 83-91.

[95] N.M. Schaeublin, L.K. Braydich-Stolle, E.L. Maurer, K. Park, R.I. MacCuspie, A.R. Afrooz, R.A. Vaia, N.B. Saleh, S.M. Hussain, Does shape matter? Bioeffects of gold nanomaterials in a human skin cell model, *Langmuir*, 28 (2012) 3248-58.

[96] J. Sabín, G. Prieto, J.M. Ruso, P.V. Messina, F.J. Salgado, M. Nogueira, M. Costas, F. Sarmiento, Interactions between DMPC liposomes and the serum blood proteins HSA and IgG, *J. Phys. Chem. B*, 113 (2009) 1655-1661.

[97] M.J. Grogan, L. Rotkina, H.H. Bau, In situ liquid-cell electron microscopy of colloid aggregation and growth dynamics, *Physical Review E* 83, 061405 (2011) 1-5.

[98] J.A. Champion, S. Mitragotri, Role of target geometry in phagocytosis, *Proc. Natl. Acad. Sci. USA*, 103 (2006) 4930-4934.

[99] J.A. Champion, Y.K. Katare, S. Mitragotri, Particle shape: A new design parameter for micro- and nanoscale drug delivery carriers, *J. Control Release*, 121 (2007) 3-9.

[100] M. Goldberd, R. Langer, X. Jia, Nanostructured materials for applications in drug delivery and tissue engineering, *J. Biomater. Sci. Polym. Ed*,18 (2007) 241-268.

[101] S.E. Gratton, P.A. Ropp, P.D. Pohlhaus, J.C. Luft, V.J. Madden, M.E. Napier, J.M. DeSimone, The effect of particle design on cellular internalization pathways, *Proc. Natl. Acad. Sci. USA*, 105 (2008) 11613-11618.

[102] J. Wang, J.D. Byrne, M.E. Napier, J.M. DeSimone, More effective nanomedicines through particle design, *Small*, 7(2011) 1919-1931.

[103] T.M. Allen, W.W. Cheng, J.I. Hare, K.M. Laginha, Pharmacokinetics and pharmacodynamics of lipidic nano-particles in cancer, *Anticancer Agents Med. Chem*, 6 (2006) 513-523.

[104] A. Dokoumetzidis, V. Karalis, A. Iliadis, P. Macheras, The heterogeneous course of drug transit through the body, *Trends Pharmacol Sci*, 25(2004) 140-6.

[105] A. Dokoumetzidis, V. Papadopoulou, G. Valsami, P. Macheras, Development of a reaction-limited model of dissolution: Application to official dissolution tests experiments, *Int. J. Pharm*, 355 (2008) 114-125.

[106] A. Dokoumetzidis, P. Macheras, The changing face of the rate concept in biopharmaceutical sciences: from classical to fractal and finally to fractional, *Pharm. Res*, 28 (2011) 1229-1232.

[107] L.M. Pereira, Fractal pharmacokinetics, *Comput Math Methods Med*, 11(2010), 161-84.

[108] D.A. Christian, S. Cai, D.M. Bowen, Y. Kim, J.D. Pajerowski, D.E. Discher, Polymersome carriers: from self-assembly to siRNA and protein therapeutics, *Eur. J. Pharm. Biopharm.* 71(2009) 463-474.

[109] C. Demetzos, Fractal analysis of Drug Delivery Nanosystems' aggregation. In: 3rd International Symposium on Biological applications of dendrimers. 5th-8th September, Toledo, Spain (2012).

[110] M.H, Gaber, K. Hong, S.K. Huang, D. Papahadjopoulos, Thermosensitive sterically stabilized liposomes: formulation and in vitro studies on mechanism of doxorubicin release from bovine serum and human plasma, *Pharm. Res*, 12 (1995) 1407-1416.

[111] M. Hossann, M. Wiggenhorn, A. Schwerdt, K. Wachholz, N. Teichert, H. Eibl, R.D. Issels, L.H. Lindner, In vitro stability and content release properties of phosphatidylglyceroglycerol containing thermosensitive liposomes, *Biochimica et Biophysica Acta*, 1768 (2007) 2491-2499.

[112] M. Hossann, Z. Syunyaeva, R. Schmidt, A. Zengerle, H. Eibl, R.D. Issels, L.H. Lindner, Proteins and cholesterol lipid vesicles are mediators of drug release from thermosensitive liposomes, *J. Control Release* 162 (2012) 400-406.

[113] S. Vamvakas, J. Martinaldo, R. Pita, M. Isaak, (2011). On the edge of new Technologies (advanced therapies, nanomedicines), *Drug Discovery Today: Technology* 8 1 (2011) e21-e28.

In: Recent Advances in Drug Delivery Research
Editor: Valerio Voliani
ISBN: 978-1-62948-228-6

Chapter 5

In Situ Gelling Systems for Sustained Drug Delivery

***Lívia Neves Borgheti-Cardoso*[1]*, Fabiana Testa Moura de Carvalho Vicentini*[1]*, Tais Gratieri*[2] *and Maria Vitória Lopes Badra Bentley*[1,*]**

[1]Faculdade de Ciências Farmacêuticas de Ribeirão Preto, Universidade de São Paulo Avenida do Café, s/n, Ribeirão Preto, SP, Brazil

[2]Faculdade de Ciências da Saúde, Universidade de Brasília. Campus Universitário Darcy Ribeiro, s/n, Brasília, DF, Brazil

Abstract

In situ gelling delivery systems have gained attention over the past few decades because they provide several advantages for sustaining drug delivery, which include the following: ease of application compared with solid implants (they can be injected using a syringe, forming a gel after injection); minimal invasive and pain; localized release for a site-specific action; dose reduction with possibly reduced side effects; ease of fabrication; ability to release lipophilic and hydrophilic drugs; and increased patient comfort and compliance.

Moreover, with the increased therapeutic application of bioactive macromolecules, which has been stimulated by advances in molecular biology and genomic research, the development of systems that protect proteins and nucleic acids against degradation in body fluids and that control the release of these agents are essential to therapeutic success. This chapter first discusses the advantages of *in situ* gelling delivery systems and their possible administration routes.

Four categories of *in situ* gelling delivery systems and the main components of each system are presented, and their *in vivo* mechanisms of achieving solidification are discussed.

The applications of these systems through various administration routes (such as subcutaneous, intratumoral, mucosal and ocular) are discussed, emphasizing sustained delivery. Finally, new perspectives are highlighted regarding the advantages of using these systems in gene therapy.

* Email: vbentley@usp.br.

Keywords: Drug delivery, *in situ* gelling system, sustained delivery, thermoplastic paste, *in situ* crosslinked systems, *in situ* polymer precipitation, *in situ* solidifying organogels

Introduction

The first *in situ* gelling delivery systems were developed in the early 1980s to deliver antibiotics for the treatment of periodontal diseases [1], and subsequently, these systems have gained attention because of several advantages such as local and sustained delivery and ease of application, which may decrease side effects and improve patient compliance and comfort [2]. In addition, the interest in *in situ* gelling delivery systems has increased because many new bioactive macromolecules, such as proteins and nucleic acids, have been developed due to the explosion of genomic information and molecular biology. These macromolecules are easily degraded in body fluids when administered by conventional routes; therefore, the development of delivery systems that can protect these macromolecules and that allow for localized and sustained release are essential for therapeutic success [1-4].

It is established that drugs that are degraded or denatured in body fluids [5], have short half-lives [6, 7] or have narrow therapeutic indices should not be administered by conventional oral or i.v. routes. Particularly for drugs with narrow therapeutic indices, sustained and local release is desirable to maintain tissue-level efficacy without systemic toxicity [8]. In this scenario, *in situ* gelling delivery systems have appeared as an attractive approach to administer drugs [6, 9, 10], proteins [11, 12] and nucleic acids [13-15] in a sustained manner and to achieve site-specific actions in different tissues such as subcutaneous, intratumoral, ocular and mucosal sites.

The use of *in situ* gelling delivery systems for the controlled release of drugs by the subcutaneous route has the advantage of being less invasive and painful than implants or other drug-delivery devices because the formulation can be injected through a syringe into the body prior to its gelation process, only forming a gel after injection and thus avoiding the necessity of surgical insertion, as in the case of an implant [1, 8]. This characteristic is also applicable in tissue engineering, where it is possible to deliver therapeutic molecules and cells into the tissues with less surgical trauma [16]. Furthermore, these systems provide the advantage of delivering drugs intratumorally, as the retention time of drugs within tumors is normally short [13]. Therefore, the administration and sustained release of drugs directly into a tumor is a promising approach to increase the intratumoral drug concentration and to avoid systemic side effects [13, 17]. Direct administration of chemotherapeutics into the tumor is even more important for brain tumors because of the blood–brain barrier, which limits the penetration of drugs administered systemically. Local administration into a brain tumor circumvents the blood–brain barrier and sustains a high anticancer-drug concentration at the target site [18].

Similarly, direct drug application into the eye is the ideal method to reach therapeutic levels for treating ocular diseases [19]. Several conventional systems are available to deliver drugs into the anterior segments of the eye (i.e., the cornea, conjunctiva and sclera), such as solutions, suspensions and semisolids as ointments and gels. However, all these systems present drawbacks that should be overcome. Upon instillation of an ophthalmic solution, most of the drug is rapidly eliminated from the precorneal area through nasolacrimal drainage and tear-turnover dilution. Additionally, drugs drained by the nasolacrimal duct may be absorbed systemically, resulting in undesirable side effects. Viscous solutions and ointments have been applied to improve the ocular bioavailability; however, these formulations may cause blurred vision, leading to poor patient compliance. Inserts are another system with poor patient acceptance, due to difficult self-insertion and foreign body sensation [20-23]. Increased ocular bioavailability with reduced side effects can be reached by using *in situ* gelling delivery systems [20-22, 24]. These systems are also useful for delivering drugs to the posterior segment of the eye, which is performed by direct injection into the vitreous body, thereby avoiding several complications related to this method and preventing drug degradation by proteases and neutralization by humoral and cellular components of the immune system [25].

Mucosal drug administration might be improved through *in situ* gelling delivery systems [26-29]. The application of *in situ* gelling systems to the nasal mucosa may prevent rapid drainage and rapid mucociliary clearance from the administration site, which occur with other systems, such as solutions [27]. Vaginal administration of these systems may also be advantageous because the formulations are easily applied, providing efficient spreadability and easily coating the vaginal surface; this method overcomes the common drawbacks of vaginal administration, which include a frequent dose regimen due to physiological protective mechanisms and a lack of patient compliance due to the discomfort that ointment and inserts may cause [30]. Moreover, *in situ* gelling systems may be an interesting approach for the vaginal delivery of vaccines [26]. The oral or buccal mucosa is also an easily accessible tissue with high permeability and blood flow that could be used as alternative route for drug delivery. Buccal drug delivery avoids hepatic first-pass metabolism and circumvents metabolism in the gastrointestinal tract [28, 29]. The mucoadhesive properties of certain gels make these systems even more suited for drug delivery to the buccal mucosa [31].

The *in vivo* gel formation can be achieved by different mechanisms. In this chapter, *in situ* gelling delivery systems will be divided in four types based on the mechanism of solidification: (1) thermoplastic paste, (2) *in situ* crosslinked systems, (3) *in situ* polymer precipitation and (4) *in situ* solidifying organogels [1, 2]. In this chapter, these mechanisms and the main components used to prepare these systems, as well as the application routes of each system (such as subcutaneous, intratumoral, ocular and mucosal), will be discussed, emphasizing their ability to sustain delivery.

Types and Mechanisms of *in Situ* Gel Formation

Thermoplastic Paste

Mechanism of Achieving Solidification in vivo and Obtention

Thermoplastic pastes are semi-solid polymer systems that can be injected into the body in the melted form and that form a depot after cooling to body temperature (Figure 1). The requirements for such *in situ* forming devices include a low melting point, ranging from 25 to 65 °C, and an inherent viscosity in the range of 0.05 to 0.8 dL/g, measured at 25 °C.

A carrier copolymer with a viscosity below 0.05 dL/g may not be capable of delaying the release of a drug, whereas a viscosity above the threshold of 0.8 dL/g is too high for easy administration through a needle. The low molecular weight and glass transition temperature makes these systems easily injectable when heated to slightly above their melting point. These polymeric systems mostly keep their shape at room temperature, and by applying heat, they can attain different shapes [1, 2].

Bioerodible thermoplastic pastes might be prepared from monomers such as D,L-lactide, ε-caprolactone, glycolide, trimethylene carbonate, dioxanone, ortho esters and anhydrides. Polymers and copolymers of these monomers have been widely used in a number of biomedical areas and have consistently demonstrated biocompatibility [2,4].

The major limitation of thermoplastic pastes is their injection at elevated temperatures (≥ 60 °C), which is extremely painful for the patient and increases the risk of necrosis at the injection site, thereby leading to encapsulation of the depot by scar tissue, which may inhibit the drug diffusion [1, 4].

In this context, the poly(ortho esters) have appeared as a polymer class with attractive properties for thermoplastic pastes due to their high biocompatibility and superiority in relation to other polyesters, such as ε-caprolactone. Some advantages of their use are as follows: (a) low melting temperatures in the range of 25–45 °C can be designed by polymer modification to overcome the drawback of high injection temperatures; (b) degradation by surface erosion avoids an acidic microenvironment, which is deleterious for proteins and deoxyribonucleic acid (DNA); and (c) the use of organic solvents in the formulation is avoided [1].

The most successful family of poly(ortho esters) was obtained by the reaction between a diketene acetal and a polyol. The employment of 1,10-decanediol as a polyol component produced hydrophobic materials, whereas hydrophilic polymers could be obtained by using triethylene glycol. The mixture of the polymers with drugs was performed at room temperature using a three-roll mill without any solvents and the incorporation of approximately 20% (w/w) polyethyleneglycol (PEG)-monomethylether facilitated the injection of the semi-solid poly(ortho esters) through small-bore needle sizes, without requiring special equipment (e.g., a hydraulic syringe) [1]. Finally, the investigation of the release and stability of different model proteins in such systems demonstrated that protein release from semi-solid, self-catalyzed poly(ortho esters) is a complex progress that may be adjusted by the proper pH and buffering capacity of the protein solution [32].

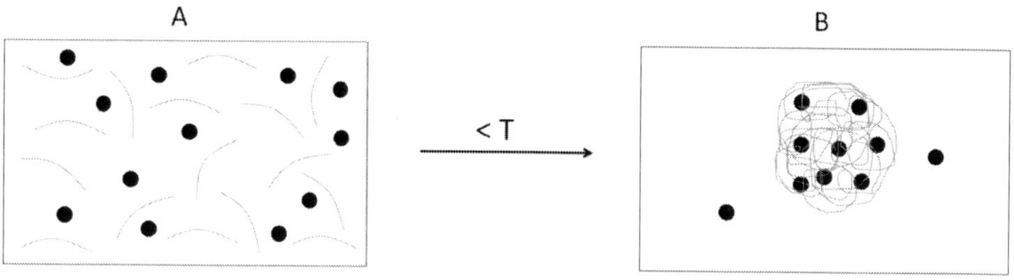

Figure 1. Schematic representation of the thermoplastic paste. (A) Polymers melting at a higher temperature. (B) Polymers cooling to body temperature, forming a gel *in situ*. (•) represents the drug.

Applications of Thermoplastic Pastes

Thermoplastic pastes can be used to create a subcutaneous drug reservoir from which the diffusion occurs into the systemic circulation. The intratumoral injection of Taxol™ and the application of pastes within tumor resection sites are examples of the thermoplastic-paste approach. Polyanhydrides, such as poly(bis(p-carboxyphenoxy) propane-sebacic acid) [33], poly(ε-caprolactone) (PCL) [34] and a thermoplastic triblock polymer system formed of poly(D,L-lactide)–*block*–poly(ethylene glycol)–*block*–poly(D,L-lactide) and blends of low-molecular-weight poly(D,L-lactide) and PCL [35] have been explored in this context.

The decrease in side effects caused by the local delivery of Taxol™ to the tumor is an advantage of using this system over systemic administration of the drug; however, some noteworthy disadvantages are associated with this polymeric system. The major limitation, as described above, is the high injection temperature. Another problem confronted was the extremely low rate of drug release, which negatively affected the polymeric paste formulation efficacy to inhibit the tumor growth [1].

The latter concern, namely, the slow release of Taxol™ from the evaluated polymeric pastes, might be caused by the high degree of crystallinity in the synthesized polymer (PCL), the high molecular weight of PCL or the compatibility of the drug for the polymer versus the aqueous phase [2]. Therefore, in an attempt to overcome this problem, blends of the polymer with water-soluble additives, such as albumin, dextran, gelatin, methylcellulose and sodium chloride, were evaluated [36].

The addition of these additives to polymeric pastes, especially gelatin or albumin, significantly improved the rate of drug release. The additives increased the water uptake and consequently produced a higher rate of drug dissolution and drug release. Additionally, the investigation of the *in vivo* efficacy of these composites, using a mouse tumor model, demonstrated tumor regression [37].

In another approach, methoxy(polyethylene glycol) (MePEG) was added to the PCL paste; this addition decreased the melting point and increased the crystallinity and the amount of water absorbed by the polymer blends but reduced the Taxol™ release rate [34]. Furthermore, this delivery system, with slight modifications in the polymer composition, was effective in inhibiting LNCaP tumor growth and prostate-specific antigen (PSA) levels in mice bearing multiple nonmetastatic tumors [38].

In Situ Crosslinked Systems

Mechanism of Achieving Solidification In Vivo and Obtention

Another category of synthetic polymeric systems comprises the *in situ* crosslinked system, in which the polymers form crosslinked networks by various means, resulting in solid polymer systems or gels. This chemical crosslinking of polymer chains might be initiated upon a change in temperature (e.g., thermosetting systems) or ion concentration, as well as by photo-irradiation (e.g., photopolymerizable systems) [2,4].

Thermosetting Systems

Thermosetting polymers are liquids that exhibit high flowability when initially constituted but that crosslink at elevated temperatures to form viscous gels. This process is known as curing and involves the establishment of covalent crosslinks between polymer chains, forming a macromolecular network. This curing is frequently initiated chemically upon heat addition, but reheating a cured polymer may lead to degradation of the polymer [2].

The polymer concentration, the hydrophobic block length and the chemical structure of the polymer affect the temperature at which the phase change occurs [39].

In contrast to thermosensitive polymers (further discussed in the next section), which exhibit a transition to the gel state due to altered polymer–water interactions above the lower critical gelation temperature, the gelation in thermosetting polymers is caused by the chemical reaction between polymeric chains, often in the presence of a catalyst or initiator [4].

A thermosetting system using multifunctional polymers was obtained by the copolymerization of either L-lactide or D,L-lactide with ε-caprolactone, employing a multifunctional polyol initiator and a catalyst (e.g., peroxides) to form polyol-terminated liquid prepolymers that were then converted to an acrylic ester-terminated pre-polymer. The curing of the liquid acrylic-terminated pre-polymer was initiated by the addition of either benzoyl peroxide or *N,N*-dimethyl-*p*-toluidine before injection into the body. After introduction of the initiator, the polymer system was injected, and polymer solidification occurred, with an estimated reaction time between 5 and 30 min [40].

The advantage of using this system was its facile syringeability; it is liquid outside the body and cures once inside the body [41]. Nevertheless, a few disadvantages have limited the system application. First is the burst effect in the drug release, which is due to the lag time for polymer solidification. This process may be explained by the fact that the crosslinking reaction inside the body is in process and the polymer is in liquid form; thus, the drug may rapidly diffuse out of the system, causing the burst. Consequently, this high drug concentration at the reaction site might cause side effects. Second, the heat that is released upon curing (up to 94 °C) due to the exothermic nature of the crosslinking reaction can cause necrosis to the surrounding tissues [2, 42]. Finally, the introduction of free radical-producing agents such as benzoyl peroxide into the body might induce tumor promotion [43-45].

Photopolymerizable Systems

Typically, these systems are formed by biocompatible, biodegradable and polymerizable macromers or prepolymers, which are photocured *in situ,* usually in the presence of photoinitiators, such as ethyl eosin, camphorquinone and derivatives of acetophenone. Macromers usually comprise at least one biodegradable region, one water-soluble region and two regions that can be polymerized by free radicals, and the rate of polymerization is significantly affected by factors such as the intensity of light, the choice of the photoinitiator and the number of reactive double bonds that are presented [4].

Photopolymerizable, degradable biomaterials would provide many benefits over chemically initiated thermoset systems. Photoinitiated reactions offer rapid polymerization rates at physiological temperatures and spatial control of the polymerization site, once the cure can be activated by a fiber optic cable. Moreover, because the starting materials are moldable putties or liquid solutions, the systems are readily placed in complex-shaped volumes and are consequently reacted to form polymers of the required magnitudes [2]. However, low tissue penetration of the initiating light and the formation of reactive oxygen species at high initiator concentrations limit their application in a clinical setting [4].

An example of a photopolymerizable, biodegradable hydrogel consists of a macromer (PEG-oligo-glycolyl-acrylate), a photosensitive initiator (eosin dye) and a light source (ultraviolet (UV) or visible light). The exposure of macromers and photoinitiator mixture to the light source leads to macromer crosslinking and forms a network [46]. This type of system is attractive for drug delivery applications because of its compatibility with hydrophilic drugs and the human body and because of the versatile control of the drug diffusion. However, these hydrogels are limited to surgical sites that are accessible to a light source because they form with difficulty after injection into the body [47-49].

The release rate of proteins from the above-mentioned photopolymerized hydrogel was dependent on their molecular weight and decreased as the molecular weight increased. The release was diffusionally controlled for molecules below a critical molecular weight (e.g., insulin), and for the larger molecules (e.g., immunoglobulin G), the release required the degradation of the hydrogel structure to afford larger openings within the gel and to allow for diffusion. Thus, to achieve prolonged release, this delivery system is best suited for large drug molecules [2].

Generally, the degradation rate, swelling ratio and mechanical strength of the network microstructure are strongly affected by the macromer concentration, light source intensity or exposure time.

Ion-Mediated Crosslinking

Interactions of electrolytes with di- or trivalent polymers can also cause gel formation due to the crosslinking of polymer chains by ionic interactions [4]. Ion-mediated gelation has been described for a number of polymers, e.g., alginates/calcium ions or chitosan/phosphate ions [50-52].

Alginates are natural polymers that form a gel upon contact with divalent cations, such as Ca^{2+}, and have been widely investigated for drug delivery. These polymers can be used directly as a drug carrier or as a carrier of other delivery systems such as liposomes [53, 54] or nanoparticles [1].

This strategy involving the triggered release of Ca^{2+} from liposomal compartments was employed using a precursor fluid containing liposomes suspended in aqueous sodium alginate, which remained fluid at room temperature but gelled when heated to 37 °C. This process is due to Ca^{2+} release and the formation of crosslinked Ca-alginate.

Alternatively, thermally triggered Ca^{2+} release from liposomes was used to activate protein crosslinking catalyzed by enzymes that also form hydrogels. This approach might be convenient for developing rapidly gelling injectable biomaterials, which can be stored at room temperature and injected into a body tissue or cavity in a minimally invasive manner, and clearly improves the half-life of the liposomes [55]. The disadvantages of using this system are a short shelf life due to the slow leakage of Ca^{2+} from the liposomes and the large amount of drug released during the initial release burst [2].

Oster, C.G. et al. [56] developed drug-loaded nanoparticles that are capable of forming a hydrogel in the presence of ions. The authors assumed that the ion-mediated gelation was caused by the positive surface charge of the nanoparticles, which were formulated using a biodegradable amine-modified branched polyester (the amine-modified poly(vinyl alcohols)-g-poly(D,L-lactide-co- glycolide). The hydrogel formation *in situ* allows for loading the depot with additional drugs, which could lead to a controlled initial dose followed by sustained release out of the particles. The degradation profile of the polymer and the electrostatic interactions of the drug with the polymer that control the drug release from these devices can be adjusted by varying the degree of amine-modification and the poly(lactide-co-glycolide) acid (PLGA) side chain length of the polymer used [1]. Finally, considering the crosslinking of thiol functional groups in different polymers without the requirement of radical-initiated polymerization, investigators immobilized thiol groups on water-soluble polymers such as chitosan and deacylated gellan gum (DGG) for *in situ* hydrogel formation [57,58]. Unfortunately, the gelation process required several hours to occur, which is too long for *in situ* use.

Applications of in Situ Crosslinked Systems

Unlike thermosensitive polymers, which will be further discussed in the next section, gelation in thermosetting polymers occurs because of a chemical reaction between polymeric chains, often in the presence of a catalyst or initiator [4]. However, the application of thermoset systems for the *in vivo* delivery of drugs is difficult because of the limitations and adverse effects associated with this type of crosslinked system [59]. In particular, the reaction conditions for *in vivo* applications are stringent, including a limited range of temperatures that are physiologically acceptable, the necessity of nontoxic monomers and/or solvents, environments rich in humidity and oxygen, the requirement for rapid processing and clinically suitable rates of polymerization [60].

Qiu et al. [61] developed a poly(ethylene glycol)-based copolymer containing multiple thiol (–SH) groups and crosslinked by vinylsulfones forming thioether bonds, which results in a hydrogel (DepoGele) that contains more than 90% water and is therefore capable of entrapping proteins. The subcutaneous injection of the polymer hydrogel formulation containing erythropoietin into rabbits facilitated the sustained release of this hormone, thereby maintaining the plasma erythropoietin levels for at least 2 weeks [57, 58, 61, 62]. Additionally, safety studies demonstrated that the gel caused a minimal inflammatory cell response when injected subcutaneously into rats, rabbits and dogs. However, the requirement for surgical excision after drug release (if the polymers are not biodegradable) is a potential drawback of this system [1].

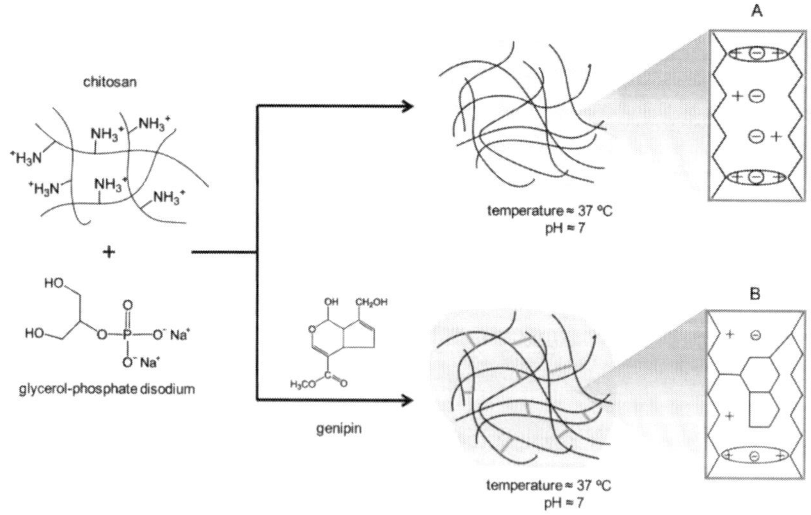

Figure 2. Schematic representation of the possible mechanism of chitosan-based hydrogel formation under the specified physiological conditions via (A) ionic crosslinking and (B) simultaneous ionic and covalent crosslinking (Reprinted with permission from [63]. Copyright (2013) American Chemical Society).

Even with the drawbacks reported, improved thermosetting crosslinking systems have been synthesized by adding genipin, a naturally occurring chemical crosslinking agent, to a chitosan solution that was previously neutralized with a glycerophosphate disodium salt complex (i.e., the ionic crosslinker). In the developed systems, the genipin concentration was used to modulate the network structure and performance (Figure 2). The study demonstrated that these hydrogels could be used under physiological conditions and that they remained localized at the injection site for at least 1 week after dorsal injection into an adult Wistar rat, while providing enhanced network properties and exhibiting improved mechanical properties and chemical stability [63].

Such promising biocompatible systems may be used in future applications apart from subcutaneous injections. Consequently, further investigations to determine the ophthalmic and mucosal biocompatibility and mucoadhesive properties of the modified formulations appear to be necessary.

In Situ Polymer Precipitation

Mechanism of Achieving Solidification In Vivo and Obtainment

In situ polymer precipitation is another approach to produce injectable systems that can solidify *in situ*. The polymer precipitation can be induced by solvent removal or by changes in the temperature or pH (Figure 3) [1, 2].

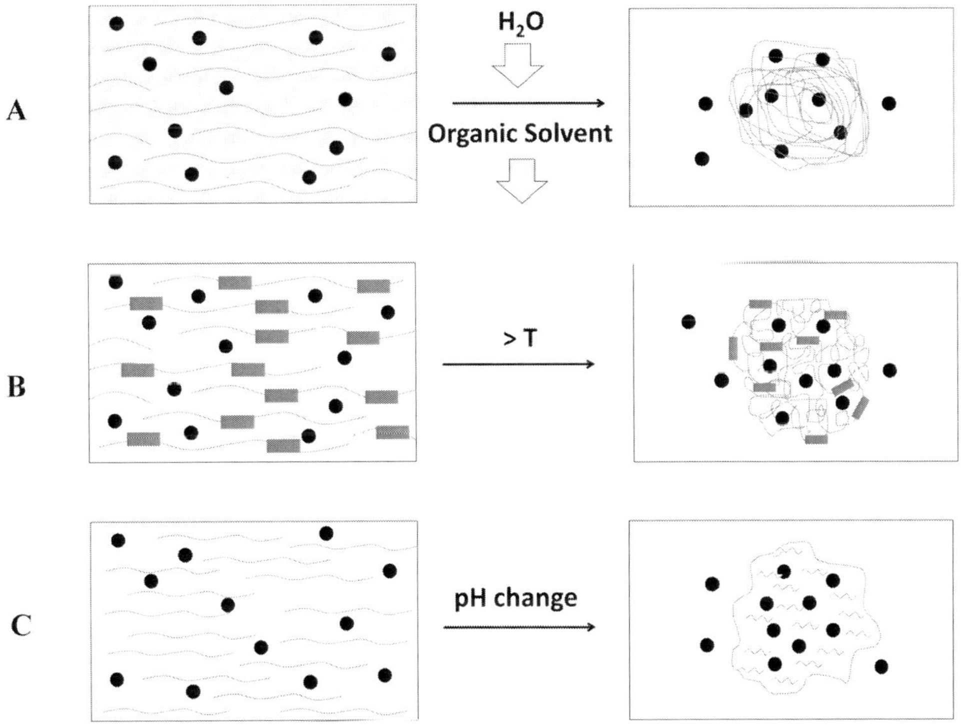

Figure 3. Schematic representation of *in situ* polymer precipitation. (A) Polymer precipitation induced by solvent removal, (B) change in temperature and (C) change in pH. (•) represents the drug (Adapted from [64,65], Copyright (2013), with permissiom from Elvesier).

Solvent Removal

The *in situ* gel formation by solvent removal occurs when a water insoluble biodegradable polymer such as poly(DL-lactide-co-glycolide), poly(DL-lactide) and poly(DL-lactide-co-ε-caprolactone) is dissolved in a water-miscible biocompatible organic solvent. The main solvents that have been used in this strategy are N-methyl-2-pyrrolidone (NMP) and dimethyl sulfoxide (DMSO) due to their pharmaceutical precedence [66]. Other utilized solvents are propylene glycol, acetone, tetrahydrofuran, 2-pyrrolidone, triacetin and glycofurol [1, 2]. Upon injection, the solvent spreads into the body while the water infiltrates into the polymeric matrix. Because the polymer is water insoluble, it precipitates and forms a gel at the site of injection [1, 2, 67]. The drug may be dissolved or dispersed into the polymeric solution. After the injection, when the solvent dissipates from the polymer-drug mixture and the water enters into the matrix, the drug may be trapped or encapsulated within the gel. The drug release follows the common rules for the diffusion or dissolution of an active agent within a polymeric matrix [67]. However, during the first few hours after injection into the body, burst release of the drug may occur, which is one of the main drawbacks of these systems [2].

To diminish the burst drug release, four parameters that influence the rate of polymer precipitation have been studied, which include (i) the molecular weight of the polymer, (ii) the solvent used, (iii) the concentration of polymer in the solvent and (iv) the presence of additives [2]. The first three parameters were evaluated by Lambert and Peck [66] using the PLGA systems for fluorescein isothiocyanate (FITC)-bovine serum albumin release. The burst effect was eliminated by low molecular weight PLGA, which allowed for a greater concentration of polymer in DMSO or NMP. The influence of the solvent choice was not clearly explained; however, it has been demonstrated that a greater burst effect is observed when the capacity of solvent to dissolve the polymeric system is higher [66]. The solvent choice is important because the agent not only acts as a solvent but also serves as a plasticizer for the polymer, which influences the gel properties [68]. The addition of an additive, such as the poly(lactide-co-glycolide)polyethylene glycol block copolymer, also reduces the burst effect because the additive coagulates to form a gel [69].

Another challenge of this strategy is the use of solvents that have questionable toxicity. Several studies have shown that polymer solutions have a high acute myotoxic potential and that they consequently may cause damage at the injection site [67, 68, 70]. The high viscosity of the polymer solution is another disadvantage of these systems because it can cause injection problems [70].

Change in the Temperature

Polymer precipitation due to changes in the environmental temperature occurs because the solubility of several polymers is temperature dependent. These polymers undergo an unusual entropy process when in solution, and this behavior promotes a phase separation when the temperature is raised to a critical value, called the "lower critical solution temperature". At this temperature, the hydrogen bonding between polymer-polymer and water-water is more favorable than polymer-water interactions; therefore, the hydrated polymer dehydrates and changes to a more hydrophobic structure [71, 72]. The drug release rates can be influence by the gel viscosity and the size of the aqueous channels [7, 24]

Many polymers undergo solubility changes based on temperature changes; these polymers include poly(N-isopropyl acryl amide) (poly-NIPAAM) [72], poloxamers [26, 27], triblock copolymer (ABA-type) composed of PLGA (A-block) and PEG (B-block) (PLGA–PEG–PLGA) [6] and chitosan [13, 73]. Depending on the polymer concentration in solution, these polymers may be found in the liquid form at room temperature and form a gel when heated to 37 °C; therefore, the polymers undergo *in situ* gelling upon injection into or contact with the body [13, 26, 27]. The gelation temperature (T_{gel}) must be adjusted to achieve an ideal system. If the T_{gel} is lower than 25 °C, then a gel might be formed at room temperature, which causes problems in manufacturing, handling and administration; by contrast, if the T_{gel} is higher than 37 °C, then the liquid form will exist at body temperature, which can harm the depot formation at the injection site [30]. Thermosensitive polymers are particularly advantageous because they do not require organic solvents, externally applied triggers or copolymerization agents for their gelation at physiological conditions [74].

Poly-NIPAAM is a prototype of thermosensitive polymers, which have the lower critical solution temperature of 32 °C, and it has been studied as an *in situ* gelling system [72]. However, poly-NIPAAM is not appropriate for biomedical application because it is cytotoxic and non-biodegradable [1, 75].

Triblock poly(ethylene oxide)–poly(propylene oxide)–poly(ethylene oxide) copolymers, PEO–PPO–PEO, known as poloxamers or pluronics, are thermosensitive polymers with broader applications [24, 30, 75]. They have low toxicity and are biocompatible. The type and concentration of these polymers affect the gelling temperature [30]. As demonstrated by Ricci and colleagues, the presence of additives and the increased polymer concentration promote a decreased sol-gel transition temperature [76]. Poloxamer 407 (P407), also called Pluronic® F127, is one of the most studied members of this family of block polymers. To improve its residence time, strength and mucoadhesiveness, several mucoadhesive substances such as carbophil, sodium alginate, or chitosan have been incorporated into these systems [77].

Chitosan is another thermosensitive polymer considered interesting for biomedical applications because it is nontoxic, biocompatible and biodegradable [13]. Chitosan is composed of β-(1–4)-linked glucosamine residues, and both the T_{gel} and the gelation time are dependent on the chitosan concentration. The drug release profiles from chitosan gels are also influenced by the chitosan concentration; an increased chitosan concentration promotes a decreased pore size in the gel matrix, and consequently, a slower drug release is observed [8].

Change in pH

The precipitation of other polymers is induced by changes in pH. These polymers have basic or acidic groups that either release or accept protons based on changes in the environmental pH [75]. When they are charged, electrostatic repulsion occurs between the polymeric chains, and the polymer exists in solution form. With the change in pH, the polymer's charge is neutralized, and it becomes a gel [8]. Ionizable polymers that have pKa values between 3 and 10 have utility for pH-responsive formulations [78].

Examples of pH-responsive polymers are polyvinylacetal diethylaminoacetate (AEA) [64, 79] and carbopol [2]. They are liquid at acidic pH values and form a gel when the pH is increased to around neutral [2, 64, 79]. During gel formation, the drug that is dissolved in the water phase can be loaded into the gel and released in a sustained manner. The polymer concentration affects both the rate of gel formation and the amount of drug loaded into the gel. These systems also pose the disadvantage of burst release [64, 79]. In addition, chitosan undergoes changes in its characteristics, depending on the pH. When chitosan is at a pH below its pKa (pH 6.2), it is in solution form due to the protonation of amine groups present on its chain, resulting in electrostatic repulsion. However, when the pH is as high as 6.2, the chitosan becomes a gel due to neutralization of its amine groups, which allow for hydrogen bonding and hydrophobic interactions between the chains [8].

An important concern about *in situ* gelling induced by pH is that the solutions are not neutral when obtained, which can cause local irritation upon injection and degrade proteins and peptides [4]. In additional, changes in pH alone did not yield satisfactory controlled release; therefore, the polymers have been modified to prepare a more suitable gelling system [80].

Applications of in Situ Polymer Precipitation

One of the first developed *in situ* gelling delivery systems was the Eligard delivery system (ATRIX Laboratories, Inc.). The system approved by the FDA consists of a liquid biodegradable polymer formulation that forms a solid implant after subcutaneous administration for delivery of leuprolide acetate, which is a luteinizing hormone–releasing hormone (LHRH) agonist useful for treating prostate cancer by suppression of serum testosterone [1, 12]. Eligard is composed of a poly (DL-lactide-co-glycolide) polymer dissolved in NMP, and the gel is formed *in situ* by solvent removal. The drug is physically mixed with the formulation immediately before injection. The system can sustain the drug delivery over various periods, e.g., 1, 3, 4 and 6 months. To facilitate sustained delivery of the drug for a specific duration, the Eligard system is formulated by varying the molecular weight of the polymer and the solvent concentration. In clinical trials, Eligard formed a gel subcutaneously and promoted 98% and 94% of sustained suppression of serum testosterone (< 20 ng/dL) in patients treated with 1- and 3-month formulation, respectively [12]. The subcutaneous administration of leuprolide acetate via an *in situ* gelling delivery system prevents its degradation by gastrointestinal enzymes [5]. Moreover, the system efficiently delivers the LHRH agonist, and various clinical trials for treating prostate cancer using Eligard are underway, as listed in Table 1.

Several studies are using *in situ* gelling systems induced by temperature changes for the sustained delivery of drugs. A gel formed by Poloxamer 407 was efficient for sustained release of lidocaine. Lidocaine is a local anesthetic, the use of which is restricted because of the short duration of its effects. Therefore, the sustained release promoted by the gel formed *in situ* extended the anesthetic effect and decreased the necessity for frequent administration in certain therapeutic applications, such as tooth extraction, minor surgery and sutures [7].

Table 1. Clinical trials to treat prostate cancer using Eligard

Intervention	Clinical trial phase	Reference
Drug: Eligard 22.5 mg	Phase 4	[81]
Drug: Docetaxel (Taxotere®) Chemotherapy Drug: Leuprolide acetate (Eligard®) Hormonal Therapy	Phase 3	[82]
Drug: Depo-Eligard®	Phase 4	[83]
Drug: Leuprolide acetate Eligard 22.5 mg	Phase 3	[84]
Drug: Docetaxel Drug: Leuprolide acetate (Eligard®) Radiation: Intensity-Modulated Radiotherapy	Phase 2	[85]

Poloxamers are also adequate for sustained intratumoral delivery of drugs, and different systems have been developed. Formulations composed of Pluronic F127 (18–23%) can solubilize β-lapachone (which has a low water solubility) and have an appropriate gel temperature range and gel strength at 37 °C that assures the permanence of the gel intratumorally for a prolonged period and that reduces systemic toxicity [9]. A mixture of methylated-b-cyclodextrin/Poloxamer 407 was also developed to deliver β-lapachone. A gel is formed when the temperature is above 29 °C, thereby facilitating *in situ* gel formation for controlled release. The intratumoral injection of this system in a mouse xenograft tumor model considerably reduced the tumor volume and increased apoptosis and DNA damage without systemic toxicity [17]. Thermogelling delivery systems based on conjugates of PEG and poly(N-isopropylamide) (PNIPAAm) were also developed to deliver anticancer drug (doxorubicin) locally for malignant gliomas [18].

In situ gel formulations of miconazole nitrate with 20% Poloxamer 407 and 10% Poloxamer 188 have been proposed for mucosal drug delivery. Such formulations have been demonstrated *in vivo* to be effective for treating vaginal candidiasis [86]. As previously discussed, poloxamers have excellent compatibility and good characteristics of prolonged release of the active ingredient. However, they have low mucoadhesive properties. Therefore, a strategy to improve the *in vivo* performance of such formulations is to combine the poloxamers with mucoadhesive polymers. A mucoadhesive *in situ* gel composed of mixtures of Poloxamer 407 and Poloxamer 188 with two different types of hydroxypropylmethyl cellulose was obtained for administering itraconazole to the vaginal mucosa. Using a texture profile analysis, the authors determined that formulations containing 20% Poloxamer 407, 10% Poloxamer 188 and 0.5% hydroxypropylmethyl cellulose offered a suitable mechanical and mucoadhesive performance and could be used as an alternative treatment for vaginal candidiasis [87].

It has been reported that these formulations not only enhance the bioavailability of drugs but also influence the immune responses to vaccines. A mouse study of a vaginal vaccine for human papillomavirus (HPV) composed of poloxamers and varying amounts of polyethylene oxide (PEO) revealed that vaccine vehicles affect the systemic and local antibody responses to HPV 16 L1 virus-like particles (VLPs). At 42 days after the first intravaginal coadministration, cholera toxin and HPV 16 L1 VLP in poloxamer/PEO 1.0% exhibited 31- and 39-fold higher titers compared with the PBS-based HPV 16 L1 VLP groups administered by the intravaginal and intramuscular routes, respectively. The authors of this study also observed that the mucoadhesiveness of poloxamer/PEO-based delivery systems increased with increasing concentrations of PEO, but formulations with PEO concentrations higher than 1.0% were considered too viscous to be delivered into the vagina [26].

An *in situ* gelling delivery system induced by temperature was also obtained using a copolymer PLGA–PEG–PLGA for sustained delivery of naltrexone hydrochloride after administration by the subcutaneous route. This drug is an opioid antagonist approved by the FDA to treat alcohol dependence. Its oral administration is not indicated because of the extensive first-pass metabolism in the liver; side effects such as pain, nausea and vomiting; and mainly the poor compliance of addicted patients. Therefore, a formulation able to sustain delivery is essential for the therapeutic application of naltrexone hydrochloride. Thus, after a single administration, the drug is released over several weeks, and first-pass metabolism and side effects are eliminated. Therefore, the developed thermogelling system is a promising strategy because it releases the drug over a period of 17 days and eliminates the drawbacks of oral administration [6]. Growth hormone also requires a sustained delivery system to improve patient compliance because of the necessity of frequent administration due to its short half-life. The subcutaneous application of an *in situ* gelling system composed of copolymer PLGA–PEG–PLGA sustained the delivery of growth hormone for 28 days [88]. Sustained delivery after the subcutaneous application of systems composed of copolymer PLGA–PEG–PLGA were also obtained for testosterone (sustained delivery for 3 months) [89], indomethacin (sustained delivery for 30 days) and 5-fluorouracil (sustained delivery for 5 days) [10].

Systems formed with copolymer PLGA-PEG-PLGA were also used to deliver drugs intratumorally. The release of paclitaxel through the ReGel® (Oncogel®) system was sustained for almost 6 weeks in a continuous manner. Compared with the systemic administration of a commercial paclitaxel product (Taxol®), the intratumoral administration of Oncogel® was demonstrated to be highly effective, without side effects and dose sparing [90].

Intratumoral injection of chitosan solution neutralized with a polyol counterionic dibase salt such as b-glycerophosphate (BST-Gel™ platform technology developed at Biosyntech Inc., Laval, QC, Canada), which is in a liquid form at room temperature and in a gel form at body temperature, was evaluated for the local delivery of paclitaxel. Similar to the Oncogel®, this system was as efficient as four intravenous injections of Taxol® in suppressing the growth of EMT-6 cancer cells in mice, however, with fewer side effects [73].

Chitosan was also used to release insulin in a pulsatile manner, which is important to reach the desirable therapeutic effect. The system was rationally developed utilizing the thermogelling and pH-responsive characteristics of chitosan, and it is glucose-sensitive due to the incorporation of glucose oxidase, which is a molecule that precisely interacts with glucose and converts glucose to gluconic acid in presence of oxygen, resulting in a lowered pH. Consequently, this system efficiently released insulin in a pulsatile manner because the increased level of glucose in the body occurs with the formation of the acid, which reduces the pH, causes changes in the pore size of the gel and consequently facilitates insulin release. In addition, this system had the advantages of *in situ* gelling due to the thermogelling characteristics of chitosan [11].

Chitosan has also been widely used in topical ophthalmic delivery systems, in which its mucoadhesive properties provide prolonged retention of the formulation at the ocular surface, thereby reducing the frequency of administration. In addition, *in situ* hydrogels can be easily instilled as drops, which improves compliance. After administration, the hydrogels undergo a sol-to-gel transition within the cul-de-sac of the eye. An *in situ* forming gel composed of a thermogelling polymer (Poloxamer) and chitosan, which acted as a mucoadhesive agent, demonstrated that chitosan enhances the texture properties and mechanical strength of poloxamer formulations and exhibits concentration-dependent, mucoadhesive properties. The formulation, which is a solution at room temperature, is easily instilled. After a 10 min instillation of a formulation composed of poloxamer/chitosan 16:1 into human eyes, 50–60% of the gel was still in contact with the corneal surface, which represented a fourfold increased retention in comparison with a conventional solution [91]. Moreover, it has been observed that chitosan acts as a permeation enhancer. When incorporating fluconazole into the same formulation described above, the authors observed a sustained release and an approximately 3.5-fold higher total amount of drug permeated across the corneas of rabbits *in vivo* compared with simple aqueous solutions of the drug. *Ex vivo* permeation studies using porcine corneas revealed that the analyzed formulations enhanced drug permeation independently of the chitosan concentration in the range from 0.5 to 1.5% w/w [92].

Not only thermogelling agents have been applied to ophthalmic formulations but also different polymers with diverse mechanisms for *in situ* gelation. Sodium alginate (an ion-sensitive gelling agent), poloxamer (a temperature-sensitive gelling agent) and Polyox (a pH-sensitive gelling agent) have been employed experimentally for the formation of *in situ* hydrogel with hydroxyl propyl methyl cellulose (HPMC) K4M acting as a thickening agent and moxifloxacin hydrochloride, a fluoroquinolone antibiotic.

The maximum concentration (Cmax) of moxifloxacin in aqueous humor and the time required for maximum concentration (Tmax) achievement were evaluated after formulation instillation into rabbits *in vivo*. The formulations were reported to be therapeutically effective, stable and non-irritating, and they exhibited better-sustained drug release compared with conventional eye drops [21].

Carbopol, a well-known pH-dependent polymer, has also been developed for ophthalmic use. Formulations can include Carbopol as a gelling agent alone or in combination with other mucoadhesive polymers or viscosity-enhancing agents [93-97]. An *in situ* pH-triggered gelling system containing baicalin reportedly has anti-cataract and anti-inflammatory effects and is composed of Carbopol (R) 974P (0.3%, w/v) combined with hydroxypropylmethyl cellulose E4M (0.6%, w/v) (a viscosity-enhancing agent); this formulation demonstrated a significantly enhanced gel strength under physiological conditions. It was demonstrated that the formulation promoted sustained drug release over a period of 8 h. Authors also reported that the Cmax and area under the curve (AUC) values were 3.6-fold and 6.1-fold higher, respectively, than those of the control solution [93]. Similarly, a pH-triggered *in situ* gelling system for the ophthalmic delivery of levofloxacin was developed by combining Carbopol 940 with HPMC. The developed formulation was demonstrated to be stable and non-irritating and provided sustained release over an 8 h period [95].

The strategy of using *in situ* forming gels for topical ophthalmic administration as a method of prolonging the formulation's retention time to improve the drug permeation (and, therefore, the bioavailability) can be used for the mucosal (e.g., buccal and vaginal) administration of drugs. As discussed previously, these systems prevent leakage and increase the contact between the formulation and the mucosal surface [26-29].

A triamcinolone acetonide-loaded hydrogel composed of Poloxamer 407 (Molecular weight 12,600), which was modified to include vinyl end groups (for preparing the hydrogel via an irradiation crosslinking reaction) and carbopol (introduced to improve the mucoadhesive properties) was prepared and evaluated on the wounded skin and buccal mucosa of rats. After 15 days, it was observed that the inflammatory response in the buccal mucosa was milder than that in the other groups treated with saline, triamcinolone acetonide solution or blank hydrogel. The researchers also observed that the wound surface was entirely covered with regenerating epithelial cells. The results indicated that the developed hydrogel exhibited sustained drug release while preventing significant histopathological changes in the skin and buccal tissues [28]. This is an example of a combination of mechanisms of *in situ* gelling, which have gained attention during recent years because of improved gel properties.

In Situ Solidifying Organogels

Mechanism of Achieving Solidification In Vivo and Obtention

Organogels are formed *in vivo* by the swelling of water-insoluble amphiphilic lipids in water, which leads to the formation of several types of lyotropic liquid crystals (LLCs) [2]. Both the swelling rate and the type of LLC formed influence the drug release [98]. The nature of the formed LLCs depends on the lipids' structural properties, temperature, amount of water in the system and characteristics of the added drug [99, 100]; therefore, changes in these parameters can alter the formation of LLCs. The packing ratio (*cpp*) is a useful parameter to predict the type of LLC formed by an amphiphile because it relates the molecule shape to properties that influence the curvature of the polar-apolar interface and, consequently, the type of aggregate formed [101]. The cpp can be described by Equation 1:

$$cpp = \frac{Vh}{Ao.Lc} \tag{1}$$

where *cpp* represents the packing ratio, *Vh* is the hydrophobic chain volume, *Ao* is the polar head group area, and *Lc* is the chain length [101].

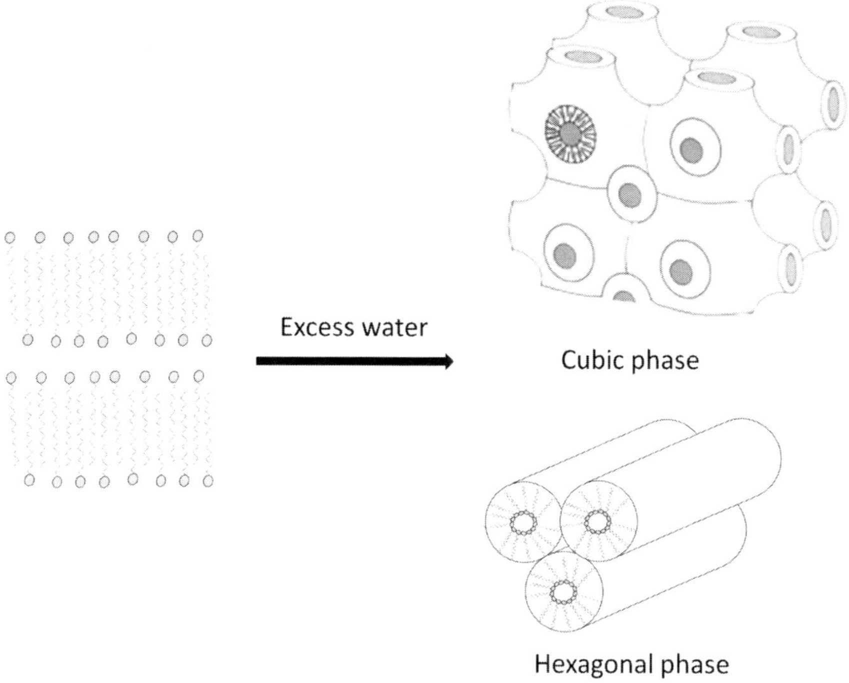

Figure 4. Schematic representation of LLC (cubic and hexagonal phase) formed from precursor fluid formulation of amphiphilic lipids after excess water.

Cubic and hexagonal phases are the primary viscous LLC formed from precursor fluid formulations such as lamellar phase containing amphiphilic lipids that swell in the presence of excess water (Figure 4). These formulations are able to sustain the release of drugs [102-105]. Studies have shown that the hexagonal phase promotes a faster and greater drug release compared with the cubic phase. The more sustained delivery of the cubic phase is thought to be controlled by the structure of this phase (pore size, tortuosity of the water channels, stiffness and high viscosity) because the drug has to diffuse through the microstructure to reach the external solution [104].

The cubic phase consists of three-dimensional curved lipid bilayers separated by water channels. It is physically stable in excess water and is highly viscous [98]. The formation of a cubic structure or a rigid gel from a less viscous phase in excess water is explained by cpp. The obtained phases are influenced mainly by *Vh* and *Ao* because *Lc* is considered constant, as with the increase in the water content or the addition of components, there is no change in the chain length [106]. The increased water content promotes an increased *Vh* because the polar head groups of the amphiphiles move more freely and perpendicularly to the plane of the water channels, while the *Ao* remains constant due to the strong interactions (hydrogen bonds) between the polar head groups. Therefore, as Vh increases whereas Ao and Lc are constant, the cubic phase is formed from less viscous phases [107]. The cpp values are usually > 1 and ≥ 1 for hexagonal and cubic phase, respectively [108].

The hexagonal phase is characterized by long-dimensional cylindrical structures, which may exist in two forms: (i) the reverse phase, in which the polar head groups of the amphiphile are in the inner cylinder portion and the non-polar groups are located around the cylinder, and (ii) the normal phase, in which the polar head groups of the amphiphile are located in the outer cylinder [109].

The main amphiphilic lipid used to obtain organogels is glycerol monooleate (monoolein) [102, 104]. Other lipids used are glycerol monopalmitostearate, glycerol monolinoleate [2] and phytantriol [104, 110]. Monoolein is a non-toxic, biodegradable and biocompatible material. It is composed of a hydrocarbon chain attached by an ester bond to a glycerol backbone. The remaining two hydroxyl groups of the glycerol confer polar characteristics [111]. The formation of LLC from monoolein occurs by the hydration of its polar domains by a hydrophilic solvent, such as water, through hydrogen bonds, while the tails assemble based on Van der Waals interactions [112]. LLCs obtained from monoolein-based systems are efficient at protecting drugs [113], improving the drug solubility and controlling the drug release [112, 114-116]. LLCs are also suited to transmucosal drug delivery because of their bioadhesive nature [117].

In addition to these advantages, these *in situ* gelling systems are useful because the costs of production are comparatively low; moreover, the raw materials are inexpensive compared with biodegradable polymers [118].

As discussed above, amphiphilic lipids are the main components for achieving an *in situ* gelling system; however, other components are necessary to render the system injectable or fluid to facilitate local administration. Therefore, the fluid precursor formulation can be obtained by mixing amphiphilic lipids with a low concentration of water and vegetable oils [2] or other compounds such as propylene glycol [103] or oleic acid and phospholipids [119]. The water content normally is lower than 30%, as demonstrated in the ternary phytantriol-water-ethanol system [110]. The presence of oil or organic compounds in these formulations is important to reduce the viscosity of the systems and to improve their syringeability [2, 103]. In contrast to certain amphiphilic lipids that require temperatures of up to 60 °C for 30 min to be melted [2], monoolein requires temperatures of 42 °C [102]; therefore, monoolein is more appropriate to overcome drug instability problems in the preparation of formulations.

Applications of In Situ Solidifying Organogels

Organogels are applicable to local and sustained drug release [100, 113] and can deliver both water-soluble drugs, such as chlorpheniramine maleate, pseudoephedrine hydrochloride [98] and tramadol HCL [119], and low water-soluble/insoluble drugs, such as salicylic acid [102]. However, there are few published studies regarding *in situ* gelling systems based on LLC. Because of their advantages, these systems deserve further research because they are potentially beneficial to several drug-based therapies.

Monoolein-based systems have been analyzed for the sustained release of various drugs. The hydrophilic drugs chlorpheniramine maleate and pseudoephedrine hydrochloride were delivered in a sustained manner from monoolein systems, and 60% and 100% of the drugs, respectively, were released within 24 h [98]. Phenylpropanolamine hydrochloride and theophylline were also completely released within 24 h and 60 h, respectively, whereas propranolol hydrochloride and diltiazem hydrochloride were not completely released within 100 h [106]. The subcutaneous administration of these systems released tramadol HCL and promoted pain relief for more than 10 h compared with the 3 to 4 h of analgesic activity of the commercially available tramadol HCl solution [119].

As discussed above, temperature can influence the obtained LLCs and, consequently, the drug release. In this scenario, the transition temperature of two systems (phytantriol + vitamin E acetate and monoolein + oleic acid) were defined. Phytantriol containing 3% (w/w) vitamin E acetate provided the most appropriate phase-transition behavior. At 30 °C, this system exhibits only the cubic phase, and at 40 °C, it exhibits only the hexagonal phase, with the cubic + hexagonal phase transition region falling between the two. The release of glucose is more rapid from the cubic phase than from the hexagonal phase. This study revealed that the phytantriol-based system can be administered subcutaneously and forms different LLCs when stimulated by the temperature (cool or hot pack) at the injection site. Consequently, the drug-delivery behavior is changed [100]. However, the phase transition induced by temperature is limited by the lack of specificity in the heat source [4]. To overcome this inconvenience, hydrophobized gold nanorods were incorporated into the liquid crystalline system; this strategy provides remote heating through resonance upon photoirradiation by a specific light source. The heating triggers the phase transition and, consequently, a change in the rate of drug release [120].

Other Organogels

Certain gels formed *in situ* from amphiphilic compounds and vegetable oils are not characterized as LLCs; however, they are also classified as organogels based on their components. Organogels containing mixtures of glyceryl palmitostearate (Precirol ATO 5) and polyglycolyzed apricot kernel oil (Labrafil 1944 CS) were obtained [121]. A system containing 10% Precirol was evaluated *in vivo* for its biocompatibility, biodegradability and ability to release steroid contraceptives (i.e., levonorgestrel and ethinyl estradiol) after subcutaneous injection. The gel obtained *in situ* was biocompatible and biodegradable between 5 and 6 weeks. In addition, it sustained release of the steroid contraceptives in female rats, promoting estrous cycle suppression [122].

Amphiphilic derivatives of l-alanine were demonstrated to form gels *in situ* when mixed with vegetable oils, and low amounts of organic solvents approved for parenteral use [123]. The resulting implants exhibited high biocompatibility following subcutaneous administration and degraded over several weeks, depending on the nature of the l-alanine derivative [124].

Hence, *in situ*-forming organogels obtained by mixing *N*-stearoyl l-alanine (m)ethyl esters (SAM) with a vegetable oil and a biocompatible hydrophilic solvent were analyzed by subcutaneous injection in rats for the delivery of leuprolide, which is a luteinizing hormone-releasing hormone agonist used to treat various conditions, such as prostate cancer, precocious puberty and endometriosis. A gradual drug release was observed for 14 to 25 days [125]. The same system was also used for sustained release of rivastigmine, which is a cholinesterase inhibitor used against Alzheimer's disease. After subcutaneous injection into rats, the formulation containing dispersed rivastigmine prolonged the drug release within the therapeutic range for 11 days. Peak plasma levels were maintained below the toxic threshold and were observed to be up to five times lower than when the control formulation was used [126]. Based on the results, the authors suggested that compared with the current once-per-day oral administration of rivastigmine, subcutaneous injections would provide a simplified dosing regimen that might alleviate the caregiver responsibilities and the treatment-related adverse effects caused by high variations in the plasma drug concentrations [126]. Similarly, additional studies employing SAM in pharmaceutical oils revealed that the SAM/soybean oil mixtures were immediately converted into gels at body temperature when the SAM concentration was higher than 5% (w/v). After subcutaneous injection into mice, the organogel underwent a rapid mass loss within the first 2 weeks, followed by a more moderate degradation, almost disappearing after 6 weeks [127]. Both the slowed degradation and the lack of toxicity indicate that such formulations can potentially be used as injectable systems for sustained drug delivery.

New Perspectives

The progress in molecular biology and genomic research has revolutionized medicine. Gene therapy developed from these discoveries has the potential to markedly change the management and treatment of human diseases. However, its clinical use is limited by various challenges specially related to delivery. The primary barriers to nucleic acid delivery are as follows: (i) rapid degradation by endogenous enzymes; (ii) difficulty in achieving cellular uptake; and (iii) insufficient bioavailability [128]. Therefore, the widespread use of gene therapy for disease prevention and treatment requires the development of clinically suitable, safe and effective drug delivery systems [129]. As discussed above, *in situ* gelling delivery systems are able to protect drugs and to promote local and sustained delivery. Therefore, the combination of gene therapy with *in situ* gelling delivery systems yields the highest therapeutic benefit without side effects [14].

Different types of *in situ* gelling systems have been studied for gene delivery [3, 13-15, 130-132]. Krebs et al. (2009) developed three different systems for the sustained release (1-2 weeks *in vitro*) of small interfering RNA (siRNA): calcium crosslinked alginate (*in situ* gelling induced by divalent cations such as Ca^{2+}), photocrosslinked alginate (*in situ* gelling induced by exposure to UV light in the presence of a photoinitiator) and collagen (*in situ* gelling induced by temperature and pH) [131]. Chitosan-based systems (*in situ* gelling induced by temperature) were also developed to deliver a potential anti-cancer gene (plasmid of pigment epithelium-derived factor) to the tumor site to treat malignant bone cancer [14] and to deliver siRNA intratumorally [13]. These systems exhibited local and sustained delivery of nucleic acids. However, the nucleic acids were released in a naked form, which has a short *in vivo* half-life and low gene efficiency.

The release of nucleic acids complexed with cationic carriers such as polyethylenimine (PEI) appears to be an interesting method for overcoming this drawback. Therefore, *in situ* gelling delivery systems incorporating or conjugating PEI [130, 132] have been developed. Monoolein-based systems (*in situ* gelling induced by formation of LLC after absorption of body fluids) were developed, and the results revealed that PEI incorporation allowed for complexation with siRNA. In addition, the *in vitro*-released siRNA was complexed with PEI, which is essential to avoid siRNA degradation and to facilitate its cellular uptake [133]. The release of naked DNA was also prevented by using a thermogelling system to deliver DNA compacted inside the nanoplexes. This system consists of cationic pentablock copolymers with poly(diethylaminoethyl methacrylate) blocks covalently attached to parent triblock pluronic copolymers and has a high transfection efficiency, being appropriate for long-term, sustained gene delivery [3].

Another promising strategy for increasing the transfection efficient is to co-deliver drugs and genes [15]. Zhang and colleagues developed an injectable thermogelling poly(diethylaminoethyl methacrylate) (PDEAEM)-Pluronic F127-PDEAEM pentablock copolymer vector system to release DNA and paclitaxel for cancer therapy. The schematic illustration of this system's formation is displayed in Figure 5. The transfection efficiency of this system was considerably enhanced by co-delivering DNA and paclitaxel when tested for sustained delivery to SKOV3 human ovarian carcinoma cells. The study was conducted using the barrier gel *in vitro* as a tumor mimic. In addition, paclitaxel demonstrated its effect as an anti-cancer drug to promote cell death [15].

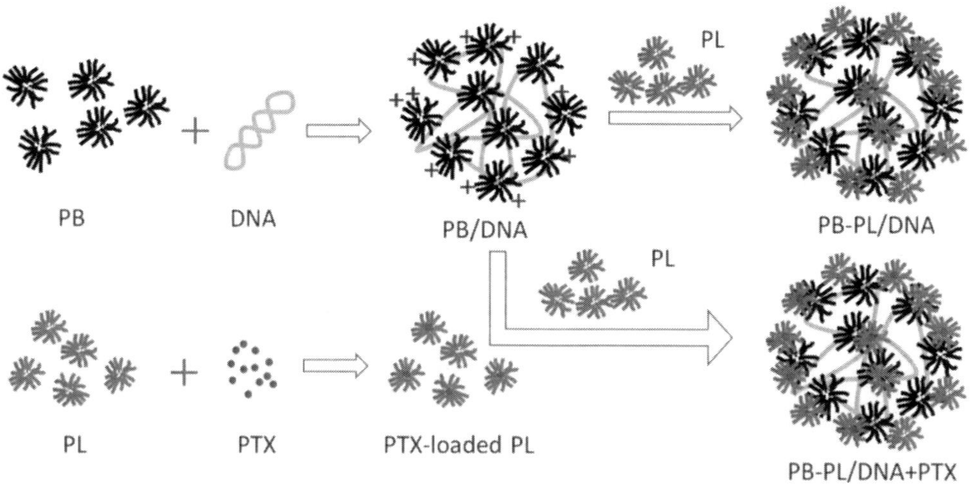

Figure 5. Schematic illustration of the system for releasing both paclitaxel and DNA. The pentablock copolymer micelles (PB) condense plasmid DNA into polyplexes of PB/DNA via ionic interactions. Excess positive charges on the surface of PB/DNA were shielded by further addition of a free Pluronic F127 (PL) micellar solution via self-assembly. Paclitaxel (PTX) was encapsulated in PL and further mixed with plain PL to self-assemble into PB/DNA, thus producing a vector containing both DNA and PTX payloads, PB-PL/DNA + PTX (Reprinted from [15], Copyright (2013), with permission from Elsevier).

These investigations have demonstrated that *in situ* gelling delivery systems are promising systems for delivering nucleic acids in gene therapy. However, more studies are necessary to optimize the developed systems. The formulations should be able to release nucleic acids in a sustained and localized manner and to efficiently promote cellular uptake, endosomal escape, transportation through the cytoplasm (siRNA) and into the nucleus (DNA) and gene expression.

Conclusion

In situ gelling delivery systems are an interesting strategy for the localized and sustained release of drugs, proteins and nucleic acids. The use of these systems for drug administration by alternative delivery routes, e.g., subcutaneous, intratumoral, ocular and mucosal, represents a promising alternative for delivering various types of drugs, especially biopharmaceuticals and genes, that are either degraded by conventional routes, have short half-lives or must be released in a sustained manner to achieve the desired therapeutic effect. *In situ* gelling delivery systems can be obtained by several compounds that can gel *in situ* after contact with the body, as triggered by one of the four types of mechanisms. The concentration of the gel-forming compounds, as well as the other components added to create the formulation, influence the gel formation and the gel characteristics. Each *in situ* gelling system has particular advantages and disadvantages, and therefore, it is necessary to choose the best system that fits appropriately with the drug and the desirable therapeutic effect. Alternatively, as demonstrated by recent research, different approaches could be combined to optimize the *in situ* gelling characteristics and, consequently, the drug release profile. Further research should address the synthesis of new polymers and amphiphilic lipids, as well as chemical modifications of pharmaceutical excipients, to improve and modulate the *in situ* gelling formation for both administration routes and therapeutic requirements. In this context, it is expected that more of these systems will enter the market in the near future.

Abbreviations

intravenous (i.v.); deoxyribonucleic acid (DNA); poly(ε-caprolactone) (PCL); methoxy(polyethylene glycol) (McPEG); prostate-specific antigen (PSA); ultraviolet (UV); poly(lactide-co-glycolide) acid (PLGA); deacylated gellan gum (DGG); N-methyl-2-pyrrolidone (NMP); dimethyl sulfoxide (DMSO); fluorescein isothiocyanate (FITC); poly(N-isopropyl acryl amide) (poly-NIPAAM); polyethyleneglycol (PEG); gelation temperature (T_{gel}); triblock poly(ethylene oxide)–poly(propylene oxide)–poly(ethylene oxide) copolymers (PEO–PPO–PEO); polyvinylacetal diethylaminoacetate (AEA); luteinizing hormone–releasing hormone (LHRH); poly(N-isopropylamide) (PNIPAAm); human papillomavirus (HPV); polyethylene oxide (PEO); virus-like particles (VLPs); maximum concentration (Cmax); time required for maximum concentration (Tmax); area under the curve (AUC); hydroxyl propyl methyl cellulose (HPMC); lyotropic liquid crystals (LLCs); packing ratio (*cpp*); hydrophobic chain volume (*Vh*); polar head group area (*Ao*); chain length (*Lc*); glyceryl palmitostearate (Precirol ATO 5); polyglycolyzed apricot kernel oil (Labrafil 1944

CS); N-stearoyl l-alanine (m)ethyl esters (SAM); small interfering RNA (siRNA); polyethylenimine (PEI); poly(diethylaminoethyl methacrylate) (PDEAEM); pentablock copolymer micelles (PB); Pluronic F127 (PL); Paclitaxel (PTX).

References

[1] Packhaeuser CB, Schnieders J, Oster CG, Kissel T. *In situ* forming parenteral drug delivery systems: an overview. *Eur. J. Pharm. Biopharm.* 2004 Sep;58(2):445-55.

[2] Hatefi A, Amsden B. Biodegradable injectable *in situ* forming drug delivery systems. *J. Control Release* 2002 Apr 23;80(1-3):9-28.

[3] Agarwal A, Unfer RC, Mallapragada SK. Dual-role self-assembling nanoplexes for efficient gene transfection and sustained gene delivery. *Biomaterials* 2008 Feb;29(5):607-17.

[4] Agarwal P, Rupenthal ID. Injectable implants for the sustained release of protein and peptide drugs. *Drug Discov. Today* 2013 Apr;18(7-8):337-49.

[5] Bauer FJ, Dziki W, Lu YMF, Taylor EV, Wang Z, inventors; Oral formulation for hydrophilic drugs.WO1999043299 A2. 1999.

[6] Khodaverdi E, Tekie FS, Mohajeri SA, Ganji F, Zohuri G, Hadizadeh F. Preparation and investigation of sustained drug delivery systems using an injectable, thermosensitive, *in situ* forming hydrogel composed of PLGA-PEG-PLGA. *AAPS PharmSciTech* 2012 Jun;13(2):590-600.

[7] Ricci EJ, Lunardi LO, Nanclares DM, Marchetti JM. Sustained release of lidocaine rom Poloxamer 407 gels. *Int. J. Pharm.* 2005 Jan 20;288(2):235-44.

[8] Ta HT, Han H, Larson I, Dass CR, Dunstan DE. Chitosan-dibasic orthophosphate hydrogel: a potential drug delivery system. *Int. J. Pharm.* 2009 Apr 17;371(1-2):134-41.

[9] Cunha-Filho MS, Alvarez-Lorenzo C, Martinez-Pacheco R, Landin M. Temperature-sensitive gels for intratumoral delivery of beta-lapachone: effect of cyclodextrins and ethanol. *ScientificWorldJournal* 2012;2012:126723.

[10] Qiao M, Chen D, Ma X, Liu Y. Injectable biodegradable temperature-responsive PLGA-PEG-PLGA copolymers: synthesis and effect of copolymer composition on the drug release from the copolymer-based hydrogels. *Int. J. Pharm.* 2005 Apr 27;294(1-2):103-12.

[11] Kashyap N, Viswanad B, Sharma G, Bhardwaj V, Ramarao P, Ravi Kumar MN. Design and evaluation of biodegradable, biosensitive *in situ* gelling system for pulsatile delivery of insulin. *Biomaterials* 2007 Apr;28(11):2051-60.

[12] Sartor O. Eligard: leuprolide acetate in a novel sustained-release delivery system. *Urology* 2003 Feb;61(2 Suppl 1):25-31.

[13] Han HD, Mora EM, Roh JW, Nishimura M, Lee SJ, Stone RL, et al. Chitosan hydrogel for localized gene silencing. *Cancer Biol. Ther.* 2011 May 1;11(9):839-45.

[14] Ta HT, Dass CR, Larson I, Choong PF, Dunstan DE. A chitosan hydrogel delivery system for osteosarcoma gene therapy with pigment epithelium-derived factor combined with chemotherapy. *Biomaterials* 2009 Sep;30(27):4815-23.

[15] Zhang B, Jia F, Fleming MQ, Mallapragada SK. Injectable self-assembled block copolymers for sustained gene and drug co-delivery: an *in vitro* study. *Int. J. Pharm.* 2012 May 1;427(1):88-96.
[16] Sakai S, Moriyama K, Taguchi K, Kawakami K. Hematin is an alternative catalyst to horseradish peroxidase for in situ hydrogelation of polymers with phenolic hydroxyl groups in vivo. *Biomacromolecules* 2010 Aug 9;11(8):2179-83.
[17] Seoane S, Diaz-Rodriguez P, Sendon-Lago J, Gallego R, Perez-Fernandez R, Landin M. Administration of the optimized beta-Lapachone-poloxamer-cyclodextrin ternary system induces apoptosis, DNA damage and reduces tumor growth in a human breast adenocarcinoma xenograft mouse model. *Eur. J. Pharm. Biopharm.* 2013 Aug;84(3):497-504.
[18] Arai T, Joki T, Akiyama M, Agawa M, Mori Y, Yoshioka H, et al. Novel drug delivery system using thermoreversible gelation polymer for malignant glioma. *J. Neurooncol.* 2006 Mar;77(1):9-15.
[19] Jain SP, Shah SP, Rajadhyaksha NS, Singh PSP, Amin PD. *In situ* ophthalmic gel of ciprofloxacin hydrochloride for once a day sustained delivery. *Drug Dev. Ind. Pharm.* 2008 Apr;34(4):445-52.
[20] Basaran B, Bozkir A. Thermosensitive and pH induced *in situ* ophthalmic gelling system for ciprofloxacin hydrochloride: hydroxypropyl-beta-cyclodextrin complex. *Acta Pol. Pharm.* 2012 Nov;69(6):1137-47.
[21] Nanjwade BK, Deshmukh RV, Gaikwad KR, Parikh KA, Manvi FV. Formulation and evaluation of micro hydrogel of Moxifloxacin hydrochloride. *Eur. J. Drug Metab. Pharmacokinet* 2012 Jun;37(2):117-23.
[22] Gupta S, Vyas SP. Carbopol/chitosan based pH triggered *in situ* gelling system for ocular delivery of timolol maleate. *Sci. Pharm.* 2010;78(4):959-76.
[23] Srividya B, Cardoza RM, Amin PD. Sustained ophthalmic delivery of ofloxacin from a pH triggered *in situ* gelling system. *J. Control Release* 2001 Jun 15;73(2-3):205-11.
[24] Ma WD, Xu H, Nie SF, Pan WS. Temperature-responsive, Pluronic-g-poly(acrylic acid) copolymers *in situ* gels for ophthalmic drug delivery: rheology, *in vitro* drug release, and *in vivo* resident property. *Drug Dev. Ind. Pharm.* 2008 Mar;34(3):258-66.
[25] Turturro SB, Guthrie MJ, Appel AA, Drapala PW, Brey EM, Perez-Luna VH, et al. The effects of cross-linked thermo-responsive PNIPAAm-based hydrogel injection on retinal function. *Biomaterials* 2011 May;32(14):3620-6.
[26] Park JS, Oh YK, Kang MJ, Kim CK. Enhanced mucosal and systemic immune responses following intravaginal immunization with human papillomavirus 16 L1 virus-like particle vaccine in thermosensitive mucoadhesive delivery systems. *J. Med. Virol.* 2003 Aug;70(4):633-41.
[27] Park JS, Oh YK, Yoon H, Kim JM, Kim CK. *In situ* gelling and mucoadhesive polymer vehicles for controlled intranasal delivery of plasmid DNA. *J. Biomed. Mater. Res.* 2002 Jan;59(1):144-51.
[28] Choi SG, Baek EJ, Davaa E, Nho YC, Lim YM, Park JS, et al. Topical treatment of the buccal mucosa and wounded skin in rats with a triamcinolone acetonide-loaded hydrogel prepared using an electron beam. *Int. J. Pharm.* 2013 Apr 15;447(1-2):102-8.
[29] Martin L, Wilson CG, Koosha F, Uchegbu IF. Sustained buccal delivery of the hydrophobic drug denbufylline using physically cross-linked palmitoyl glycol chitosan hydrogels. *Eur. J. Pharm. Biopharm.* 2003 Jan;55(1):35-45.

[30] Ibrahim E, Ismail S, Fetih G, Shaaban O, Hassanein K, Abdellah NH. Development and characterization of thermosensitive pluronic-based metronidazole *in situ* gelling formulations for vaginal application. *Acta Pharm.* 2012 Mar;62(1):59-70.

[31] Nagai T, Machida Y. Buccal delivery systems using hydrogels. *Adv. Drug Deliv. Rev.* 1993;11:179-91.

[32] van de Weert M, van Steenbergen MJ, Cleland JL, Heller J, Hennink WE, Crommelin DJ. Semisolid, self-catalyzed poly(ortho ester)s as controlled-release systems: protein release and protein stability issues. *J. Pharm. Sci.* 2002 Apr;91(4):1065-74.

[33] Walter KA, Cahan MA, Gur A, Tyler B, Hilton J, Colvin OM, et al. Interstitial taxol delivered from a biodegradable polymer implant against experimental malignant glioma. *Cancer Res.* 1994 Apr 15;54(8):2207-12.

[34] Winternitz CI, Jackson JK, Oktaba AM, Burt HM. Development of a polymeric surgical paste formulation for taxol. *Pharm. Res.* 1996 Mar;13(3):368-75.

[35] Zhang X, Jackson JK, Wong W, Min W, Cruz T, Hunter WL, et al. Development of biodegradable polymeric paste formulations for taxol: an *in vitro* and *in vivo* study. *Int. J. Pharm.* 1996;137(2):199-208.

[36] Dordunoo SK, Oktaba AMC, Hunter W, Min W, Cruz T, Burt HM. Release of taxol from poly(e-caprolactone) pastes: effect of water-soluble additives. *J. Control Release* 1997;44(1):87-94.

[37] Pitt CG. Poly-e-caprolactone and its copolymers. In: Chasin M, Langer R, editors. Biodegradable Polymers as Drug Delivery Systems. New York: Marcel Decker; 1990. p.71-120.

[38] Jackson JK, Gleave ME, Yago V, Beraldi E, Hunter WL, Burt HM. The suppression of human prostate tumor growth in mice by the intratumoral injection of a slow-release polymeric paste formulation of paclitaxel. *Cancer Res.* 2000 Aug 1;60(15):4146-51.

[39] Deligkaris K, Tadele TS, Olthuis W, van den Berg A. Hydrogel-based devices for biomedical applications. *Sens Actuators B Chem.* 2010 Jun 3;147(2):765-74.

[40] Moore LA, Norton RL, Whitman SL, Dunn RL. An injectable biodegradable drug delivery system based on acrylic terminated poly e-caprolactone. *Proceedings of 21st Annual Meeting of the Society of Biomaterials*, CA. 1995.

[41] Dunn RL, English JP, Cowsar DR, Vanderbelt DP, inventors; Biodegradable *in-situ* forming implants and methods for producing the same. *US patent* 5 340 849. 1994.

[42] Biehl G, Harms J, Hanser U. Experimental studies on heat development in bone during polymerization of bone cement. Intraoperative measurement of temperature in normal blood circulation and in bloodlessness. *Arch. Orthop. Unfallchir* 1974;78(1):62-9.

[43] Gimenez-Conti IB, Binder RL, Johnston D, Slaga TJ. Comparison of the skin tumor-promoting potential of different organic peroxides in SENCAR mice. *Toxicol Appl Pharmacol.* 1998 Mar;149(1):73-9.

[44] Zhao J, Lahiri-Chatterjee M, Sharma Y, Agarwal R. Inhibitory effect of a flavonoid antioxidant silymarin on benzoyl peroxide-induced tumor promotion, oxidative stress and inflammatory responses in SENCAR mouse skin. *Carcinogenesis* 2000 Apr;21(4):811-6.

[45] Saleem M, Alam A, Ahmed S, Iqbal M, Sultana S. Tephrosia purpurea ameliorates benzoyl peroxide-induced cutaneous toxicity in mice: diminution of oxidative stress. *Pharm. Pharmacol. Commun.* 1999;5(7):455-61.

[46] Hubbell JA, Pathak CP, Sawhney AS, Desai NP, Hill JL, inventors; Photopolymerizable biodegradable hydrogels as tissue contacting materials and controlled release carriers. *US patent* 5 410 016. 1995.
[47] Annavajjula D, Yim K, Rowe SC, Rocovick SC, Hubbell JA. A Novel Drug Delivery System for Recombinant Human Growth Hormone with Photopolymerized Hydrogels. Proceedings of 28th International Symposium on Controlled Release of Bioactive Materials and Fourth Consumer and Diversified Products Conference 2001,2:985-986.
[48] Sawhney AS, Pathak CP, Hubbell JA. Bioerodible hydrogels based on photopolymerized poly(ethylene glycol)-co-poly(alpha- hydroxy acid) diacrylate macromers. *Macromolecules* 1993;26(4):581-7.
[49] Philbrook M, Lehnert S, Warnock D, Duan S, Enscore D, Roth L. Tissue-adherent depot for prevention of local tumor recurrence. *Proceedings of 27th International Symposium on Controlled Release of Bioactive Materials* 2000:510-511.
[50] Chenite A, Chaput C, Wang D, Combes C, Buschmann MD, Hoemann CD, et al. Novel injectable neutral solutions of chitosan form biodegradable gels *in situ*. *Biomaterials* 2000 Nov;21(21):2155-61.
[51] Leloup O, Renaud MA, Chaput C, Chenite A, Desrosiers EA, Shive M. Intramuscular Implantations of Thermogelling Chitosan-based Materials. *Proceedings of 28th International Symposium on Controlled Release of Bioactive Materials and Fourth Consumer & Diversified Products Conference* 2001,1:261-262.
[52] Cohen S, Lobel E, Trevgoda A, Peled A. A novel *in situ*-forming ophthalmic drug delivery system from alginates undergoing gelation in the eye. *J. Control Release* 1997;44(2-3):201-8.
[53] Viegas TX, Reeve LE, Henry RL, inventors; Medical uses of *in-situ* formed gels. *US patent* 5 318 780. 1994.
[54] Cui H, Messersmith PB. Thermally triggered gelation of alginate for controlled release. In: McCulloch I, Shalaby SW, editors. Tailored Polymeric Materials For Controlled Delivery Systems. Washington, DC: American Chemical Society 1998:203-11.
[55] Westhaus E, Messersmith PB. Triggered release of calcium from lipid vesicles: a bioinspired strategy for rapid gelation of polysaccharide and protein hydrogels. *Biomaterials* 2001 Mar;22(5):453-62.
[56] Oster CG, Wittmar M, Unger F, Barbu-Tudoran L, Schaper AK, Kissel T. Design of amine-modified graft polyesters for effective gene delivery using DNA-loaded nanoparticles. *Pharm. Res.* 2004 Jun;21(6):927-31.
[57] Bernkop-Schnurch A, Hornof M, Zoidl T. Thiolated polymers--thiomers: synthesis and *in vitro* evaluation of chitosan-2-iminothiolane conjugates. *Int. J. Pharm.* 2003 Jul 24;260(2):229-37.
[58] Krauland AH, Leitner VM, Bernkop-Schnurch A. Improvement in the *in situ* gelling properties of deacetylated gellan gum by the immobilization of thiol groups. *J. Pharm. Sci.* 2003 Jun;92(6):1234-41.
[59] Peter SJ, Nolley JA, Widmer MS, Merwin JE, Yaszemski MJ, Yasko AW, et al. *In vitro* degradation of a poly(propylene fumarate) / b-tricalcium phosphate composite orthopedic scaffold. *Tissue Eng.* 1997;3:207-15.
[60] Burkoth AK, Anseth KS. A review of photocrosslinked polyanhydrides: *in situ* forming degradable networks. *Biomaterials* 2000 Dec;21(23):2395-404.

[61] Qiu B, Stefanos S, Ma J, Lalloo A, Perry BA, Leibowitz MJ, et al. A hydrogel prepared by *in situ* cross-linking of a thiol-containing poly(ethylene glycol)-based copolymer: a new biomaterial for protein drug delivery. *Biomaterials* 2003 Jan;24(1):11-8.

[62] Qiu B, Stefanos S, Leibowitz M, Sinko P, Stein S. A Novel Injectable Polymer Hydrogel System - Depogel for Controlled Delivery of Small and Large Molecule Drugs. *Proceedings of 28th International Symposium on Controlled Release of Bioactive Materials and Fourth Consumer & Diversified Products Conference* 2001;2:1009-1010.

[63] Moura MJ, Faneca H, Lima MP, Gil MH, Figueiredo MM. *In Situ* Forming Chitosan Hydrogels Prepared via Ionic/Covalent Co-Cross-Linking. *Biomacromolecules* 2011 Sep;12(9):3275-84.

[64] Aikawa K, Matsumoto K, Uda H, Tanaka S, Shimamura H, Aramaki Y, et al. Hydrogel formation of the pH response polymer polyvinylacetal diethylaminoacetate (AEA). *Int. J. Pharm.* 1998;167:97-104.

[65] Le Renard PE, Jordan O, Faes A, Petri-Fink A, Hofmann H, Rufenacht D, et al. The *in vivo* performance of magnetic particle-loaded injectable, *in situ* gelling, carriers for the delivery of local hyperthermia. *Biomaterials* 2010 Feb;31(4):691-705.

[66] Lambert WJ, Peck KD. Development of an *in situ* forming biodegradable poly-lactide-coglycolide system for the controlled release of proteins. *J. Control Release* 1995;33:189-95.

[67] Dunn RL, English JP, Cowsar DR, Vanderbelt DP, inventors; Biodegradable *in-situ* forming implants and methods of producing the same.*US Pat.* 4 938 763. 1999.

[68] Shah NH, Railkar AS, Chen FC, Tarantino R, Kumar S, Murjani M, et al. A biodegradable injectable implant for delivering micro and macromolecules using poly (lactic-co-glycolic) acid (PLGA) copolymers. *J. Control Release* 1993;27:139-47.

[69] Chandrashekar BL, Zhou M, Jarr EM, Dunn RL, inventors; Controlled release liquid delivery compositions with low initial drug burst.*US Pat.* 6 143 314. 2000.

[70] Kranz H, Brazeau GA, Napaporn J, Martin RL, Millard W, Bodmeier R. Myotoxicity studies of injectable biodegradable *in-situ* forming drug delivery systems. *Int. J. Pharm.* 2001 Jan 5;212(1):11-8.

[71] Hoffman AS. Applications of thermally reversible polymers and hydrogels in therapeutics and diagnostics*. *J. Control Release* 1987;6:297-305.

[72] Stile RA, Burghardt WR, Healy KE. Synthesis and Characterization of Injectable Poly(*N*-isopropylacrylamide)-Based Hydrogels That Support Tissue Formation *in Vitro*. *Macromolecules* 1999;32:7370-9.

[73] Ruel-Gariepy E, Shive M, Bichara A, Berrada M, Le GD, Chenite A, et al. A thermosensitive chitosan-based hydrogel for the local delivery of paclitaxel. *Eur. J. Pharm. Biopharm.* 2004 Jan;57(1):53-63.

[74] Kempe S, Mader K. *In situ* forming implants - an attractive formulation principle for parenteral depot formulations. *J. Control Release* 2012 Jul 20;161(2):668-79.

[75] Qiu Y, Park K. Environment-sensitive hydrogels for drug delivery. *Adv. Drug Deliv. Rev.* 2001 Dec 31;53(3):321-39.

[76] Ricci EJ, Bentley MV, Farah M, Bretas RE, Marchetti JM. Rheological characterization of Poloxamer 407 lidocaine hydrochloride gels. *Eur. J. Pharm. Sci.* 2002 Nov;17(3):161-7.

[77] Ur-Rehman T, Tavelin S, Grobner G. Chitosan *in situ* gelation for improved drug loading and retention in poloxamer 407 gels. Int J Pharm 2011 May 16;409(1-2):19-29.

[78] Schmaljohann D. Thermo- and pH-responsive polymers in drug delivery. *Adv. Drug Deliv. Rev.* 2006 Dec 30;58(15):1655-70.

[79] Aikawa K, Mitsutake N, Tanaka S, Shimamura H, Aramaki Y, Tsuchiya S. Drug release from pH-response polyvinylacetal diethylaminoacetate hydrogel, and application to nasal delivery. *Int. J. Pharm.* 1998;168:181-8.

[80] Wu J, Su ZG, Ma GH. A thermo- and pH-sensitive hydrogel composed of quaternized chitosan/glycerophosphate. *Int. J. Pharm.* 2006 Jun 6;315(1-2):1-11.

[81] Clinical Trials [Internet]. 2013 [updated 2013 Mar 4]. Available from: http://clinicaltrials.gov/ct2/show/NCT01511874?term=eligard&rank=4.

[82] Clinical Trials [Internet]. 2013 [updated 2012 Jan 25]. Available from: http://clinicaltrials.gov/ct2/show/study/NCT00283062?term=eligard&rank=5.

[83] Clinical Trials [Internet]. 2013 [updated 2013 Feb 13]. Available from: http://clinicaltrials.gov/ct2/show/NCT01793077?term=eligard&rank=9.

[84] Clinical Trials [Internet]. 2013 [updated 2013 Jan 16]. Available from: http://clinicaltrials.gov/ct2/show/NCT00378690?term=eligard&rank=23.

[85] Clinical Trials [Internet]. 2013 [updated 2012 Nov 1]. Available from: http://clinicaltrials.gov/ct2/show/NCT00452556?term=eligard&rank=35.

[86] Karavana SY, Senyigit ZA, Hilmioglu-Polat S, Metin DY, Zekioglu O, Baloglu E. Mucoadhesive *In Situ* Gel Formulations of Miconazole Nitrate for the Treatment of Mucosal Candidiasis. *Lat. Am. J. Pharm.* 2012 Aug;31(6):821-9.

[87] Karavana SY, Rencber S, Senyigit ZA, Baloglu E. A New *in-Situ* Gel Formulation of Itraconazole for Vaginal Administration. *Pharmacol. Pharm.* 2012;3:417-26.

[88] Chen S, Singh J. Controlled release of growth hormone from thermosensitive triblock copolymer systems: *In vitro* and *in vivo* evaluation. *Int. J. Pharm.* 2008 Mar 20;352(1-2):58-65.

[89] Chen S, Singh J. Controlled delivery of testosterone from smart polymer solution based systems: *in vitro* evaluation. *Int. J. Pharm.* 2005 May 13;295(1-2):183-90.

[90] Zentner GM, Rathi R, Shih C, McRea JC, Seo MH, Oh H, et al. Biodegradable block copolymers for delivery of proteins and water-insoluble drugs. *J. Control Release* 2001 May 14;72(1-3):203-15.

[91] Graticri T, Gelfuso GM, Rocha EM, Sarmento VH, de Freitas O, Lopez RFV. A poloxamer/chitosan *in situ* forming gel with prolonged retention time for ocular delivery. *Eur. J. Pharm. Biopharm.* 2010 Jun;75(2):186-93.

[92] Gratieri T, Gelfuso GM, de Freitas O, Rocha EM, Lopez RFV. Enhancing and sustaining the topical ocular delivery of fluconazole using chitosan solution and poloxamer/chitosan *in situ* forming gel. *Eur. J. Pharm. Biopharm.* 2011 Oct;79(2):320-7.

[93] Wu HY, Liu ZD, Peng JJ, Li L, Li N, Li JW, et al. Design and evaluation of baicalin-containing *in situ* pH-triggered gelling system for sustained ophthalmic drug delivery. *Int. J. Pharm.* 2011 May 30;410(1-2):31-40.

[94] Wu CJ, Qi HY, Chen WW, Huang CY, Su C, Li WM, et al. Preparation and evaluation of a Carbopol (R)/HPMC-based *in situ* gelling ophthalmic system for puerarin. Yakugaku Zasshi 2007;127(1):183-91.

[95] Mohanambal E, Arun K, Sathali AAH. Formulation and Evaluation of pH-triggered *in situ* Gelling System of Levofloxacin. *Indian J. Pharm. Educ.* 2011 Jan;45(1):58-64.

[96] Manjappa AS, Nanjwade BK, Manvi FV, Murthy RSR. Sustained Ophthalmic *In Situ* Gel of Ketorolac Tromethamine: Rheology and *In Vivo* Studies. *Drug Dev. Res.* 2009 Sep;70(6):417-24.

[97] Cao F, Zhang XL, Ping QN. New method for ophthalmic delivery of azithromycin by poloxamer/carbopol-based *in situ* gelling system. *Drug Deliv.* 2010 Sep;17(7):500-7.

[98] Chang CM, Bodmeier R. Swelling of and drug release from monoglyceride-based drug delivery systems. *J. Pharm. Sci.* 1997 Jun;86(6):747-52.

[99] Chang CM, Bodmeier R. Low viscosity monoglyceride-based drug delivery systems transforming into a highly viscous cubic phase. *Int. J. Pharm.* 1998 Oct 30;173(1-2):51-60.

[100] Fong WK, Hanley T, Boyd BJ. Stimuli responsive liquid crystals provide 'on-demand' drug delivery *in vitro* and *in vivo*. *J. Control Release* 2009 May 5;135(3):218-26.

[101] Mitchell DJ, Ninham BW. Micelles, Vesicles and Micro-Emulsions. *J. Chem. Soc. Faraday Trans.* 1981;77:601-29.

[102] Lara MG, Bentley MV, Collett JH. *In vitro* drug release mechanism and drug loading studies of cubic phase gels. *Int. J. Pharm.* 2005 Apr 11;293(1-2):241-50.

[103] Phelps J, Bentley MV, Lopes LB. *In situ* gelling hexagonal phases for sustained release of an anti-addiction drug. *Colloids Surf B Biointerfaces* 2011 Oct 15;87(2):391-8.

[104] Rizwan SB, Hanley T, Boyd BJ, Rades T, Hook S. Liquid crystalline systems of phytantriol and glyceryl monooleate containing a hydrophilic protein: Characterisation, swelling and release kinetics. *J. Pharm. Sci.* 2009 Nov;98(11):4191-204.

[105] Scherlund M, Welin-Berger K, Brodin A, Malmsten M. Local anaesthetic block copolymer system undergoing phase transition on dilution with water. *Eur. J. Pharm. Sci.* 2001 Aug;14(1):53-61.

[106] Chang CM, Bodmeier R. Binding of drugs to monoglyceride-based drug delivery systems. *Int. J. Pharm.* 1997 Feb 28;147(2):135-42.

[107] Amar-Yuli I, Garti N. Transitions induced by solubilized fat into reverse hexagonal mesophases. *Colloids Surf B Biointerfaces* 2005 Jun 25;43(2):72-82.

[108] Mezzenga R, Grigorov M, Zhang ZD, Servais C, Sagalowicz L, Romoscanu AI, et al. Polysaccharide-induced order-to-order transitions in lyotropic liquid crystals. *Langmuir* 2005 Jul 5;21(14):6165-9.

[109] Borné J, Nylander T, Khan A. Phase Behavior and Aggregate Formation for the Aqueous Monoolein System Mixed with Sodium Oleate and Oleic Acid. *Langmuir* 2001;17(25):7742-51.

[110] Han K, Pan X, Chen M, Wang R, Xu Y, Feng M, et al. Phytantriol-based inverted type bicontinuous cubic phase for vascular embolization and drug sustained release. *Eur. J. Pharm. Sci.* 2010 Dec 23;41(5):692-9.

[111] Kulkarni CV, Wachter W, Iglesias-Salto G, Engelskirchen S, Ahualli S. Monoolein: a magic lipid? *Phys. Chem. Chem. Phys.* 2011 Feb 28;13(8):3004-21.

[112] Libster D, Aserin A, Garti N. Interactions of biomacromolecules with reverse hexagonal liquid crystals: drug delivery and crystallization applications. *J. Colloid Interface Sci.* 2011 Apr 15;356(2):375-86.

[113] Sadhale Y, Shah JC. Biological activity os insulin in GMO gels and the effect of agitation. *Int. J. Pharm.* 1999;191:65-74.

[114] Lopes LB, Ferreira DA, de Paula D, Garcia MT, Thomazini JA, Fantini MC, Bentley, MV. Reverse hexagonal phase nanodispersion of monoolein and oleic acid for topical delivery of peptides: *in vitro* and *in vivo* skin penetration of cyclosporin A. *Pharm. Res.* 2006 Jun;23(6):1332-42.

[115] Lopes LB, Lopes JL, Oliveira DC, Thomazini JA, Garcia MT, Fantini MC, Collett, JH, Bentley, MV. Liquid crystalline phases of monoolein and water for topical delivery of cyclosporin A: characterization and study of *in vitro* and *in vivo* delivery. *Eur. J. Pharm. Biopharm.* 2006 Jun;63(2):146-55.

[116] Yariv D, Efrat R, Libster D, Aserin A, Garti N. *In vitro* permeation of diclofenac salts from lyotropic liquid crystalline systems. *Colloids Surf B Biointerfaces* 2010 Jul 1;78(2):185-92.

[117] Geraghty PB, Attwood D, Collett JH, Dandiker Y. The *in vitro* release of some antimuscarinic drugs from monoolein/water lyotropic liquid crystalline gels. *Pharm. Res.* 1996 Aug;13(8):1265-71.

[118] Matschke C, Isele U, van Hoogevest P, Fahr A. Sustained-release injectables formed *in situ* and their potential use for veterinary products. *J. Control Release* 2002 Dec 13;85(1-3):1-15.

[119] Malonne H, Fontaine J, Moes A. *In vitro/in vivo* characterization of a tramadol HCl depot system composed of monoolein and water. *Biol. Pharm. Bull.* 2000 May;23(5):627-31.

[120] Fong WK, Hanley TL, Thierry B, Kirby N, Boyd BJ. Plasmonic nanorods provide reversible control over nanostructure of self-assembled drug delivery materials. *Langmuir* 2010 May 4;26(9):6136-9.

[121] Gao ZH, Shukla AJ, Johnson JR, Crowley WR. Controlled release of a contraceptive steroid from biodegradable and injectable gel formulations: *in vitro* evaluation. *Pharm. Res.* 1995 Jun;12(6):857-63.

[122] Gao ZH, Crowley WR, Shukla AJ, Johnson JR, Reger JF. Controlled release of contraceptive steroids from biodegradable and injectable gel formulations: *in vivo* evaluation. *Pharm. Res.* 1995 Jun;12(6):864-8.

[123] Couffin-Hoarau AC, Motulsky A, Delmas P, Leroux JC. *In situ*-forming pharmaceutical organogels based on the self-assembly of L-alanine derivatives. *Pharm. Res.* 2004 Mar;21(3):454-7.

[124] Motulsky A, Lafleur M, Couffin-Hoarau AC, Hoarau D, Boury F, Benoit JP, et al. Characterization and biocompatibility of organogels based on L-alanine for parenteral drug delivery implants. *Biomaterials* 2005 Nov;26(31):6242-53.

[125] Plourde F, Motulsky A, Couffin-Hoarau AC, Hoarau D, Ong H, Leroux JC. First report on the efficacy of L-alanine-based *in situ*-forming implants for the long-term parenteral delivery of drugs. *J. Control Release* 2005 Nov 28;108(2-3):433-41.

[126] Vintiloiu A, Lafleur M, Bastiat G, Leroux JC. *In Situ*-forming oleogel implant for rivastigmine delivery. *Pharm. Res.* 2008 Apr;25(4):845-52.

[127] Wang KK, Jia QA, Han F, Liu HZ, Li SM. Self-assembled L-alanine derivative organogel as *in situ* drug delivery implant: characterization, biodegradability, and biocompatibility. *Drug Dev. Ind. Pharm.* 2010 Dec 10;36(12):1511-21.

[128] Wong SY, Pelet JM, Putnam D. Polymer systems for gene delivery-past, present, and future. *Prog. Polym. Sci.* 2007 Aug;32(8-9):799-837.

[129] Niidome T, Huang L. Gene therapy progress and prospects: Nonviral vectors. *Gene Ther* 2002 Dec;9(24):1647-52.

[130] Kim YM, Park MR, Song SC. Injectable polyplex hydrogel for localized and long-term delivery of siRNA. *ACS Nano* 2012 Jul 24;6(7):5757-66.

[131] Krebs MD, Jeon O, Alsberg E. Localized and sustained delivery of silencing RNA from macroscopic biopolymer hydrogels. *J. Am. Chem. Soc.* 2009 Jul 8;131(26):9204-6.

[132] Nguyen K, Dang PN, Alsberg E. Functionalized, biodegradable hydrogels for control over sustained and localized siRNA delivery to incorporated and surrounding cells. *Acta Biomater*. 2013 Jan;9(1):4487-95.

[133] Borgheti-Cardoso LN. Sistemas de liberação de geleificação *in situ* para veiculação de siRNA: desenvolvimento, caracterização e estudos *in vitro* e *in vivo* em modelo animal [Master´s thesis]. Ribeirão Preto, Brazil: Faculdade de Ciências Farmacêuticas de Ribeirão Preto – Universidade de São Paulo; 2012.

In: Recent Advances in Drug Delivery Research
Editor: Valerio Voliani

ISBN: 978-1-62948-228-6

Chapter 6

Solid Lipid Nanoparticles Prepared by the Phase Inversion Temperature Method as Carriers for Idebenone

M. G. Sarpietro[1], M. L. Accolla[2], G. Puglisi[1], F. Castelli[1] and L. Montenegro[1*]

[1]Dipartimento di Scienze del Farmaco,
Università di Catania, Catania, Italy
[2]Dipartimento di Scienze della Salute,
Università 'Magna Græcia' di Catanzaro, Germaneto (CZ), Italy

Abstract

Solid lipid nanoparticles (SLN) are regarded as a promising alternative to other colloidal drug carriers to improve drug delivery after topical and systemic administration. Although different methods have been developed to prepare SLN, most of them show some drawbacks.

Recently, we developed a novel method to prepare SLN from micro-emulsions with low surfactant content based on the phase inversion temperature (PIT), to overcome the disadvantages of other preparation techniques and to allow an easy scale-up. Since these SLN were intended both for topical and systemic therapy, we chose as drug to be loaded idebenone (IDE), a synthetic derivative of ubiquinone with a potent antioxidant activity, that could be beneficial in the treatment of both skin oxidative damages and neurodegenerative diseases such as Parkinson's and Alzheimer diseases. Biological studies performed on primary cultures of astrocytes obtained from rat cerebral cortex showed that the antioxidant activity of IDE-loaded SLN was stronger than free IDE without any cytotoxic effect. Further *in vitro* studies on a model of blood brain barrier showed that loading IDE into SLN could allow its parenteral administration in aqueous vehicles, thus avoiding the use of organic solvents to solubilize IDE, a poor water-soluble compound. *In vitro* skin permeation experiments performed on these IDE-loaded SLN suggested that they could allow IDE targeting to the upper skin layers.

[*] Corresponding Author address: Email: lmontene@unict.it.

In this chapter, to elucidate the interaction mechanisms of IDE-loaded SLN with biological barriers, their interactions with a model of biological membranes consisting of multilamellar liposomes were investigated by differential scanning calorimetry (DSC) analyses. IDE-loaded SLN prepared by the PIT method were analyzed to evaluate their morphology and their technological properties. All SLN showed a spherical shape and good properties in terms of mean size (< 100 nm) and stability upon storage at room temperature, avoiding the use of great amount of surfactants and of purification steps required by conventional micro-emulsion procedures. Results of DSC studies pointed out IDE-loaded SLN ability to interact with phopholipid bilayers depending on their composition while free IDE was not absorbed by the biological membrane model used.

In conclusion, SLN obtained by the PIT method could be useful to increase both IDE topical and systemic bioavailability, thus improving its antioxidant activity.

Keywords: Idebenone, solid lipid nanoparticles; PIT; DSC; skin permeation; blood brain barrier

Abbreviations

SLN = Solid Lipid Nanoparticles;
IDE = Idebenone;
PIT = Phase Inversion Temperature;
DSC = Differential Scanning Calorimetry;
MLV Multilamellar Vesicles;
BBB = Blood Brain Barrier;
FRDA = Friedreich Ataxia;
CNS = Central Nervous System;
ROS = Reactive Oxygen Species;
APPH = 2, 2′- azobis 2-amidinopropane hydrochloride;
FD4 = fluorescein-dextran 4000;
DMPC = dimyristoylphosphatidylcholine;
HLB = Hydrophilic Lipophilic Balance;
P.I. = Polidispersity Index;
CP = Cetyl Palmitate.

Introduction

In the last decades, a great deal of attention has been focused on the design of colloidal carriers as drug delivery systems, such as liposomes [1], microemulsions [2], dendrymers [3], polymeric nanoparticles [4] and solid lipid nanoparticles (SLN) [5]. The latter are emerging as a promising alternative approach to other colloidal carriers because of their advantages including controlled drug release, drug targeting, ability to incorporate both lipophilic and hydrophilic drugs, improved bioavailability, biocompatibility, improved drug stability, multiple administration routes (oral, parenteral, topical), easy scale-up and manufacturing, and low production costs [5, 6].

SLN consist of physiological solid lipids dispersed in aqueous surfactant solutions that stabilize the lipid dispersion by preventing particle aggregation. The main drawbacks of SLN are related mostly to their preparation as high pressures and/or rapid temperature changes, generally involved in these techniques, can lead to drug leaking during storage, co-existence of lipid polymorphs, drug degradation, gelation phenomena and need of purification steps. Although high-pressure hot homogenization is widely used to prepare SLN, because it provides small particles, the high temperatures used may increase the degradation rate of the drug and the carrier and may retard lipid crystallization due to the formation of a supercooled melt [7]. Thermal stresses and high pressures can be avoided by using the solvent emulsification/evaporation technique [8] but the need of using organic solvents limits its pharmaceutical application. SLN preparation based on dilution in cold water of oil-in-water microemulsions allows to overcome some of the problems connected to other techniques [9]; however the high surfactant concentrations required to prepare the initial microemulsions could represent an important disadavantage of this technique [6].

Recently, we developed a novel technique to prepare SLN from o/w microemulsions with low surfactant content by using the phase inversion temperature (PIT) method [10]. This method allowed us to obtain SLN with good technological properties such as small particle size, low polidispersity index and good stability upon storage at room temperature, avoiding the use of great amount of surfactants and purification steps as required by conventional microemulsion procedures. Since these SLN were designed as topical and systemic drug delivery, we chose to load in these nanoparticles idebenone (Figure 1), a potent antioxidant regarded as useful in the treatment of both skin [11] and cerebral impairments [12].

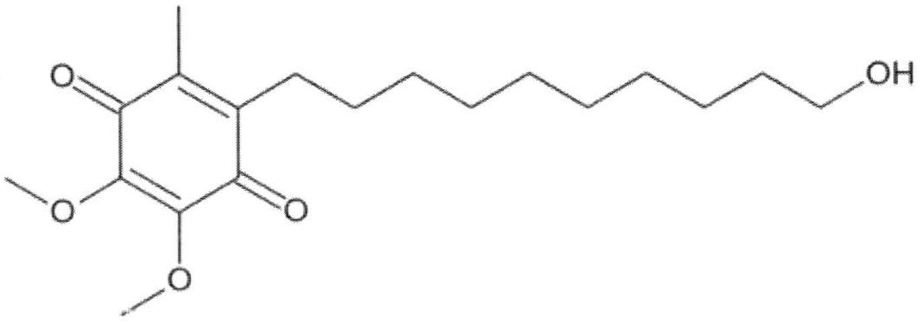

Figure 1. Chemical structure of idebenone.

Takeda Pharmaccuticals Company Ltd originally developed Idebenone (IDE), a synthetic analogue of co-enzyme Q_{10} with a shorter carbon side chain and subsequent increased water solubility [13], for the treatment of Alzheimer's disease but since 1999 IDE has been studied as a possible therapeutic agent for Friedreich ataxia (FRDA). *In vitro* studies showed IDE ability to interact with the mitochondrial respiratory chain as an electron carrier, providing support for mitochondrial function and ATP production [14]. Furthermore, due to its ability to inhibit lipid peroxidation in mitochondria, IDE acts as an antioxidant, protecting membranes from oxidative damages [15]. Trials on IDE clinical efficacy showed an improvement of neurological functions and of cardiac hypertrophy in patients with FRDA [16, 17]. Being IDE a very lipophilic drug with low water solubility, only an oral dosage form is on the pharmaceutical market for the treatment of neurological diseases, but its bioavailability at the level of the Central Nervous System (CNS) is poor (0.4% of the dose reaches the brain), due to IDE reduced absorption [18].

Studies on IDE activity as topical antioxidant showed that this co-enzyme Q_{10} analogue was more potent than tocopherol and co-enzyme Q_{10} itself [19]. Therefore, topical supplementation with IDE is regarded as a useful treatment to reduce reactive oxygen species (ROS) induced skin damages by improving skin antioxidant capacity [20].

Recently, to improve IDE bioavailability after parenteral administration, we prepared IDE-loaded SLN by the PIT method using cetyl palmitate as solid lipid and three different non-ionic emulsifiers, oleth-20 (unsaturated acyl chain), ceteth-20 (saturated linear acyl chain), and isoceteth-20 (saturated, branched acyl chain) [10]. Due to their lipophilic characteristics and their small particle size, SLN could reach the CNS, overcoming the blood-brain barrier (BBB) by endocytosis or transcytosis mechanisms, or they could permeate the tight junctions between endothelial cells [21, 22]. Furthermore, SLN retention in brain blood capillaries and their absorption into capillary walls could provide a higher drug concentration gradient, leading to enhanced drug transport across the endothelial cells [21, 22].

Our *in vitro* studies on IDE-loaded SLN performed on primary cultures of astrocytes, obtained from rat cerebral cortex, showed no cytoxic effect and a stronger activity than free IDE in inhibiting APPH-induced ROS production depending on the type of surfactant used to prepare these SLN. As shown in Figure 2, IDE-loaded SLN containing ceteth-20 as emulsifier provided the highest inhibition (100%) of ROS production. Further *in vitro* experiments on a model of BBB consisting of MDCKII-MDR1 monolayers, pointed out that IDE permeation from IDE-loaded SLN was lower than that of free IDE, regardless of different SLN compositions [23]. The use of FD4 and diazepam as markers of the paracellular pathway and the transcellular pathway, respectively, showed that IDE could permeate via a transcellular pathway. However, it was noteworthy that the amount of IDE permeated from these SLN was similar to the amount that in previous *in vitro* experiments on astrocyte cell cultures showed an antioxidant activity higher than free IDE.

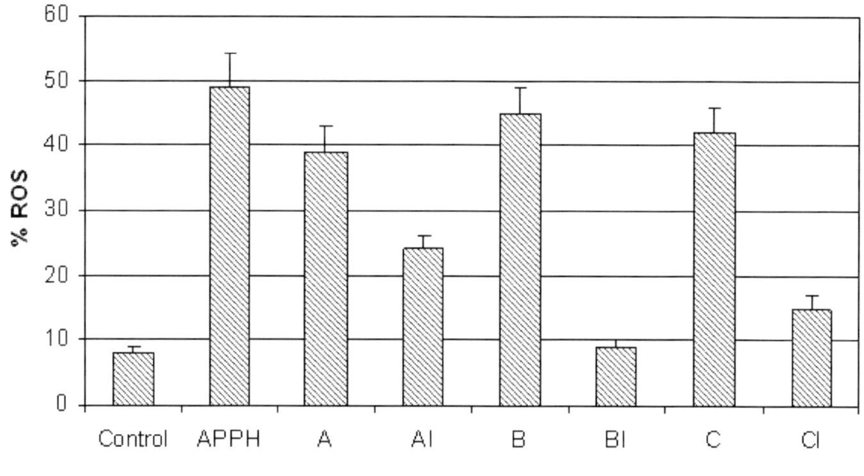

Figure 2. Inhibition of APPH-induced ROS production in astrocyte cultures by unloaded SLN and SLN loading IDE 0.7% w/w. Results were obtained treating astrocyte cultures with APPH and then adding the SLN under investigation. Control = no treatment; APPH = treatment with APPH 20 mM alone; A = unloaded SLN containing isoceteth-20; AI = IDE-loaded SLN containing isoceteth-20; B = unloaded SLN containing ceteth-20; BI = IDE-loaded SLN containing ceteth-20; C = unloaded SLN containing oleth-20; CI = IDE-loaded SLN containing oleteth-20.

These results suggest that IDE loading into SLN may represent an advantageous strategy to prepare IDE aqueous vehicles suitable for parenteral administration, avoiding the use of co-solvents that could induce adverse side effects. Due to their small size (<100 nm), these SLN could be supposed to have a prolonged blood circulation, thus increasing the time for which the drug remains in contact with BBB and for the drug to be taken up by the brain [24-25].

IDE-loaded SLN, prepared by the PIT method with a composition similar to that described for drug delivery to the brain, were investigated to assess their suitability as IDE topical delivery system [26]. *In vitro* permeation and penetration studies performed on newborn pig skin showed that no IDE permeation occurred from these SLN while an IDE accumulation into the upper skin layers (stratum corneum and epidermis) was observed, depending on both drug loading and SLN composition [26]. When SLN containing ceteth-20 or isoceteth-20 as surfactant were applied on the skin, the highest IDE content was found in the epidermis while IDE accumulated into the horny layer when SLN loading high amount of IDE were prepared using oleth-20 as surfactant (Figure 3). The results of our *in vitro* skin permeation and penetration studies suggest that loading IDE into these SLN could provide a useful tool to improve IDE bioavailability after topical administration, providing an IDE targeting to the upper skin layers, where the drug is supposed to exert its antioxidant activity.

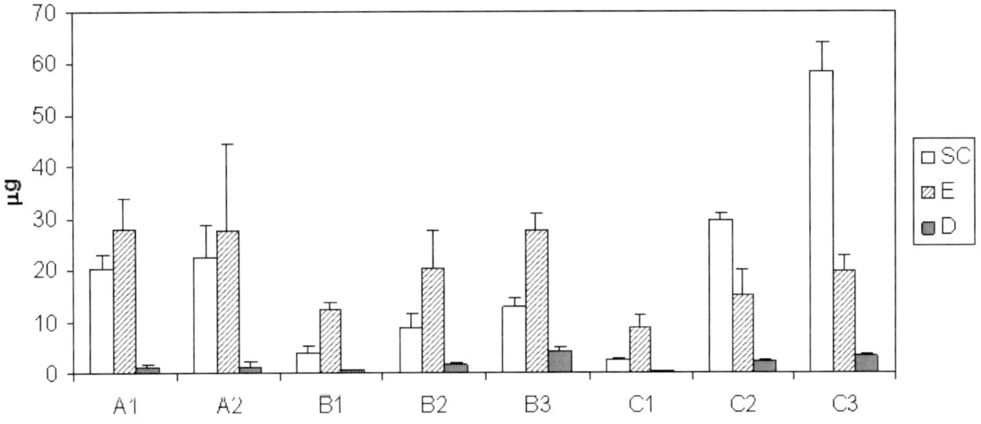

Figure 3. *In vitro* skin penetration in different skin layers of IDE from SLN loading different percentages of IDE. SC = stratum corneum; E = epidermis; D = dermis. A = SLN containing isoceth-20; B = SLN containing ceteth-20; C = SLN containing oleth-20; 1 = IDE 0.5% w/w; 2 = IDE 0.7 % w/w; 3 = IDE 1.1 % w/w.

Other authors [27] evaluated *in vitro* IDE skin penetration/permeation from nanostructured lipid carriers. Their experiments revealed an approximately three-fold increase of both IDE skin permeation and penetration into the upper layers of the skin. The authors attributed these results both to nanoparticle penetration into the hair follicles and to the ability of the surfactants contained in these nanoparticles to disrupt the packing of the lipid bilayers in the horny layer, thus improving IDE permeation through the skin. Studies performed on SLN loaded with the lipophilic dye nile red, as a model agent, outlined the relevance of the type of drug interaction with lipid matrices for skin uptake and targeting [28]. So far, the mechanism of nanoparticle skin penetration has not yet been clarified and contradictory results about nanoparticles ability to penetrate into the stratum corneum have been reported [29-31].

Due to the complexity of both the processes involved in SLN cellular uptake and the cell membrane structure, biomimetic model cell membranes are increasingly used to investigate the biophysical interactions between SLN and biomembranes [32]. To explain the results obtained using SLN prepared by the PIT method as carriers for systemic and topical IDE delivery, in this chapter we discuss the interactions that may occur between IDE loaded SLN and biological membranes as revealed by differential scanning calorimetry (DSC) studies performed on a biomembrane model, represented by multilamellar vesicles (MLV) made of dimyristoylphosphatidylcholine (DMPC).

Differential scanning calorimetry, first developed in the early1960s, is the most common thermal analysis technique. Thermal analysis is a group of techniques that study the relationship between a sample property and its temperature. In particular, DSC measures the heat flow in and out of a sample and a reference material whilst the sample and the reference are heated, cooled or held isothermally at a given temperature [33]. DSC can detect endothermic and exothermic effects, determines peak areas (transition and reaction enthalpies) and temperatures that characterize a peak, and measures specific heat capacity [34]. Considering the ability to measure enthalpy changes and phase transitions, there are multiple applications for such a versatile tool. DSC is, in fact, used in several scientific disciplines, such as chemistry and biochemistry, environmental analysis, food chemistry and pharmacy. In the pharmaceutical field, this technique is largely employed to investigate physicochemical features of different compounds such as proteins [35] and nucleic acids [36], to determine drug purity [37], to evaluate the interaction between drugs and nucleic acids [38], and between drugs and biological compartments [39], to characterize several type of drug carriers such as hydrogels [40], microspheres [41], nanostructured lipid carriers [42], polymer-oil nanostructured carrier [43], solid lipid nanoparticles [44, 45], liposomes [46], invasosomes [47]. In addition, it is used to evaluate drug release by different delivery systems [48].

SLN Morphology and Technological Properties

DSC studies were performed on unloaded SLN and SLN loading 0.7 % w/w IDE prepared using the phase inversion temperature (PIT) method, as previously reported [10, 23, 26]. SLN composition is reported in Table 1.

Cetyl palmitate was chosen as solid lipid as it is regarded as a safe and biocompatible ingredient [49, 50]. Studies on the toxicity of SLN, whose lipid core consisted of cetyl palmitate, indicated a good tolerability of such nanocarriers with no evident cytotoxic effect [51, 52].

Non-ionic surfactants were selected because their irritation potential is considered the lowest with respect to anionic and cationic surfactants [53].

The morphology of the SLN under investigation was evaluated by transmission electron microscopy (TEM), using a transmission electron microscope (model JEM 2010, Jeol, Peabody, MA, USA). As previously reported [10], the PIT method provided spherical unloaded and IDE-loaded SLN (Figure 4), with no evident sign of aggregation. Other authors, studying cetyl palmitate SLN by electron microscopy and atomic force microscopy [54] observed an almost spherical form of the particles. On the contrary, different SLN shapes, such as cubical or platelet-like patterns, were reported for SLN prepared using well defined lipids of high purity (e.g., pure triglycerides) [55, 56]. These findings have been attributed to the tendency of chemically homogenous lipid to form more or less perfect crystals with the typical platelet-like pattern of the β-modification while chemically heterogeneous lipids in combination with heterogeneous surfactants seem to favor the formation of ideally spherical lipid nanoparticles [5].

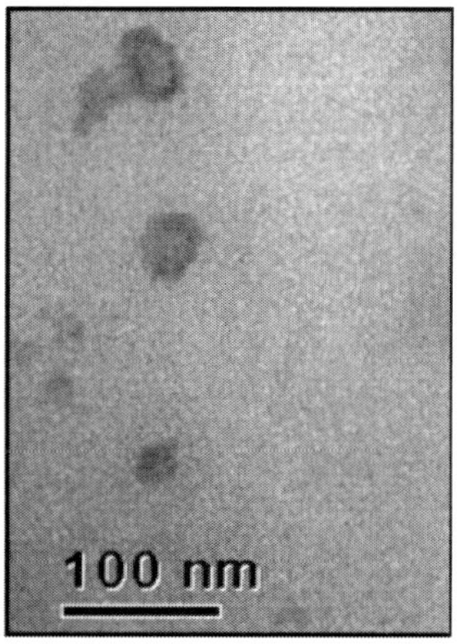

Figure 4. TEM picture of SLN prepared by the PIT method.

Table 1. Composition (% w/w) of unloaded and IDE-loaded SLN

SLN	Ceteth-20	Isoceteth-20	Oleth-20	GO	CP	IDE	Water*
A	---	10.6	---	3.5	7	---	q b 100
AI	---	10.6	---	3.5	7	0.7	q b 100
B	8.7	---	---	4.4	7	---	q b 100
BI	8.7	---	---	4.4	7	0.7	q b 100
C	---	---	7.5	3.7	7	---	q b 100
CI	---	---	7.5	3.7	7	0.7	q b 100

* Water containing 0.35 % w/w imidazolidinyl urea and 0.05 % w/w methylchloroisothiazolinone and methylisothiazolinone as preservatives. GO = glyceryl oleate; CP = cetyl palmitate.

Mean particle size and polidispersity index were determined by dynamic light scattering using a Zetasizer Nano ZS 90 (Malvern, Germany), which performed particle sizing by means of a 4 mW laser diode operating at 670 nm, scattering light at 90°. Table 2 shows that all SLN had small sizes ranging from 36 to 60 nm, and a single peak in size distribution. As reported in the literature [57, 58], submicron particle sizes are easily achieved since the microemulsion already contains droplets in the nano-size range. The conventional microemulsion based SLN preparation requires the dilution in cold water of a hot microemulsion to produce SLN [9], thus providing formulations with lipid contents considerably lower compared with the high pressure homogenization technique. Unlike the conventional technique based on the dilution of microemulsions, the PIT method did not require a dilution step and specific equipment to form SLN.

Table 2. Particle size (size ± S.D.), polidispersity index (poly ± S.D.), and phase inversion temperature (PIT) values of unloaded and IDE loaded SLN

SLN	Size ± S.D. (nm)	Poly ± S.D.	PIT (°C)
A	40.5 ± 0.6	0.31 ± 0.01	80
AI	36.6 ± 0.5	0.32 ± 0.01	80
B	60.8 ± 4.5	0.53 ± 0.12	80
BI	34.2 ± 0.4	0.22 ± 0.01	78
C	37.1 ± 0.8	0.23 ± 0.01	78
CI	36.9 ± 0.4	0.26 ± 0.01	78

IDE incorporation into SLN B produced a significant decrease of particle size while IDE addition to SLN A or C did not affect particle size. A lower polidispersity index (P.I.) after loading the active ingredient into SLN B was observed, as well.

These results could be due to different interactions between IDE and the surfactant layers, depending on the type of surfactant used to prepare these SLN. Since isoceteth-20 has a branched acyl chain while oleth-20 and ceteth-20 have linear acyl chains, unsaturated and saturated respectively, a different packing of the surfactant molecules at the interface could be expected, leading to a different IDE ability to penetrate the tail group region of the surfactant layer and to affect particle curvature radius. In our experiments, the slight differences in surfactant lipophilicity (HLB values: oleth-20 15.3, isoceteth-20 15.5, ceteth-20 15.7) did not seem to affect significantly SLN particle size.

To assess their stability, SLN were stored in airtight jars, and then kept in the dark at room temperature and at 37° C for two months, separately. At fixed time intervals (24 hours, one week, two weeks, three weeks, one month, and two months) after their preparation, mean particle size and polidispersity index of the samples were determined.

A correlation between the HLB temperature (or PIT temperature) and the surfactant HLB has been previously reported [59]. As the surfactant HLB increases the HLB, temperature increases as well and the higher the HLB temperature, the greater the formulation stability. Since we prepared these SLN using surfactants with similar HLB values, similar PIT values and similar stability for these formulations could be expected.

In our experiments, although PIT values were very close for all the SLN prepared (Table 2), their stability during storage at room temperature for two months was different since particle size of IDE-loaded SLN A increased while no significant change was observed for all the other formulations (Figure 5).

The lower stability of IDE-loaded SLN A could be due to the branched structure of the surfactant used to prepare these SLN that could lead to a lower intercalation of IDE between the tail group regions of the surfactant layer, with a resulting looser packing of the surfactant layer that would increase aggregation phenomena. During storage at 37°C, less stability in terms of particle size for all the formulations tested was observed (data not shown), likely due to an increase of energy into the system leading to particle aggregation and size growth, as previously reported in the literature [5].

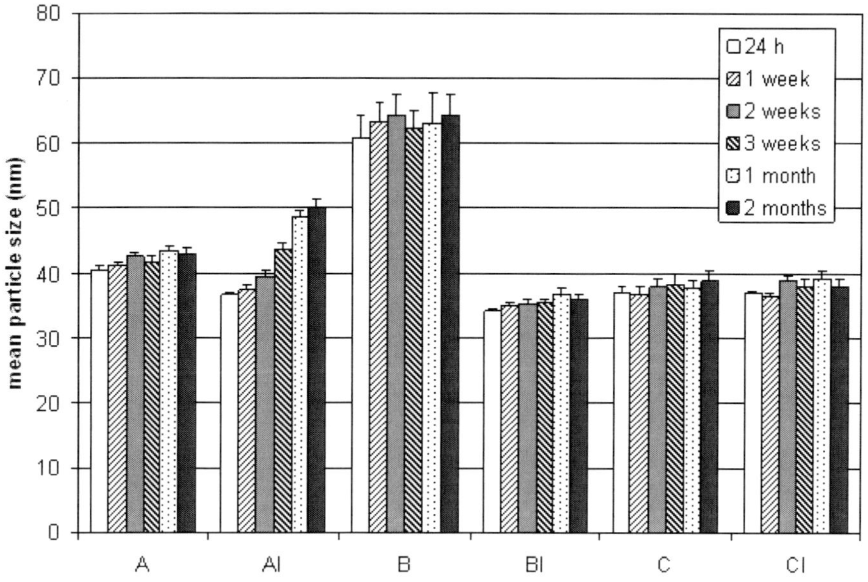

Figure 5. Mean particle size of unloaded (A, B and C) and IDE-loaded (AI, BI and CI) SLN during storage at room temperature for 2 months.

Interaction Mechanisms of SLN with Biological Membranes

The permeation of both unloaded and IDE loaded SLN within a biomembrane model, consisting of multilamellar vesicles (MLV) of dimyristoylphosphatidylcholine (DMPC), was investigated by DSC using a Mettler Toledo STAR^e system (Switzerland) equipped with a DSC-822^e calorimetric cell, and Mettler TA-STAR^e software.

Preliminarily, the calorimetric characterization of these SLN was carried out to identify their calorimetric signals, and these curves served as references in the subsequent permeation study. 100 μL of SLN was placed into 160 μL calorimetric pan, hermetically sealed and submitted to at least three subsequent heating and cooling calorimetric scans in the temperature range 5 - 65°C (2 °C/min in heating mode and 4 °C/min in cooling mode).

When submitted to heating scans, the SLN lipid core absorbs heat to change its physical state, and DSC detects this heat variation and outputs a thermogram, i.e., a calorimetric curve with a characteristic peak temperature.

Unloaded SLN thermograms had not relevant differences to each other (see Figure 6 for an example). They were characterized by a main peak at 42.0°C, a wide shoulder at 32.0°C and a very small shoulder at 46.5°C. SLN thermogram was quite different from that of cetyl palmitate (CP) in aqueous medium, in fact, CP calorimetric curve showed a main peak at 50.5°C and a very broad peak at 39.0°C. The reduction of peak temperature that occurred in SLN with respect to the lipid in bulk is widely documented in literature [60-62] and was due both to the high specific surface area of the nanosized particles and to the lipid interaction with the other components of the SLN [63].

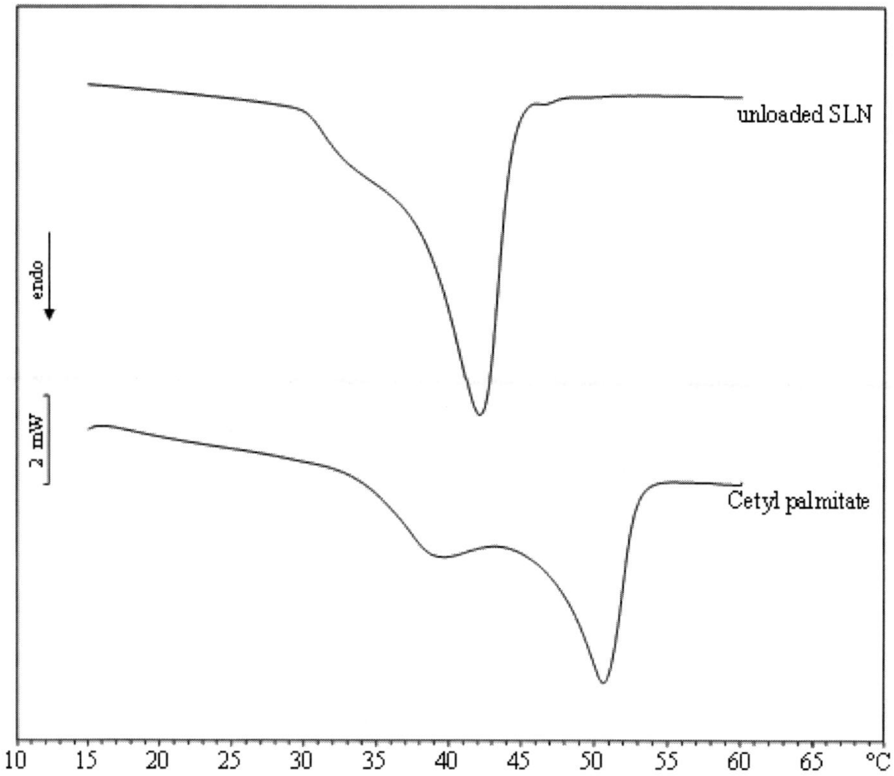

Figure 6. Calorimetric curves, in heating mode, of unloaded SLN and Cetyl palmitate in aqueous medium.

To study unloaded and IDE loaded SLN interactions with the biomembrane model, MLV consisting of DMPC were obtained as previously described [64].

To analyze the interaction of IDE with liposomes, MLV loaded with increasing molar fractions (0.015, 0.03, 0.06, 0.09 and 0.12) of IDE with respect to DMPC were also prepared by adding a solution of IDE in chloroform/methanol (1:1, v:v) to the same tubes where DMPC aliquots were distributed. The DSC analysis of unloaded and IDE loaded MLV was performed placing 120 μL of the MLV sample into the calorimetric pan, hermetically closed and submitted to the following cycles: a heating scan from 5 to 37 °C (2 °C/min); a cooling scan from 37 to 5 °C (4 °C/min); for at least three times.

SLN permeation of SLN within MLV was studies by placing 26 μL of SLN into the calorimetric pan where 94 μL of MLV was added. The calorimetric pan was closed and submitted to the following scans: (i) a heating scan from 5 to 55 °C (2 °C/min); a cooling scan from 55 to 37 °C (4 °C/min); (iii) an isotherm scan of 60 min at 37 °C; (iv) a cooling scan from 37 to 5 °C (4 °C/min). This procedure was repeated continuously for at least eight times. The temperature of 37°C was chosen for the isotherm scans as it is very close to the physiological temperature, and in this condition the MLV are in a disordered liquid crystalline phase that favors interaction and uptake of foreign molecules.

DSC analysis of the uptake of IDE by the MLV was carried out by weighting an amount of IDE corresponding to 0.06 molar fraction with respect to DMPC in the calorimetric pan, and by adding 120 μL of MLV. The calorimetric pan was closed and submitted to the same scans described for DSC analysis of the permeation of SLN within MLV.

Figure 7 shows the thermogram of IDE loaded SLN compared to that of unloaded SLN. The thermograms were different. In particular, in IDE loaded SLN A and SLN B the wide shoulder at 32.0°C became less evident instead the small shoulder at 46.5°C increased becoming a small peak. In IDE loaded SLN C the shoulders at 32.0°C and 46.5°C disappeared and the main peak split in two peaks at 41.0 and 42.6°C.

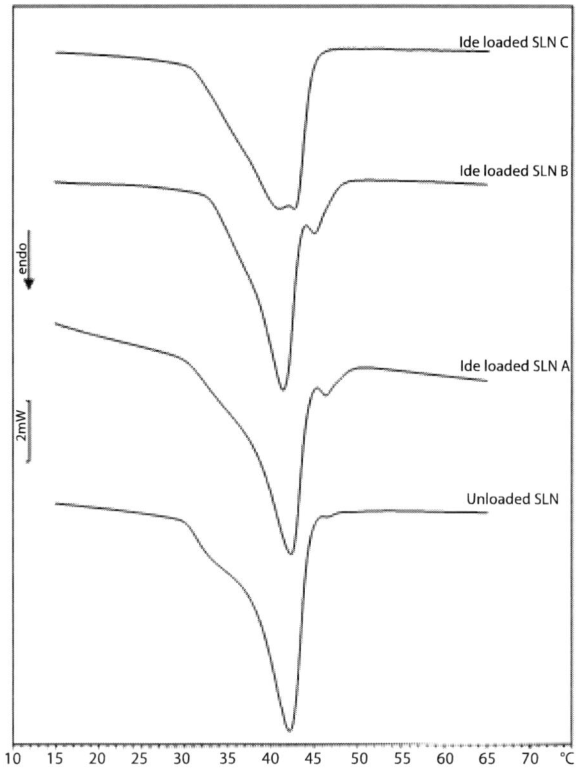

Figure 7. Calorimetric curves, in heating mode, of unloaded and IDE loaded SLN.

To investigate the different calorimetric signals of IDE loaded SLN with respect to unloaded SLN, especially to ascertain that the shoulder at higher temperature in IDE loaded SLN was due to IDE inside the SLN, some experiments were carried out. IDE was analyzed in the solid form, in aqueous medium, and after being submitted to the same experimental conditions used for SLN preparation and the obtained calorimetric curves are shown in Figure 8.

Solid IDE had a sharp melting peak at 53.2°C; instead, when it was put in an aqueous medium, the melting event occurred at 45.7°C. IDE subjected to the same experimental conditions of the SLN preparation showed a flat thermogram in the range of temperature used for SLN thermal analysis. Finally, solid IDE was put in contact with unloaded SLN and submitted to the same calorimetric cycle of the permeation analysis. As an example, in Figure 9 the results obtained with SLN B are shown and compared with those of unloaded and IDE loaded SLN B.

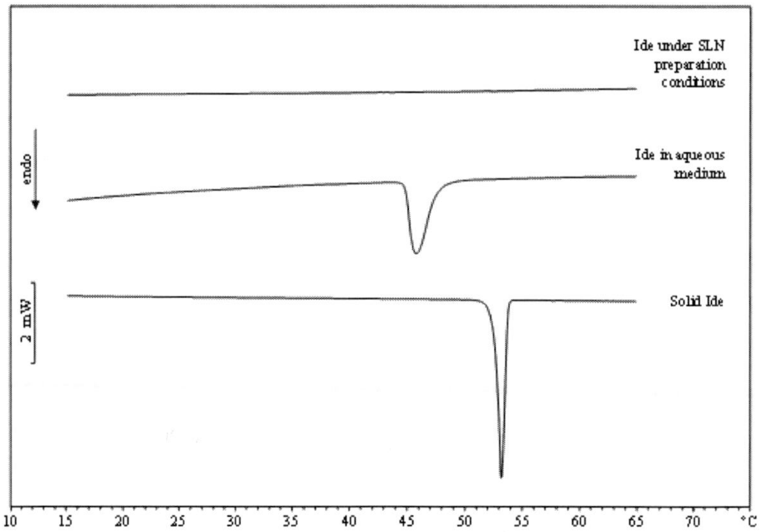

Figure 8. Calorimetric curves, in heating mode, of solid IDE, IDE in aqueous medium and IDE submitted to the same conditions of SLN preparation.

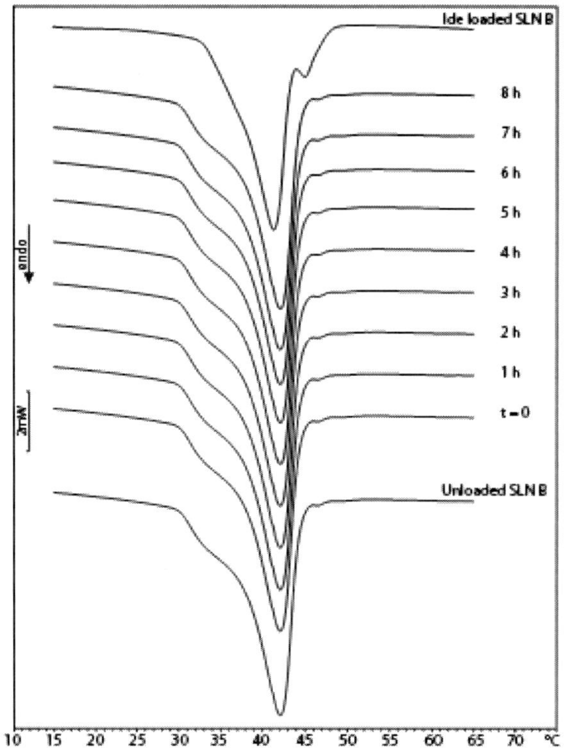

Figure 9. Calorimetric curves, in heating mode, of unloaded SLN B left in contact with solid IDE, for increasing incubation time. Calorimetric curves of unloaded and IDE loaded SLN B are used as reference curves.

It was clear that the presence of IDE outside of SLN did not give rise to any calorimetric signal and did not modify the SLN calorimetric curves. Therefore, the presence of IDE within the SLN was responsible for the different signals that were observed in the thermograms of IDE loaded SLN compared to unloaded SLN.

Moreover, the surfactant unsaturation influenced IDE localization within the SLN that gave rise to different calorimetric signals (small peak at 46.5°C for SLN A and SLN B; split peak at 41 and 42.6°C for SLN C).

The interaction of IDE with liposomes was performed to evaluate how the drug affected the thermotropic behavior of the biomembrane model. DMPC liposomes showed a characteristic thermogram with two peaks, a small one called pretransition peak at 17.0°C, due to the transition from the gel to the ripple phase, and a sharp main peak that occurred at the melting temperature (T_m) of 25.0°C for the transition from the ripple to liquid crystalline phase [65, 66]. MLV were loaded with different concentrations of IDE, in particular with 0.015, 0.03, 0.06, 0.09, and 0.12 molar fractions with respect to DMPC. These samples were submitted to DSC analysis and the resulting thermograms (Figure 10) demonstrated the interaction between IDE and MLV, in particular IDE caused the disappearance of the pretransition peak, the widening and the shift of the main transition peak toward lower temperature in a concentration-dependent manner. At 0.12 molar fraction a phase separation was observed, so at high concentrations IDE was not evenly distributed in MLV. These findings are in agreement with those of Fresta et al. [67].

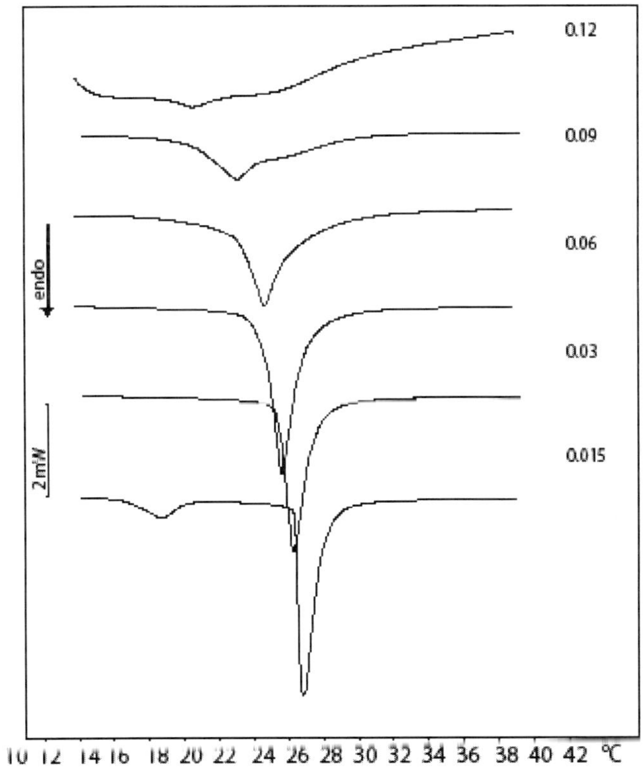

Figure 10. Calorimetric curves, in heating mode, of unloaded and loaded MLV with different molar fractions of IDE.

To study the permeation of both unloaded and IDE loaded SLN within the DMPC, SLN and the biomembrane model (unloaded MLV) were put in contact at 37°C and the calorimetric scan was performed immediately after the contact and hourly to monitor the progress of the permeation.

The thermograms of unloaded SLN, unloaded MLV, IDE loaded MLV and loaded SLN (in the case of the analysis of IDE loaded SLN) were used as references.

First, unloaded SLN were analyzed to evaluate the capability of the carrier to penetrate the phospholipid bilyers. As shown in Figure 11, in the first scan, MLV and SLN maintained their characteristic curves. However, already after one hour of incubation (second scan), the pretransition peak disappeared and the main MLV peak split into a shoulder and a smaller peak. This peak occurring at the same T_m of unloaded MLV (25.0°C) was caused by the melting of the empty inner layers of the MLV; instead the shoulder at a lower temperature was due to the melting of the outer MLV layers that already contained SLN. Increasing the incubation time, the shoulder and the peak merged into a single peak, indicating that SLN also passed in the inner layers, and then achieved a homogeneous distribution in the MLV. The peak of the SLN remained almost unchanged for the whole time of the experiment. Therefore SLN were able to penetrate the outer bilayers and then the inner layers of MLV maintaining their structural integrity.

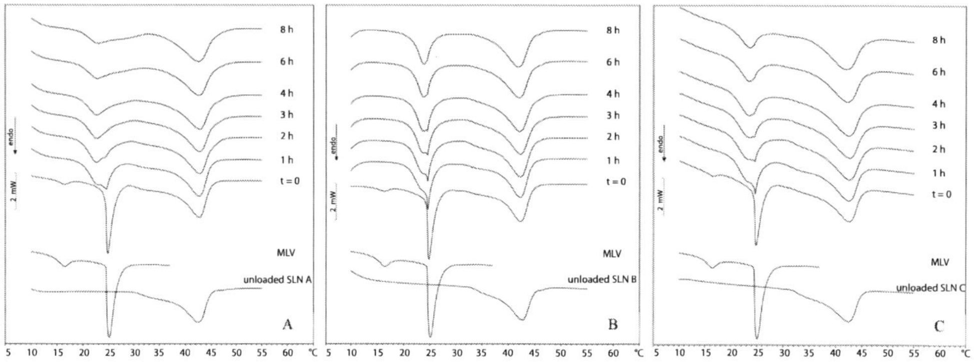

Figure 11. Calorimetric curves, in heating mode, of MLV put in contact with (A) unloaded SLN A, (B) unloaded SLN B and (C) unloaded SLN C at increasing incubation time. The calorimetric curves of starting substances put in contact (MLV and unloaded SLN), are used as references.

Afterwards, the permeation of IDE loaded SLN within the MLV was assessed to evaluate the eventual release of IDE from SLN to the biomembrane model. Preliminarily, uptake of IDE by the biomembrane model was evaluated. To this aim, an exact amount of solid IDE (corresponding to 0.06 molar fraction) was put in contact with unloaded MLV in the calorimetric pan and submitted to calorimetric scans. The obtained calorimetric curves are shown in Figure 12 and were compared with those of unloaded and IDE loaded (0.06 molar fraction) MLV. From this experiment it was evident that IDE was not absorbed by phospholipid bilayers, in fact the thermograms remained almost unchanged with respect to that of unloaded MLV. Likely, IDE was not able to cross the aqueous medium because of its lipophilicity (Log P 3.49, calculated using Advanced Chemistry Development Software Solaris V. 4.67).

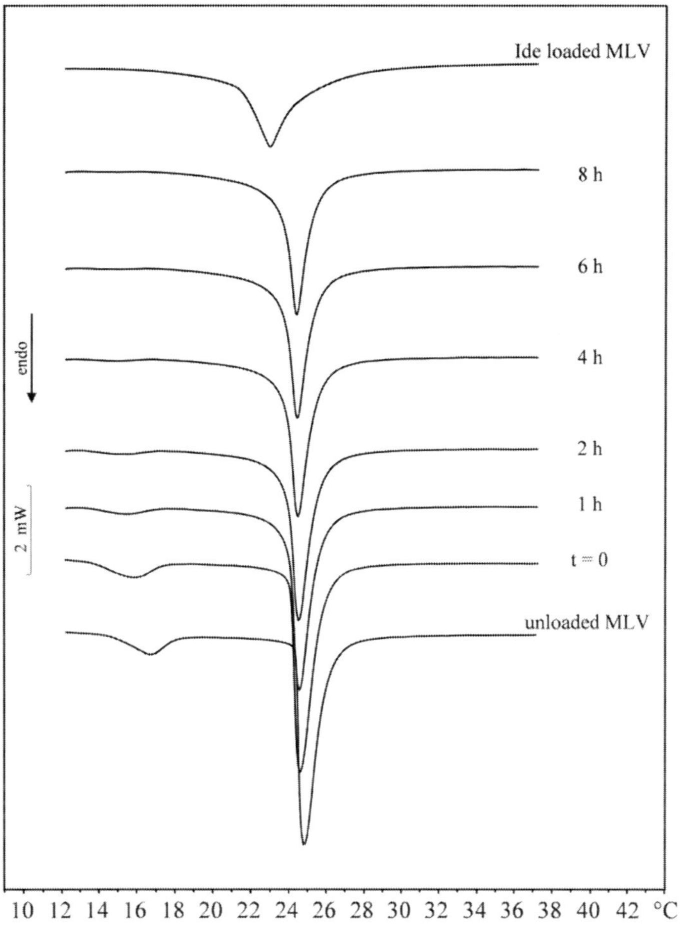

Figure 12. Calorimetric curves, in heating mode, of MLV put in contact with solid IDE (0.06 molar fraction) at increasing incubation time. The calorimetric curves of unloaded and IDE loaded (0.06 molar fraction) MLV are used as references.

On the contrary, IDE loaded SLN were able to release the drug to MLV bilayers as shown by the thermograms reported in Figure 13. In fact, with regard to the calorimetric signals of MLV, the pretransition peak disappeared and in the first scan the main peak was broaden; in the second scan a shoulder at lower temperature appeared; then, the shoulder and main peak merged forming a unique broad peak. Variations of IDE loaded SLN were also observed. In particular, the shoulder at 32.0°C reduced gradually and the small peak that was attributed to the presence of IDE within the SLN A and SLN B disappeared; with regard to SLN C the peaks at 41.0 and 42.6°C immediately formed a unique peak. These results confirmed that SLN released IDE as soon as they came in contact and entered the MLV.

To corroborate these findings, the same experiment without MLV was carried out, placing in the calorimetric pan only IDE loaded SLN. In Figure 14, the obtained thermograms for IDE loaded SLN C are shown, as an example. The thermograms did not change in all the scans and the calorimetric signal caused by IDE in SLN did not modify, indicating that IDE was released by SLN only when they were in contact with liposomes. In addition, a greater release of IDE from SLN C than from SLN A and SLN B was achieved as demonstrated by the greater enlargement of the peak of MLV interacting with SLN C.

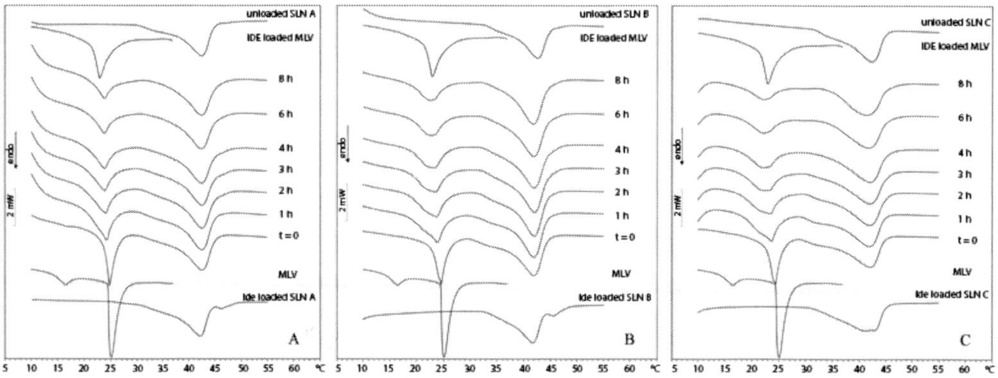

Figure 13. Calorimetric curves, in heating mode, of MLV put in contact with (A) IDE loaded SLN A, (B) IDE loaded SLN B and (C) IDE loaded SLN C at increasing incubation time. The calorimetric curves of starting substances put in contact (MLV and IDE loaded SLN), IDE loaded MLV and unloaded SLN are used as references.

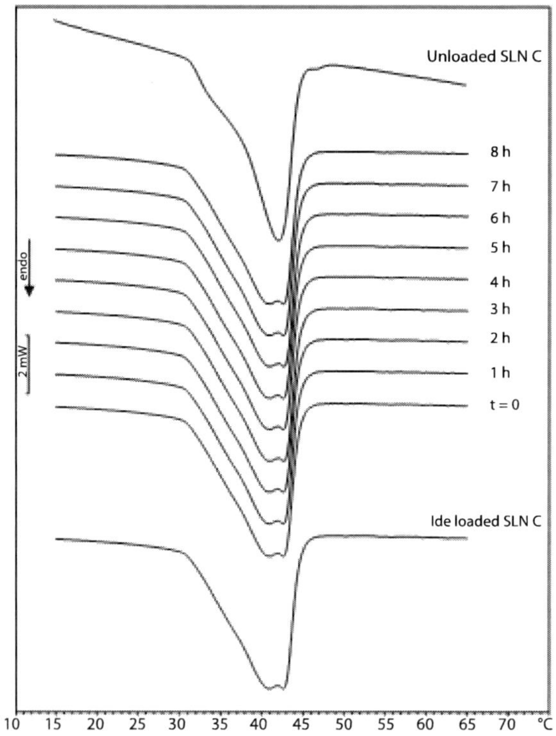

Figure 14. Calorimetric curves, in heating mode, of IDE loaded SLN C left at 37°C for incresing incubation time. The reference curves represent the cases of total (unloaded SLN C curve) and absent (IDE loaded SLN C curve) release of IDE.

All these experiments revealed that free IDE was not absorbed by the biological membrane model used while SLN could penetrate phospholipid bilayers and therefore, they could be regarded as suitable carriers for IDE, releasing the drug within the biomembrane model. The comparison of the calorimetric results with those obtained from IDE skin penetration/permeation experiments points out the possibility of using DSC studies to predict IDE loaded SLN ability to interact with the upper skin layers, depending on the surfactant used to prepare these SLN. In particular, both DSC and skin penetration/permeation studies showed that the greatest amount of IDE released into MLV bilayers and penetrated into the stratum corneum, respectively, was detected when SLN containing oleth-20 as surfactant were used.

On the other hand, when IDE permeation from these SLN was assessed using a model of BBB consisting of MDCKII-MDR1 monolayers, a similar permeation of IDE was observed, regardless of the SLN used.

These results could be likely due to a greater similarity of the biomembrane model used to the horny layer, consisting of an approximately equimolar mixture of several lipids, ceramides, cholesterol, free fatty acids and minor amounts of cholesterol sulphate [68]. Therefore, further studies are ongoing to assess the feasibility of using DSC studies as a tool to predict IDE skin permeation from SLN prepared by PIT method by determining the calorimetric behavior of these SLN loaded with different amount of IDE.

Conclusion

In this chapter, we discussed the interactions between unloaded and idebenone loaded SLN, prepared by the PIT method, and a model of biological membranes consisting of MLV, studied by differential scanning calorimetry. All the SLN investigated showed good technological properties in terms of particle size, polidispersity index and stability upon storage at room temperature for two months. DSC studies highlighted their ability to interact with the biomembrane model and these interactions were different depending on the surfactant used for their preparation. In particular, the results of calorimetric studies suggest that the greatest IDE accumulation in the upper skin layers, observed in previous *in vitro* skin permeation/penetration experiments [26], could be attributed to a better interaction of SLN containing oleth-20 with the skin barrier. On the contrary, free IDE was not absorbed by the biological membrane model used, suggesting that these SLN could represent a promising delivery system for IDE targeting to the upper skin layers. SLN interactions with a biomembrane model consisting of MLV made of DMPC did not account for IDE permeation data across a model of BBB. Therefore, to explain these results further experiments are planned using different models both of biomembranes and of BBB. In conclusion, IDE loaded SLN ability to interact with biomembranes pointed to their suitability as carriers to improve both IDE topical and systemic bioavailability.

References

[1] T. Kozako, N. Arima, M. Yoshimitsu, S.I. Honda, S. Soeda, Liposomes and nanotechnology in drug development: focus on oncotargets, *Int. J. Nanomed.* 7 (2012) 4943-51.

[2] M.J. Lawrence, G.D. Rees, Microemulsion-based media as novel drug delivery systems, *Adv. Drug Del. Rev.* 64 (2012) 175–193.
[3] R. M. Pearson, S. Sunoqrot, H. J. Hsu, J. W. Bae, S. Hong, Dendritic nanoparticles: the next generation of nanocarriers? *Ther. Deliv.* 3 (2012) 941-59.
[4] C. Vauthier, K. Bouchemal, Methods for the preparation and manufacture of polymeric nanoparticles, *Pharm. Res.* 26 (2009) 1025-1058.
[5] W. Mehenert, K. Mäder, Solid lipid nanoparticles. Production, characterization and applications, *Adv. Drug Del. Rev.* 64 (2012) 83–101.
[6] S. Kumar, J.K. Randhawa, High melting lipid based approach for drug delivery: Solid lipid nanoparticles, *Mat. Sci. Eng. C-Mater.* 33 (2013) 1842–1852.
[7] H. Bunjes, B. Siekmann, K. Westesen, Emulsions of supercooled melts – a novel drug delivery system. In: S. Benita (Ed.), *Submicron Emulsions in Drug Targeting and Delivery,* Harwood Academic Publishers, Amsterdam, 1998, 175-204.
[8] B. Siekmann, K. Westesen, Investigations on solid lipid nanoparticles prepared by precipitation in o/w emulsions, *Eur. J. Pharm. Biopharm.* 43 (1996) 104-109.
[9] M.R. Gasco, *Method for producing solid lipid microspheres having a narrow size distributio*n, United States Patent (1993) USS 188837.
[10] L. Montenegro, A. Campisi, M. G. Sarpietro, C. Carbone, R. Acquaviva, G. Raciti, G. Puglisi, In vitro evaluation of idebenone-loaded solid lipid nanoparticles for drug delivery to the brain, *Drug Dev. Ind. Pharm.* 37 (2011) 737-746.
[11] P. Farris, Idebenone, green tea, and Coffeeberry® extract: new and innovative antioxidants, *Dermatol. Ther.* 20 (2007) 322–329.
[12] T. Meyer, G. Buyse, Idebenone: An emerging therapy for Friedreich ataxia, *J. Neurol.* 256 (2009) 25–30.
[13] E. Wieland, E. Schutz, V.W. Armstrong, F. Kuthe, C. Heller, M. Oellerich, Idebenone protects hepatic microsomes against oxygen radical-mediated damage in organ preservation solutions, *Transplantation* 60 (1995) 444–451.
[14] M. Suno, A. Nagaoka, Inhibition of lipid peroxidation by a novel compound (CV-2619) in brain mitochondria and mode of action of the inhibition, *Biochem. Biophys. Res. Comm.* 125 (1984) 1046–1052.
[15] M. Suno, A. Nagaoka, Inhibition of lipid peroxidation by a novel compound, idebenone (CV-2619), *Jpn. J. Pharmacol.* 35 (1984) 196–198.
[16] G. Buyse, L. Mertens, G. Di Salvo, I. Matthijs, F. Wiedemann, B. Eyskens, W. Goossens, N. Goemans, G.R. Sutherland, J.L. Van Hove, Idebenone treatment in Friedreich's ataxia: neurological, cardiac and biochemical monitoring, *Neurology* 60 (2003) 1679–1681.
[17] L. Schols, M. Vorgerd, M. Schillings, G. Skipka, J. Zange, Idebenone in patients with Friedreich's ataxia, *Neurosci. Lett.* 306 (2001) 169–172.
[18] J.C. Gillis, P. Benefield, D. McTavish, Idebenone. A review of its pharmacodynamic and pharmacokinetic properties, and therapeutic use in age-related cognitive disorders, *Drugs Aging* 5 (1994) 133–152.
[19] D. McDaniel, B. Neudecker, J. Dinardo, J.A. Lewis II, H.I. Maibach, Idebenone: a new antioxidant-Part I. Relative assessment of oxidative stress protection capacity compared to commonly known antioxidants, *J. Cosmet. Dermatol.* 4 (2005) 10–17.

[20] D. McDaniel, B. Neudecker, J. DiNardo, J.A. Lewis II, H.I. MaibachClinical efficacy assessment in photodamaged skin of 0.5% and 1.0% idebenone, *J. Cosmet. Dermatol.* 4 (2005) 167–173.

[21] M.D. Joshi, R.H. Muller, Lipid nanoparticles for parenteral delivery of actives, *Eur. J. Pharm. Biopharm.* 71 (2009) 161-172.

[22] I.P. Kaur, R. Bhandari, S. Bhandari, V. Kakkar, Potential of solid lipid nanoparticles in brain targeting, *J. Control. Release* 127 (2008) 97-109.

[23] L. Montenegro, A. Trapani, A. Latrofa, G. Puglisi, In vitro evaluation on a model of blood brain barrier of idebenone-loaded solid lipid nanoparticles, *J. Nanosci. Nanotechnol.* 12 (2012) 330-337.

[24] Y. Chen, G. Dalwadi, H.A.E. Benson, Drug delivery across the blood–brain barrier, *Cur. Drug Deliv.* 1 (2004) 361–376.

[25] S.H. Gohla, A. Dingler, Scaling up feasibility of the production of solid lipid nanoparticles (SLN™), *Pharmazie* 56 (2001) 61–63.

[26] L. Montenegro, C. Sinico, I. Castangia, C. Carbone, G. Puglisi, Idebenone-loaded solid lipid nanoparticles for drug delivery to the skin: in vitro evaluation, *Int. J. Pharm.* 434 (2012) 169-174.

[27] B. Li, Z.Q. Ge, Nanostructured lipid carriers improve skin permeation and chemical stability of Idebenone, *AAPS Pharm. Sci. Tech.* 13 (2012) 276-83.

[28] S. Lombardi Borgia, M. Regehly, R. Sivaramakrishnan, W. Mehnert, H.C. Korting, K. Danker, B. Röder, K.D. Kramer, M. Schäfer-Korting, Lipid nanoparticles for skin penetration enhancement—correlation to drug localization within the particle matrix as determined by fluorescence and parelectric spectroscopy, *J. Control. Release* 110 (2005) 151– 163.

[29] J. Lademann, H. Richter, S. Schanzer, F. Knorr, M. Meinke, W. Sterry, A. Patzelt, Penetration and storage of particles in human skin: perspectives and safety aspects, *Eur. J. Pharm. Biopharm.* 77 (2011) 465–468.

[30] [30] J. Lademann, H. Richter, A. Teichmann, N. Otberg, U. Blume-Peytavi, J. Luengo, B. Weiss, U.F. Schaefer, C.M. Lehr, R. Wepf, W. Sterry, Nanoparticles—an efficient carrier for drug delivery into the hair follicles, *Eur. J. Pharm. Biopharm.* 66 (2007) 159–164.

[31] S.H. Nam, X.Y. Ji, J.S. Park, Investigation of tacrolimus loaded nanostructured lipid carriers for topical drug delivery, *Bull. Korean Chem. Soc.* 32 (2011) 956–960.

[32] M.H. Chiu, E.J. Prenner, Differential scanning calorimetry: an invaluable tool for a detailed thermodynamic characterization of macromolecules and their interactions, *J. Pharm. Bioallied Sci.* 3 (2011) 39–59.

[33] ICTAC Nomenclature of Thermal Analysis adopted by the ICTAC Council on 29 August 2006. Available from: http://www.ictac.org

[34] H. Fortunato, DSC: history, instruments and devices. In: R. Pignatello (Ed.), *Drug-biomembrane interaction studies. Application of calorimetric techniques.* Woodhead Publishing Limited, 2013 in press.

[35] T. Chen, D.M. Oakley, Thermal-analysis of proteins of pharmaceutical interest, *Thermochim. Acta* 248 (1995) 229-244.

[36] G. E. Plum, K. J Breslauer, Calorimetry of proteins and nucleic acids, *Curr. Opin. Struc. Biol.* 5 (1995) 682-690.

[37] D. Giron, C. Goldbronn, Place of DSC purity analysis in pharmaceutical development, *J. Therm. Anal.* 44 (1995) 217-251.

[38] I. Haq, Part II: The Thermodynamics of Drug–Bipolymer Interaction. Thermodynamics of drug–DNA interactions, *Arch. Biochem. Biophys.* 403 (2002) 1–15.

[39] C. Carbone, R. Pignatello, DSC in Drug-biomembrane interaction studies. In: R. Pignatello (Ed.) *Drug-biomembrane interaction studies. Application of calorimetric techniques*. Woodhead Publishing Limited, 2013, in press.

[40] I. M. El-Sherbiny, H. D. C. Smyth, Poly(ethylene glycol)–carboxymethyl chitosan-based pH-responsive hydrogels: photo-induced synthesis, characterization, swelling, and in vitro evaluation as potential drug carriers, *Carbohyd. Res.* 345 (2010) 2004–2012.

[41] A. Berthold, K. Cremer, J. Kreuter, Preparation and characterization of chitosan microspheres as drug carrier for prednisolone sodium phosphate as model for anti-inflammatory drugs, *J. Control. Release* 39 (1996) 17-25.

[42] C.-Y. Zhuang, N. Li, M. Wang, X.-N. Zhang, W.-S. Pan, J.-J. Peng, Y.-S. Pan, X. Tang, Preparation and characterization of vinpocetine loaded nanostructured lipid carriers (NLC) for improved oral bioavailability, *Int. J. Pharm.* 394 (2010) 179–185.

[43] M. Narvekar, H. Y. Xue, H. L. Wong, A novel hybrid delivery system: Polymer-oil nanostructured carrier for controlled delivery of highly lipophilic drug all-trans-retinoic acid (ATRA), *Int. J. Pharm.* 436 (2012) 721– 731.

[44] R.H. Muller, S.A. Runge, V. Ravelli, A.F. Thunemann, W. Mehnert, E.B. Souto, Cyclosporine-loaded solid lipid nanoparticles (SLN): Drug–lipid physicochemical interactions and characterization of drug incorporation. *Eur. J. Pharm. Biopharm.* 68 (2008) 535–544.

[45] L. Montenegro, M. G. Sarpietro, S. Ottimo, G. Puglisi, F. Castelli, Differential scanning calorimetry studies on sunscreen loaded solid lipid nanoparticles prepared by the phase inversion temperature method, *Int. J. Pharm.* 415 (2011) 301-306.

[46] D. Paolino, D. Cosco, L. Racanicchi, E. Trapasso, C. Celia, M. Iannone, E. Puxeddu, G. Costante, S. Filetti, D. Russo, M. Fresta, Gemcitabine-loaded PEGylated unilamellar liposomes vs GEMZAR: biodistribution, pharmacokinetic features and in vivo antitumor activity, *J. Control. Release* 144 (2010) 144-150.

[47] N. Dragicevic-Curic, M. Friedrich, S. Petersen, D. Scheglmann, D. Douroumis, W. Plass, A. Fahr, Assessment of fluidity of different invasomes by electron spin resonance and differential scanning calorimetry, *Int. J. Pharm.* 412 (2011) 85–94.

[48] M. G. Sarpietro, F. Castelli, Transfer kinetics from colloidal drug carriers and liposomes to biomembrane models: DSC studies. *J. Pharm. Bioallied Sci.* 3 (2011) 77-88.

[49] J. J. Wang, K. S. Liu, K. C. Sung, C.Y. Tsai, J. Y. Fang, Lipid nanoparticles with different oil/fatty ester ratios as carriers of buprenorphine and its prodrugs for injection, *Eur. J. Pharm. Sci.* 38 (2009) 138–146.

[50] R. Yang, R. Gao, F. Li, H. He, X. Tang, The influence of lipid characteristics on the formation, in vitro release, and in vivo absorption of protein-loaded SLN prepared by the double emulsion process, *Drug Dev. Ind. Pharm.* 37 (2011) 139-148

[51] N. Schöler, H. Hahn, R. H. Müller, O. Liesenfeld, Effect of lipid matrix and size of solid lipid nanoparticles (SLN) on the viability and cytokine production of Macrophages, *Int. J. Pharm.* 231 (2002) 167–176.

[52] R. H. Müller, S. Maassen, C. Schwarz, W. Mehnert, Solid lipid nanoparticles (SLN) as potential carrier for human use: interaction with human granulocytes, *J. Control. Release* 47 (1997) 261–269.
[53] I. Effendy, H.I. Maibach, Surfactants and experimental irritant contact dermatitis, *Contact Dermatitis* 33 (1995) 217-25.
[54] A. Dingler, R.P. Blum, H. Niehus, R.H. Müller, S. Gohla, Solid lipid nanoparticles (SLN™/Lipopearls™) - a pharmaceutical and cosmetic carrier for the application of vitamin E in dermal products, *J. Microencapsul.* 16 (1999) 751–767.
[55] K. Westesen, B. Siekmann, M.H.J. Koch, Investigations on the physical state of lipid nanoparticles by synchroton radiation X-ray diffraction, *Int. J. Pharm.* 93 (1993) 189–199.
[56] B. Siekmann, K. Westesen, Submicron-sized parenteral carrier systems based on solid lipids, Pharm. *Pharmacol. Lett.* 1 (1992) 123–126.
[57] M.R. Gasco, Solid lipid nanospheres from warm micro-emulsions, *Pharm. Tech. Eur.* 9 (1997) 52–58.
[58] L. Boltri, T. Canal, P.A. Esposito, F. Carli, Lipid nanoparticles: Evaluation of some critical formulation parameters, *Proc. Intern. Symp. Control. Rel. Bioact. Mater.* 20 (1993) 346–347.
[59] P. Izquierdo, J. Feng, J. Esquena, T.F. Tadros, J.C. Dederen, M.J. Garcia, N. Azemar, C. Solans, The influence of surfactant mixing ratio on nano-emulsion formation by the PIT method, *J. Colloid. Interface Sci.* 285 (2005) 388-394.
[60] D. Hou, C. Xie, K. Huang, C. Zhu, The production and characteristics of solid lipid nanoparticles (SLNs), *Biomaterials* 24 (2003) 1781-1785.
[61] J. Liu, T. Gong, C. Wang, Z. Zhong, Z. Zhang, Solid lipid nanoparticles loaded with insulin by sodium cholate-phosphatidylcholine-based mixed micelles: preparation and characterization, *Int. J. Pharm.* 340 (2007) 153-162.
[62] B. Siekmann, K. Westesen, Thermoanalysis of the recrystallization process of melt-homogenized glyceride nanoparticles, *Colloids Surf. B* 3 (1994) 159–175.
[63] D. Chirio, M. Gallarate, E. Peira, L. Battaglia, L. Serpe, M. Trotta, Formulation of curcumin-loaded solid lipid nanoparticles produced by fatty acids coacervation technique, *J. Microencapsul.* 28 (2011) 537-548.
[64] V. Librando, Z. Minniti, M. L. Accolla, O. Cascioc, F. Castelli, M. G. Sarpietro, Calorimetric evaluation of interaction and absorption of polychlorinated biphenyls by biomembrane models, *Chemosphere* 91 (2013) 791–796.
[65] H. Matsuki, M. Goto, K. Tada, N. Tamai, Thermotropic and barotropic phase behavior of phosphatidylcholine bilayers, *Int. J. Mol. Sci.* 14 (2013) 2282-2302.
[66] K.M.G. Taylor, R.M. Morris, Thermal analysis of phase transition behaviour in liposomes, Thermochim. Acta 248 (1995) 289–301.
[67] M. Fresta, C.A. Ventura, E. Mezzasalma, G. Puglisi, A calorimetric study on the idebenone-phospholipid membrane interaction, *Int. J. Pharm.* 163 (1998) 133-143.
[68] P. Garidel, Insights in the biochemical composition of skin as investigated by micro infrared spectroscopic imaging, *Phys. Chem. Chem. Phys.* 5 (2003) 2673-2679.

In: Recent Advances in Drug Delivery Research
Editor: Valerio Voliani
ISBN: 978-1-62948-228-6

Chapter 7

Polyphenol Conjugate: Synthesis and Potential Biomedical Applications

***O. Vittorio**[*1, 2], **G. Cirillo**[3,4], **S. Hampel**[4], **F. Iemma**[3] and **M. Kavallaris**[1, 2]*

[1]Children's Cancer Institute Australia, Lowy Cancer Research Centre, University of New South Wales, Sydney, Australia
[2]Australian Centre for Nanomedicine, University of New South Wales, Sydney, Australia
[3]Department of Pharmacy, Health and Nutritional Sciences, University of Calabria, Arcavacata di Rende (CS), Italy
[4]Leibniz Institute for Solid State and Materials Research Dresden, Germany

Abstract

Among the scientific community, the interest in antioxidant compounds is rapidly increasing due to their favorable biological properties, which makes them attractive for the biomedical, pharmaceutical, cosmetic, and food industries. Consequently, several different scientific reports and publications have devoted their attention to the understanding of the molecular mechanisms determining the biological activities, taking into consideration the cumulative evidence connecting the reactive oxygen species and most of the human degenerative disorders like cancer, neurodegeneration, atherosclerosis, and cardiovascular diseases. Among the realm of antioxidants, polyphenols represents the most relevant and their activity is mostly related to their ability in reducing oxidative damage of biological macromolecules (lipids, proteins, enzymes, carbohydrates, and DNA) inside living cells and/or tissues. Unfortunately, the serum stability of polyphenols remains one of the major challenges in their biomedical application. In order to overcome

*Children's Cancer Institute Australia, Lowy Cancer Research Centre, University of New South Wales, Sydney, Australia ; Australian Centre for Nanomedicine, University of New South Wales, Sydney, Australia. Email: OVittorio@ccia.unsw.edu.au.

this problem, many efficient chemical strategies were exploited for the functionalization of polyphenols with different polymers and nano-materials

This chapter is an overview of the different class of polyphenol conjugates, which will be analyzed in terms of synthesis and biological activity.

Keywords: Polyphenols, Bio-conjugates, Cancer

Abbreviations

3,5-dibenzylidenepiperidin-4-one (DBP);
Carbon NanoTubes (CNTs);
carvacrol-grafted chitosan nanoparticles (CHCA NPs);
catechin (CA);
chitosan/(3-chloropropyl)trimethoxysilane hybrid scaffolds (CTS/CPTMS);
electron paramagnetic resonance (EPR);
Epicatechin (EC);
Epicatechin Gallate (ECG);
Epigallocatecin (EGC);
Epigallocatechin-3 Gallate (EGCG);
eugenol-grafted chitosan nanoparticles (CHEU NPs);
Low-density lipoprotein (LDL);
low critical solution temperature (LCST);
N-isopropylacrylamide (NIPAAm);
N,N-ethylenebisacrylamide (EBA);
polymethacrylic acid (PMAA);
reactive nitrogen species (RNS);
reactive oxygen species (ROS);
starch-quercetin conjugate (ST-Q)

Introduction

In recent years evidence linking the development of human diseases and the oxidative stress has been going increase proved; consequently the interest in the application of antioxidants as medical treatments has grown [1]. The generally accepted hypothesis is that in any biological system an important balance between the formation of reactive oxygen species (ROS) and reactive nitrogen species (RNS) and their removal must be maintained. ROS and RNS are formed regularly as a result of normal organ functions, or as a result of excess oxidative stress.

Antioxidants are compounds able to protect the human body against damage by ROS and RNS and by virtue of this ability they have been found to protect against the development of several diseases such as cancer, neurodegenerative diseases, atherosclerosis, and prostaglandin-mediated inflammatory processes [2-3]. Many papers have covered the well-established physiological antioxidant roles of α-tocoferol, ferulic acid, ascorbic acid and enzymes, such as superoxide dismutase and glutathione peroxidase, myo-inositol hexaphosphoric acid and their derivatives [4]. Moreover, their superior biological properties have been extensively investigated for potential use in the food, pharmaceutical, biomedical and cosmetic industries [5-6].

Among the realm of antioxidant occurring molecules, a crucial role is played by polyphenols. These basically consist of phenolic acids and flavonoids, with a high chemical variety in relation to the number of aromatic rings and to the number and the position of phenolic groups [7]. These secondary plant metabolites, naturally present in fruit and vegetables, are part of our daily diet. In the last fifteen years polyphenols have generated great interest among the scientific community, in particular after the publication of several epidemiological studies showing an inverse correlation between dietary consumption of polyphenol-rich food and incidence and mortality for cardiovascular disease and cancer. The activity of these molecules mainly related to the ability to scavenge free radicals, donate hydrogen atoms or electron, or chelate metal ions. A number of studies have devoted their attention to understanding the biochemical mechanisms involved in different biological activities of polyphenols [8]. In this regard, it should be considered that polyphenols can act as both pharmaceutical coadjuvants and/or therapeutic agents.

The antioxidant and biological properties of polyphenols are related not only to the structure of phenolic compounds, but also to their solubility properties which greatly influence their biomedical applications [9]. Several research groups have focused their attention to the chemical modification of polyphenols to improve their solubility. Recently, by-products from the wood industry, in particular sawdust from sawmills, have been proposed as a potential source of tannins, cheap antioxidants for the food industry [10]. These tannins containing many OH groups are water-soluble and they have limited solubility in lipid environments such as the cell membrane. For this reason, they do not act as effective autoxidizing agents in the lipid bi-layer. To improve this defect, chemical reactions, e.g., esterification with a fatty acid or alcohol have been proposed to improve their lipophilicity, preserving the antioxidant properties [11]. The esterification of polyphenols to modify their hydrophilic properties is one of several different chemical modifications of these antioxidant compounds.

In the present chapter, we will give an overview of the most important polyphenol conjugates, with specific attention to the naturally occurring derivatives as well as to the most innovative synthetic materials.

Polyphenol Conjugated in Plants

Deep physical-chemical and biological characterization of polyphenol conjugates extracted from different plants have been described (table 1).

Polyphenol-polysaccharide conjugates were isolated from plant extracts obtained from 17 Polish traditional medicinal plants, belonging to *Asteraceae* and *Rosaceae* families [12]. The researchers investigated the role of these polyphenolic-polysaccharide conjugates in the defence against oxidative stress induced by peroxynitrite anions in human platelets [13]. Blood platelets are involved in inflammatory responses because they can deliver various biologically active compounds like serotonin, histamine, and platelet activation factor. Moreover, $NO^{\bullet}$ and $O2^{\bullet -}$, reactive nitrogen and oxygen species, are generated in platelets.

Table 1. Natural polyphenols and polymer found in plants and their biomedical activity

Polyphenol	Bioactivity
Epigallocatechin-3-gallate Source: Green Tea	- Anticancer effects - Cardioprotective effect - Prevention of liver injury - Neuroprotection - Antiulcer properties - Prevention of decline of bone microarchitecture -Antioxidant properties
Resveratrol Source: Red Wine	- Cardioprotective effect - Protection of Endothelial functions - Reduction of blood pressure - Inhibition of vascular inflammation - Prevention of platelet aggregation - Reduction of oxidative stress - Reduction of cardiac hypertrophy - Anti-atherogenic effect
Quercetin Source: Red Wine	- Protection of Endothelial functions - Antiatherogenic effect - Anti-inflammatory effect
Polyphenol -Polysaccharide Conjugates Source: Asteraceae and Rosaceae	- Anti-inflammatory effect
Polyphenol -Polysaccharide Conjugates Source: C. Canadensis	- Protection of blood platelets function
Hydroxybenzoic and Cinnamic acid derivatives Source: Swallow root	- Antioxidant properties - Fibroblast protection - Protection against DNA damage
Semimyrtucommulone and Myrtucommulone A Source: Myrtle	- Inhibition of oxidative degradation of cholesterol and LDL - Inhibition of linoleic acid peroxidation
Amentoflavone Source: Selaginella tamariscina	- Neuroprotection on neonatal brain
Decarboxymethyl ligstroside Source: Olive Oil	- Antiulcer properties
Geraniin and Corilagin Source: Japanese Medical Plants	- Anticancer properties
Tyrosol – Hydroxytyrosol Source: Grapes – Olives	- Cardioprotective effect
Epicatechin Source: Green Tea	- Neuroprotection
Myricetin Source: Grapes	- Keratinocytes protection
Procyanidin Source: Parkia biglobosa	- Protection of Endothelial functions
Oligomeric Procyanidins Source: Larix gmelinii bark	- Antioxidant properties
Proanthocyanidins Source: Persimmon leaf	- Anti-hypertensive effect
Insoluble components of foods Source: Cereals - Vegetables and oat flour	- Antioxidant properties in gastro-intestinal tract

The reaction of $O2^{-•}$ and $NO^{•}$ leads to production of peroxynitrite ($ONOO^{-}$), which can alter the mechanism of platelet activation and their hemostatic function, inducing the oxidation of platelet thiols, as well as the carbonylation and nitration of platelet and plasma proteins [14]. The whole of these modifications can alter the platelet response, and may be an important factor involved in cardiovascular diseases and in inflammatory conditions. Authors confirmed the suitability of polyphenol-polysaccharide conjugates extracted from *C. Canadensis* in reducing the nitrative and oxidative damage induced by $ONOO^{-}$ in blood platelets.

Harish Nayaka et al. (2010) determined the phenolic acid composition in swallow root (*Decalepis hamiltonii*) free phenolic acid (SRFP), swallow root conjugated phenolic acid (SRCP) and swallow root insoluble-bound phenolic acid (SRIBP) extracts. Moreover it was demonstrated that these components possess cytoprotection activity on NIH 3T3 fibroblast cells because they showed radical scavenging ability and protection against DNA damage induced by hydroxyl radical [15].

Myrtle (*Myrtus communis* L., Myrtaceae) is widely distributed in the Mediterranean area and is used as a culinary spice and an antiseptic and anti-inflammatory agent in folk medicine. Oligomeric non-prenylated acylphloroglucinols, called semimyrtucommulone and myrtucommulone A, isolated from myrtle, represent a particular kind of natural polyphenol conjugate [16]. These compounds showed potent protective effect in simplified models of oxidative degradation of cholesterol and LDL, which play crucial role in the development of cardiovascular diseases. Importantly, it was demonstrated that myrtucommulone induces apoptosis of cancer cells via the intrinsic mitochondrial pathway and only marginally affects normal non transformed cells [17]. Serpen and colleagues analyzed the health effects of the insoluble matter in many food samples such as cereals, vegetables and oat flour, proving that antioxidant functional groups, such as phenolic acids, bond to the insoluble components of foods and they quench free radicals [18]. To confirm that the antioxidant activity of these insoluble food components was related to the presence of fiber-bound antioxidant compounds, authors evaluated the reduction of the antioxidant activity by means of alkaline hydrolysis, and as a result, a 90% reduction of the antioxidant activity was recorded. Furthermore, authors elucidated that the insoluble matters of food remain in the gastrointestinal tract for a long time and may help in quenching the soluble radicals that are continuously produced in the intestinal tract and that could be involved in the etiology of colon cancer [19].

Innovative Polyphenol Conjugates: Modification with Natural Polymers

There are many reports on the design and synthesis of bio-conjugates obtained by the covalent linkage of polyphenols with natural polymers, like proteins and polysaccharides, which could be applied in the food, biomedical and "health-care" industry.

The main limitation in the practical employment of polyphenols as preservatives in the food industry is their low stability when exposed to high temperature, light, etc. The conjugation of antioxidants to biomacromolecules can overcome this drawback, conferring a high value to both the components: the antioxidant molecule, when linked to a macromolecule, becomes more stable, while the biopolymer acquires the properties of the linked antioxidant. Several different polysaccharides and proteins have been used as starting materials for the preparation of innovative antioxidant bio-conjugates and an overview of the most significant are reported below.

By virtue of its special biocompatible and antimicrobial activity, chitosan is one of the most studied polysaccharides, and it is applied in different fields, such as wound healing and food packaging [20-21]. The synthesis of chitosan-polyphenol conjugates have been proposed by employing different synthetic approaches. Tyrosinase has been used to graft flavonoids onto chitosan macromolecules using a non-specific chemical approach as an attractive nontoxic and environmentally friendly alternative [22]. With the grafting of the flavonoid onto chitosan fibers, the antioxidant properties were enhanced when compared to the unmodified fibers. This conjugation enhanced the antibacterial activity [23] and the anticancer activity of flavonoids [24]. These authors showed increased antitumoral activity of curcumin when this was conjugated with chitosan.

The major catechins, a group of polyphenols, in green tea include: Epigallocatechin-3 Gallate (EGCG); Epigallocatecin (EGC); Epicatechin (EC); and Epicatechin Gallate (ECG). EGCG being the most abundant and best studied for its anticancer activity.

In order to improve catechin stability and activity many different natural polymers were used for their conjugation, such as chitosan, dextran, gelatin etc. Catechin- and gallic acid-chitosan conjugates, retaining the antioxidant properties of the linked polyphenol, were obtained by free radical grafting procedure [25]. This synthetic approach allowed us to work in eco-friendly conditions, because the use of organic solvents and the generation of toxic by-products were completely avoided; to initiate the grafting reaction, a water soluble redox initiator system, composed of ascorbic acid and hydrogen peroxide was employed. A possible mechanism of antioxidant insertion onto chitosan involves the interaction between the hydroxyl radicals, generated by the redox pair initiator system, with the H-atoms contained in the α-methylene (CH_2) or with the hydroxyl groups (OH) of the hydroxymethylene group or with the amino group. At those sites, the insertion of the antioxidant molecules can subsequently occur by hydroxyl radicals, generated by the interaction between redox pair components, attack H-atoms in α-methylene (CH_2) or hydroxyl groups (OH) of the hydroxymethylene group of the chitosan. In addition, the reactive amino group in chitosan is important in several of the structural modifications targeted because the deprotonated amino group acts as a powerful nucleophile (pKa 6.3) readily reacting with electrophilic reagents. Even in free radical initiated copolymerization, NH_2 groups of chitosan are involved in macroradical formation at those sites, the insertion of the antioxidant molecules can occur.

In another work, chitosan/(3-chloropropyl)trimethoxysilane hybrid scaffolds (CTS/CPTMS) were functionalized with caffeic acid by a grafting approach [26]. The conjugation of caffeic acid to CTS/CPTMS hybrid scaffold increased the compressive strength of the material and enhanced its scavenging activity, anti-cancer property, and antibacterial activity. In human osteosarcoma UMR-106 cells, the caffeic acid grafted scaffolds inhibited cell growth, alkaline phosphatase activity and cell attachment.

Pasanphan and colleagues employed electron paramagnetic resonance (EPR) to demonstrate a wide range of antioxidant activity for a chitosan-gallic acid conjugate synthesized in the presence of 1-ethyl-3-(3'-dimethylaminopropyl) carbodiimide as a coupling agent [27]. Even if the functionalization degree was only 15%, high antioxidant ability was recorded, as highlighted by the EC_{50} values (0.021 mg mL^{-1} for $^{\bullet}R$ and 0.066 mg

mL^{-1} for $^{\bullet}OH$), when compared to other chitosan derivatives, such as sulfated chitosan (EC50 = 0.1 mL^{-1} for $^{\bullet}R$ and 3.269 mg mL^{-1} for $^{\bullet}OH$).

Another study reports on the preparation of nanoparticles with both antioxidant and antibacterial properties by grafting eugenol and carvacrol (two components of essential oils) on chitosan nanoparticles [28]. Eugenol and carvacrol were firstly formulated, and then the grafting of these oils to chitosan nanoparticles was carried out via the Schiff base reaction, obtaining carvacrol-grafted chitosan nanoparticles (CHCA NPs) and eugenol-grafted chitosan nanoparticles (CHEU NPs). The scavenging activity of CHCA NPs and CHEU NPs conjugates was much higher than the free carvacrol and eugenol [28].

Besides chitosan, other polysaccharides have been exploited for the synthesis of antioxidant conjugates. Cirillo and colleagues synthesized a starch-quercetin conjugate (ST-Q) by free-radical grafting procedure using, as reported before for chitosan, ascorbic acid and hydrogen peroxide as free radical initiators. Stability tests, performed by UV-irradiation, demonstrated that the insertion of Q in starch structure increased the stability of macromolecule, as confirmed by a degradation value of 9 % compared to 24% for native starch [29]. Similarly, the conjugate was found to be stable against α-amylase degradation, with a 44% lower degradation value compared to that obtained when native starch is used. The antioxidant tests confirmed high antioxidant ability as showed by the EC_{50} values of 2.52 mg mL^{-1} for DPPH; 1.15 mg mL^{-1} for peroxynitrite and 4.31 mg mL^{-1} for lipid peroxidation assay. Results also show an enhanced ability of starch conjugate in preventing gallic acid (used as a model drug) from degradation. The amount of preserved drug by the antioxidant macromolecular system was almost 95% in all the environments tested, while native starch was less effective, with preserved gallic acid of about 30% under light stress, 43% under thermal treatment and 52% under oxidative stress. Finally, authors evaluated the enzymatic activity of the conjugate against acetylcholine esterase (EC_{50} of 12.1 mg mL^{-1}), tyrosinase (EC_{50} of 15.7 mg mL^{-1}) to prove the potential beneficial effects of ST-Q on human health.

The same synthetic procedure was exploited to obtain the covalent conjugation of catechin to alginate and inulin, linear polysaccharides widely used in food and beverage areas [30]. The characterization of the conjugates showed that the antioxidant properties of catechin are completely retained after the conjugation process. In a recent work, inulin-catechin conjugate was further engineered by adding the thermo-responsive element, N-isopropylacrylamide (NIPAAm). This polymer undergoes a sharp coil-globule transition and phase separation at a temperature of 30-32°C (low critical solution temperature – LCST) [31]. This interesting characteristic allows to modulate the antioxidant properties of the biomaterial in relation to the temperature deviation around the LCST. A hydrogel with antioxidant properties controlled by the external temperature were obtained by performing the direct polymerization of inulin with catechin (CA), NIPAAm and N,N-ethylenebisacrylamide (EBA) (used as crosslinking agent).

In a different study we described a dextran-catechin conjugate obtained by radical grafting proposed as an anticancer agent for the treatment of pancreatic ductal adenocarcinoma [32]. We observed significant cytotoxicity against pancreatic cancer cells (IC_{50} of 377.7 mg mL^{-1} for MIA PaCa-2 and 295.34 mg mL^{-1} for PL45 cells) with lower effects on non-neoplastic cells (IC_{50} of 838.33 mg $mL^{-1}$for HPNE cells), indicating its potential for low toxicity on normal tissues commonly associated with standard chemotherapy treatments.

In other works, the functionalization of carboxylic group with dicyclohexylcarbodiimide was used as a synthetic strategy to couple ferulic acid and α-tocopherol to microcrystalline cellulose [33], and ferulic acid to dextran [34]. These systems were found to be effective in inhibiting the free radical damage in rat liver microsomal membranes in the range of 0.5-6 mg/ml.

Most of the described studies exploit the conjugation of polysaccharides with antioxidants, however some examples of protein-based antioxidant conjugates can be found in the literature. An interesting study was published by Valenta and colleagues in 1998, where lysozyme was modified by the covalent attachment of caffeic acid and cinnamic acid in order to generate preservatives exhibiting a broad antimicrobial spectrum against Gram-positive and Gram-negative bacteria. Condensation reaction mediated by a water-soluble carbodiimide was employed as a synthetic strategy to obtain the constitution of amide bindings between the carboxyl groups of ligands and primary amino groups of the enzyme. It was found that the conjugates were characterized by a wider antimicrobial spectrum compared to non-modified lysozyme and the results show a concentration of 0.2% of the lysozyme-caffeic acid/lysozyme mixture (1+1) as the minimum required to exert a bacteriostatic effect for Gram-negative as well as for Gram-positive bacteria [35].

Gelatin, a degradation product of collagen, extensively used in food, adhesives and the pharmaceutical field, is another key protein modified with antioxidant moieties through different synthetic strategies. This protein is characterized by a low level of immunostimulation and cytotoxicity and it is easy to modify at the level of its amino acid groups [36].

Chung et al. proposed the use of a laccase-catalyzed oxidation to covalently conjugate catechin to gelatin through the lysine residues. As a result, the gelatin-catechin conjugate was more capable of inhibiting oxidation of LDL than unconjugated catechin. At a concentration of 70 μM the conjugate reduces the fluorescence due to the oxidative marker to 45%, while this value was 60% for free flavonoid [37].

The addition of antioxidant molecules on gelatin side chains was also obtained by radical reaction of gelatin with gallic acid and catechin. The hydrogen peroxide redox pair was used as an initiator system [38]. As reported in the case of polysaccharides, the hydroxyl radicals generated by the interaction among redox pair components, attack the sensible residues in the side chains of protein, producing radical species on the aminoacidic structure. After that, antioxidant molecules were added to the reaction mixture, obtaining the formation of antioxidant-gelatin covalent bonds. The conjugates were characterized by increased scavenging and antioxidant activities compared with the free gallic acid. An extensive biological characterization of the gelatin-gallic acid conjugate was performed in view of possible biomedical applications of this macromolecular system [39]. First, the scavenging properties towards peroxynitrite anion were tested showing that the EC_{50} value of gallic acid does not significantly change after the conjugation process. Second, the functionality of the conjugate was explored in terms of beneficial effects on human health by testing its activity on selected enzymes. Specifically, acetyl cholinesterase and α-amylase were tested to investigate putative beneficial effects of the synthesized biopolymer in the treatment of Alzheimer disease and diabetes. The recorded enzyme activity showed an EC_{50} values of 7.1 and 9.8 mg mL^{-1}, respectively for acetyl cholinesterase and α-amylase. Furthermore, the anticancer activity of the bio-conjugate was determined in prostate carcinoma and renal carcinoma cell lines by comparing its effect on cancer cell viability with pure gelatin. The results showed that the conjugate is able to reduce the viability of all the tested cancer cell lines with a considerably higher efficiency than the free drug. The same protein conjugate was employed for the preparation of composites materials by incorporation of carbon nanotubes (CNT) into the polymer. This nanocomposite was tested as an anticancer polymer therapeutic in HeLa cancer cells and results showed that the presence of CNT into the sample greatly enhances the anticancer activity by virtue of the increased uptake [40].

Another class of antioxidant conjugate is referred to antioxidant peptides [41]. These materials could be prepared through enzymatic hydrolysis from various natural proteins [42-43], synthetic peptide libraries or chemical modification of preformed peptides [44]. On a study focused on the enhancement of the antioxidant activity of hydroxycinnamic acids through conjugation with antioxidative peptides [45]. Authors concluded that Caffeic Acid-Ala-His-NH_2 was an ideal antioxidant in both hydrophilic and hydrophobic environments. In a subsequent study the same authors focused their attention on histidine residue and constructed histidine dipeptide libraries in order to increase the antioxidant potential [46]. Experimental data showed that the conjugation of caffeic acid to histidine-containing dipeptides enhanced its antioxidant activity because of the radical trapping ability of imidazole in histidine. Caffeic Acid-Pro-His-NH_2 was found to be a powerful ideal antioxidant in both hydrophilic and lipophilic systems, probably because the structure of proline enabled histidine to stabilize the hydroxyls of the polyphenol, leading to the enhanced antioxidative activities. Furthermore, proline gives a critical effect on the enhanced antioxidant activity [47].

Ouberai and colleagues in 2009 synthesized an interesting class of polyphenol-peptide conjugate [48]. These materials can have a great potential in the treatment of Alzheimer disease by virtue of their ability to inhibit the aggregation of β-amyloid peptides into toxic aggregates. The curcumin-polypeptide conjugates represent another clear example of material effective in binding amyloid peptides [49].

Polyphenol Conjugate by Synthetic Routes

The high antioxidant properties of conjugated polyphenols, as well as their enhanced chemical and physical properties, have led to the development of synthetic materials able to couple the biological functionalities of polyphenols with the chemical properties of polymeric materials (table 2).

An example on this concept is the preparation of a synthetic derivative of curcumin [50]. Despite its broad effects on the biological functions of cells, the potential use of curcumin as a therapeutic agent is severely affected by its low water solubility, poor in vivo bioavailability, and rapid metabolism. Its structure has also been widely modified to improve its pharmacokinetic profile, focusing mainly on changes in the β-diketone structure and aryl substitution pattern of the molecule [51]. Simoni et al., considering the ability of polyamine to specifically convey a bioactive functionality into mitochondria by virtue of electrostatic forces, developed a polyamine derivative of the curcumin analogue, 3,5-dibenzylidenepiperidin-4-one (DBP) [50]. The results demonstrated that the proposed bioconjugate retained all the antioxidant activity of DBP, which was accompanied by a significant loss of cytotoxicity.

Table 2. Natural and synthetic polymers modified by conjugation with polyphenols

Polyphenol	Polymers
Flavonoids	Chitosan
Catechin – Gallic acid	Chitosan
Caffeic acid	Chitosan
Eugenol and Carvacrol	Chitosan
Quercetin	Starch
Catechin	Dextran
Catechin	Alginate – Inulin
Catechin	Inulin
Ferulic acid – α-tocopherol	Cellulose
Ferulic acid	Dextran
Caffeic acid – Cinnamic acid	Lysozyme
Catechin	Gelatin
Catechin	Omopolymer
Epigallocatechin-3-gallate	Omopolymer
Quercetin	Omopolymer
Rutin	Omopolymer
Catechin	Omopolymer
Trolox	Omopolymer
Gallic acid	Gelatin
Hydroxycinnamic acids	Antioxidant Peptides
Caffeic acid	Antioxidant Peptides
Curcumin	Peptides
Curcumin	Polyamine
Catechin	poly(allylamine)
Catechin – Quercetin	Bovine Serum Albumin – α-casein
Catechin	Poly(ε-lysine)
Salicylic derivatives	Poly(melamine)
Resveratrol	poly-ε-caprolactone-co-acrylic acid
Ferulic acid	Poly(methacrylic acid)
Quercetin	Poly(methacrylic acid)
Quercetin	β-Cyclodextrin - Polyvinylpyrrolidone – Pluronic
Cinnamic acid	Epoxidized soybean oil
Catechin	Oligomeric silsesquioxane
Curcumin	Polyethylene Glycol
C. Platycladi extract	Polysaccharides
Gallic acid	Carbon Nanotubes

In a work of Li et al., resveratrol was coupled through a hydrolysable covalent bond with the carboxylic acid groups in porous poly-ε-caprolactone surface grafted with acrylic acid [52]. These authors demonstrated that this conjugation strategy preserved antioxidant properties of resveratrol. Moreover, when tested in vivo, the conjugated resveratrol showed increased DNA synthesis and alkaline phosphatase activity in osteoblasts and prevented femoral bone loss in ovariectomized rats.

Grafting procedures were also exploited for the direct co-polymerization of ferulic acid and methacrylic acid [53]. Both soluble and microparticulate systems were prepared by this innovative technique and the resulting functional polymers were found to be suitable for application as food preservatives and antimicrobial agents as a consequence of their ability to inhibit the free radical formation and the *S. Aureus* proliferation [54]. Methacrylic acid was also conjugated with quercetin and the obtained macromolecular system was found to be effective as an anticancer agent against HeLa cells, as a result of its increased stability [55].

With the aim to improve the physiological and pharmacokinetic properties of polyphenols, enzyme-catalyzed conjugation reactions were developed [56]. The biomimetic process using oxidative enzymes is of great interest for the "in situ" production of biopolymers and for further applications onto fabrics, satisfying an environmentally friendly concept by replacing chemical processes. Laccase-catalyzed enzymatic synthesis of catechin conjugate with poly(allylamine) has led to materials with improved physiological properties in comparison with unconjugated catechin [57]. Similarly, another study highlighted the ability of laccase to catalyze the conjugation of flavonoids (quercetin and catechin) with proteins (α-casein and BSA) [58]. The results showed that quercetin conjugates presented much higher antioxidant activity compared to protein-catechin conjugates (2-3 times higher). Similarly, a conjugate of catechin and poly(ε-lysine) was proposed as inhibitory agent of enzymes such as collagenase, hyaluronidase and xanthine oxidase which can be highly activated in different pathologies [59].

In different works, the conjugation of polyphenol was obtained in terms of synthesis of oligo-derivative of the antioxidant. This was the case for trolox [60], quercetin [61], catechin [62] and EGCG [63]. In the first case, poly-trolox ester nanoparticles were evaluated for their ability to either inhibit or induce cellular oxidative stress in a dose-dependent manner. This polymer delivery form demonstrated unique ability to suppress protein oxidation, a feature not seen in the free drug form, emphasizing the advantage of the delivery/dosage formulation on the regulating cellular response.

In the case of quercetin, the dissolution rate of the poorly water-soluble antioxidant drug was enhanced by fabricating its nanoparticles, complexes and solid dispersions with β-cyclodextrin, polyvinylpyrrolidone, and pluronic F127 using evaporative precipitation of nanosuspension. Similarly, a biocompatible route for the direct synthesis of water soluble polyquercetin was proposed by using horseradish peroxidase as a catalyst [64]. The resulting polymer was envisioned in order to be more thermally stable and therefore suitable for the highly regulated food industry and/or drug industry.

Regarding EGCG, the polymer obtained by its laccase-catalyzed oxidative coupling showed much higher superoxide anion scavenging activity than the EGCG monomer [63]. Catechin was polymerized by using both laccase and horseradish peroxidase as catalysts, and the obtained poly(catechin) was found to greatly scavenge superoxide anions in a concentration dependent manner, and almost completely scavenged at 200 μM, while the inhibition activity of monomeric catechin starts at 300 μM [62].

Laccase was also employed for the synthesis of polymeric derivatives of rutin, with the resulting poly(rutin) able to enhance the cell viability in the endothelium with higher protection effects against the oxidative damage in comparison to that of the rutin monomer [65].

Uyama made a detailed overview of polyphenol oligo-derivative of catechin. He focused on poly(catechin)s condensed through acetaldehyde, showing that this synthetic approach is one of the most efficient synthetic approaches to improve the physiological properties of catechin. The first tested effect was the inhibitory activities against LDL peroxidation, and it was found that catechin-acetaldehyde polycondensate showed greater activity compared to monomeric catechin and that the activity was dependent on the catechin unit concentration. The activity on xanthine oxidase was then evaluated for *p*-hydroxybenzaldehyde polycondensate; an inhibition effect higher than that recorded for monomeric catechin (which did not exhibit inhibition activity to a concentration up of 300 μM) was demonstrated. According to the author evaluation, this may be due to the interaction (hydrogen bonds and electrostatic interactions) of a phenol group in the side chain of *p*-hydroxybenzaldehyde polycondensate and xanthine oxidase [66].

Finally, an emerging research field is the conjugation of natural occurring polyphenols within nanomaterials [67]. A bio-conjugate of polyhedral oligomeric silsesquioxane and catechin, synthesized via horseradish peroxidase catalysis, has been proposed as a starting substrate to construct nanocomposites with precise control of nano-architecture and properties [68]. The conjugation of curcumin with poly(ethylene glycol) assisted magnetic iron oxide nanoparticles was achieved through a sonication mediated route, and, as a result, a synergic effect in free radical scavenging potency of the phytocompound in conjugated state was detected [69].

Recently, the synthesis of Ag nanoparticles generated by reducing $AgNO_3$ with the *C. Platycladi* extract was investigated and the antibacterial activities of the nanoparticles evaluated. Authors found that the biomolecules in the extract, played a dual role as reducing and protecting agents and that the reducing sugars and flavonoids were mainly responsible for the bioreduction of silver ions [70].

As reported for natural polymers, the conjugation of polyphenol compounds to nanomaterials was also performed by grafting procedure. In particular, the grafting of gallic acid onto CNTs was obtained by the radical insertion of gallic acid on the CNT's shell. Specific tests were performed to prove that the GA-CNT conjugate retains all the biological properties of the free polyphenol [71].

In a most recent work Cirillo et al. synthesized an innovative polymer therapeutic made of quercetin, carbon nanotubes and polymethacrylic acid [40]. The flavonoid quercetin was selected as biologically active components due to its well know anticancer activity [72]; the polymeric part polymethacrylic acid (PMAA) enhanced the flavonoid water solubility and increased its stability leading to a sustained activity over time [73]; the Carbon Nanotubes (CNT) component increased the interaction with cells by virtue of its ability to be highly internalized into living cells and tissue leading to a higher efficiency of the whole system [74]. This nano modified compound was very effective in inducing the apoptosis in cancer cells without any side effects on non-malignant cells [40].

Conclusion

Reactive oxygen species exert a multitude of biological effects covering a wide spectrum that ranges from physiological regulatory functions to damaging alterations participating in the pathogenesis of an increasing number of diseases. Several natural antioxidants have been investigated in vitro and in animal models to assess their potential therapeutic effect in conditions linked to oxidative stress. Polyphenols are the major class of antioxidant able to reduce the oxidative damages of lipids, proteins, enzymes, carbohydrates, and DNA in living cells and tissues. However, the stability of polyphenols remains one of the major challenges in their application. The recent development of innovative chemical strategies in the synthesis of polymers and nano-materials has been exploited to modify the polyphenols, thus allowing their use for medical application. In this chapter we described the main chemical strategies exploited for increasing the stability and the activity of polyphenol at physiological conditions. The combination of polyphenols with natural and synthetic polymers represents a new and promising strategy for developing more effective antioxidants.

Acknowledgments

Vice Chancellor's Fellowship University of New South Wales, NSW, Australia (O.V.)

National Health and Medical Research Council, Senior Research Fellowship, NSW, Australia (M.K.)

Regional Operative Program (ROP) Calabria ESF 2007/2013 – IV Axis Human Capital Operative Objective M2 - Action D.5 (G.C.)

References

[1] S. Reuter, S. C. Gupta, M.M. Chaturvedi, B.B. Aggarwal, Oxidative stress, inflammation, and cancer: How are they linked? *Free Radical Biology & Medicine* 49 (2010) 1603–1616.

[2] J. W. Stephens, P.M. Khanolkar and S.C. Bain, The biological relevance and measurement of plasma markers of oxidative stress in diabetes and cardiovascular disease. *Atherosclerosis* 202 (2009) 321-329.

[3] F. L. Muller, M.S. Lustgarten, Y. Jang, A. Richardson and H. Van Remmen, Trends in oxidative aging theories. *Free Radical Biol. Med.* 43 (2007) 477-503.

[4] M. S. Brewer, Natural Antioxidants: Sources, Compounds, Mechanisms of Action, and Potential Applications. *Comprehensive Reviews in Food Science and Food Safety* 10 (2010) 221–247.

[5] B. Halliwell and J.M.Gutteridge, Free radicals, antioxidants, and human disease: curiosity, cause, or consequence? *Lancet* 344 (1994) 721-724.

[6] A. Azzi, K.J.A.Davies and F. Kelly, Free radical biology – terminology and critical thinking. *FEBS Letters* 558 (2004) 3-6.

[7] L. Bravo, Polyphenols: chemistry, dietary sources, metabolism, and nutritional significance. *Nutrit. Rev*. 56 (1998) 317-333.

[8] B. Frei and J.V. Higdon, Antioxidant activity of tea polyphenols in vivo: evidence from animal studies. *J. Nutr.* 133 (2003) 3275S-3284S.

[9] R. Tsao, Chemistry and Biochemistry of Dietary Polyphenols. *Nutrients* 2 (2010)1231-1246.

[10] B. Poaty, S. Dumarçay, P. Gérardin and D. Perrin, Modification of grape seed and wood tannins to lipophilic antioxidant derivatives. *Ind. Crops Prod.* 31 (2012) 509-515.

[11] G. Jin and H. Yoshioka, Synthesis of lipophilic poly-lauronyl(+)-catechins and radical-scavenging activity. *Biosci. Biotechnol. Biochem.* 69 (2005) 440-447.

[12] L. Pawlaczyk, L. Czerchawski, W. Pilecki, E. Lamer-Zarawska and R. Gancarz, Polyphenolic-polysaccharide compounds from selected medicinal plants of Asteraceae and Rosaceae families: Chemical characterization and blood anticoagulant activity. *Carbohyd. Res.* 77 (2009) 568-575.

[13] L. Pawlaczyk, L. Czerchawski, W. Kuliczkowski, B. Karolko, W. Pilecki, W. Witkiewicz and R. Gancarz, Anticoagulant and anti-platelet activity of polyphenolic-polysaccharide preparation isolated from the medicinal plant Erigeron canadensis L. *Thromb. Res.* 127 (2011) 328-340.

[14] J. Saluk-Juszczak, B. Olas, I. Pawlaczyk, R. Gancarz and B. Wachowicz, Effects of the extract from Conyza canadensis on human blood platelet aggregation. *Gen. Physiol. Biophys* 26 (2007) 150-152.

[15] M. A. Harish Nayaka, U.V. Sathisha and S.M. Dharmesh, Cytoprotective and antioxidant activity of free, conjugated and insoluble-bound phenolic acids from swallow root (Decalepis hamiltonii) *Food Chem.* 119 (2010) 1307-1

[16] A. Rosa, M.P. Melis, M. Deiana, A. Atzeri, G. Appendino, G. Corona, A. Incani, D. Loru, and M.A. Dessì, Protective effect of the oligomeric acylphloroglucinols from Myrtus communis on cholesterol and human low density lipoprotein oxidation. *Chem. Phys. Lip.* 155 (2008). 16-23.

[17] I. Tretiakova, D. Blaesius, L. Maxia, S. Wesselborg, K. Schulze-Osthoff, J.Jr. Cinatl, M. Michaelis, O. Werz, Myrtucommulone from Myrtus communis induces apoptosis in cancer cells via the mitochondrial pathway involving caspase-9. *Apoptosis* 13 (2008) 119-31.

[18] A. Serpen, E. Capuano, V. Fogliano and V. Gökmen, New Procedure to Measure the Antioxidant Activity of Insoluble Food Components. *J. Agric. Food Chem.* 55 (2007) 7676-7681.

[19] C. F. Babbs and M.G. Steiner, Simulation of Free Radical Reactions in Biology and Medicine: A New Two- Compartment Kinetic Model of Intracellular Lipid Peroxidation." *Free Radical Biology and Medicine* 8.5 (1990): 471-85.

[20] M. Maeda, H. Murakami, H. Ohta and M. Tajima. Stimulation of IgM 15 production in human-human hybridoma HB4C5 cells by chitosan. *Biosci. Biotechnol. Biochem.* 56 (1992) 427-431.

[21] S.Y. Chae, M. Jang and J. Nah, Influence of molecular weight on oral absorption of water soluble chitosans. *J. Control. Rel.* 102 (2004) 383-394.

[22] F. Sousa, G.M. Guebitz, and V. Kokol, Antimicrobial and antioxidant properties of chitosan enzymatically functionalized with flavonoids. *Progress Biochem.* 44 (2009) 749-756.

[23] W. Xie, P. Xu, W. Wang and Q. Liu, Preparation and antibacterial activity of a water-soluble chitosan derivative. *Carbohydr. Polym.* 50 (2002).:35-40.

[24] F. Sousa, G. M. Guebitz, V. Kokol, Antimicrobial and antioxidant properties of chitosan enzymatically functionalized with flavonoids. *Process Biochemistry* 44 (2009) 749–756.

[25] M. Curcio, F. Puoci, F. Iemma, O.I. Parisi, G. Cirillo, U.G. Spizzirri, and N. Picci Covalent Insertion of Antioxidant Molecules on Chitosan by a Free Radical Grafting Procedure. *J. Agric. Food Chem.* 57 (2009) 5933-5938.

[26] J. C. Shiu, M.H. Ho, S.H. Yu, A.C. Chao, Y.R. Su, W.J. Chen, Z.C. Chiang and W.P Yang, (Preparation and characterization of caffeic acid grafted chitosan/CPTMS hybrid scaffolds. *Carbohyd. Polym.* 79 (2010).724-730.

[27] W. Pasanphan, G.R. Buettner and S. Chirachanchai, Chitosan gallate as a novel potential polysaccharide antioxidant: an EPR study. *Carbohyd. Res.* 345 (2010) 132-140.

[28] F. Chen, Z. Shi, K.G. Neoh and E.T. Kang, Antioxidant and Antibacterial Activities of Eugenol and Carvacrol-Grafted Chitosan Nanoparticles. *Biotech. Bioeng.* 104 (2009) 30-39.

[29] Cirillo, F. Puoci, F. Iemma, M. Curcio, O.I. Parisi, U.G. Spizzirri, I. Altimari and N. Picci. Starch-quercetin conjugate by radical grafting: synthesis and biological characterization. *Pharm. Dev. Technol.* 17 (2012) 466-476.

[30] U. G. Spizzirri, O.I. Parisi, F. Iemma, G. Cirillo, F. Puoci, M. Curcio and N. Picci, Antioxidant–polysaccharide conjugates for food application by eco-friendly grafting procedure. *Carbohyd. Polym.* 79 (2010) 333-340.

[31] U. G. Spizzirri, I. Altimari, F. Puoci, O.I. Parisi, F. Iemma and N. Picci, Innovative antioxidant thermo-responsive hydrogels by radical grafting of catechin on inulin chain. *Carbohyd. Polym.* 84 (2011) 517-523.

[32] O. Vittorio, G. Cirillo, F. Iemma, G. Di Turi, E. Jacchetti, M. Curcio, S. Barbuti, N. Funel, O.I. Parisi, F. Puoci and N. Picci. Dextran-catechin conjugate: a potential treatment against the pancreatic ductal adenocarcinoma. *Pharm. Res.* 29 (2012) 2601-2614.

[33] S. Trombino, R. Cassano, E. Bloise, R. Muzzalupo, S. Leta, F. Puoci and N. Picci, Design and synthesis of cellulose derivatives with antioxidant activity. *Macromol.Biosci.* 8 (2008) 86-95.

[34] R. Cassano, S. Trombino, R. Muzzalupo, L. Tavano and N. Picci. A novel dextran hydrogel linking trans-ferulic acid for the stabilization and transdermal delivery of vitamin E. *Eur. J. Pharm. Biopharm.* 72 (2009) 232-238.

[35] C. Valenta, E. Schwarz and A. Bernkop-Schnurch. Lysozyme-caffeic acid conjugates: possible novel preservatives for dermal formulations. *Int. J. Pharm.* 174 (1998) 125-132.

[36] N. R. Maddux, S.B. Joshi, D.B. Volkin, J.P. Ralston and C.R. Middaugh, Multidimensional methods for the formulation of biopharmaceuticals and vaccines. *Food Hydrocol.* 25 (2011) 1813-1827.

[37] J. E. Chung, M. Kurisawa, H. Uyama and S. Kobayashi, Enzymatic synthesis and antioxidant property of gelatin-catechin conjugates. *Biotech. Lett.* 25 (2003a) 1993-1997.

[38] U. G. Spizzirri, F. Iemma, F. Puoci, G. Cirillo, M. Curcio, O.I. Parisi and N. Picci. Synthesis of Antioxidant Polymers by Grafting of Gallic acid and Catechin on Gelatin *Biomacromolecules* 10 (2009) 1923-1930.

[39] G. Cirillo, K. Kraemer, S. Fuessel, F. Puoci, M. Curcio, U.G. Spizzirri, I. Altimari and F. Iemma. Biological Activity of a Gallic Acid-Gelatin Conjugate. *Biomacromolecules* 11 (2010) 3309-3315.

[40] G. Cirillo O. Vittorio, S. Hampel, F. Iemma, P. Parchi, M. Cecchini, F. Puoci, N. Picci,b Quercetin nanocomposite as novel anticancer therapeutic: Improved efficiency

and reduced toxicity, *European Journal of Pharmaceutical Sciences* 49 (2013) 359–365.

[41] E. Y. Park, H. Murakami and Y. Matsumura, Effects of the addition of amino acids and peptides on lipid oxidation in a powdery model system. *J. Agric. Food Chem.* 53 (2005) 8334-8341.

[42] E. Mendis, N. Rajapakse, S.K. Kim, Antioxidant Properties of a Radical-Scavenging Peptide Purified from Enzymatically Prepared Fish Gelatin Hydrolysate. *J. Agric. Food* Chem. 53 (2005) 581-587.

[43] K. C. Hsu, G.H. Lu and C.L. Jao. Antioxidative properties of peptides prepared from tuna cooking juice hydrolysates with orientase (Bacillus subtilis). *Food Res.* Int. 42 (2009) 647-652.

[44] K. Saito, D.H. Jin, T. Ogawa, K. Muramoto, E. Hatakeyama, T. Yasuhara and K. NokiharaAntioxidative properties of tripeptide libraries prepared by the combinatorial chemistry. *J. Agric. Food Chem.* 51 (2003) 3668-3674.

[45] S. Y. Kwak, H.S. Seo and Y.S. Lee, Synergistic antioxidative activities of hydroxycinnamoyl-peptides. *J. Pept. Sci.* 15 (2009) 634-641.

[46] H. S. Seo, S.Y. Kwak and Y.S. Lee. Antioxidative activities of histidine containing caffeic acid-dipeptides. *Bioorg. Med. Chem. Lett.* 20 (2010) 4266-4272.

[47] S.Y. Kwak, S. Lee, J.K. Yang, and Y.S. Lee, Antioxidative activities of caffeoyl-proline dipeptides. *Food Chem.* 130 (2012) 847-852.

[48] M. Ouberai, P. Dumy, S. Chierici and J. Garcia, Synthesis and Biological Evaluation of Clicked Curcumin and Clicked KLVFFA Conjugates as Inhibitors of β-Amyloid Fibril Formation. *Bioconjugate Chem.* 20 (2009) 2123–2132.

[49] M. Daval, S. Bedrood, T. Gurlo, C.J. Huang, S. Costes, P. C. Butler and R. Langen, The effect of curcumin on human islet amyloid polypeptide misfolding and toxicity. *Amyloid* 17 (2010) 118–128.

[50] E. Simoni, C. Bergamini, R. Fato, A. Tarozzi, S. Bains, R. Motterlini, A. Cavalli, M.L. Bolognesi, A. Minarini, P. Hrelia, G. Lenaz, M. Rosini and C. Melchiorre Polyamine Conjugation of Curcumin Analogues toward the Discovery of Mitochondria-Directed Neuroprotective Agents. *J. Med. Chem.* 53 (2010) 7264-7268.

[51] S. Padhye, D. Chavan, S. Pandey, J. Deshpande, K.V. Swamy and F.H. Sarkar, Perspectives on chemopreventive and therapeutic potential of curcumin analogs in medicinal chemistry. *Mini-Rev. Med. Chem.* 10 (2010) 372-387.

[52] Y. Li, S. Danmark, U. Edlund, A. Finne-Wistrand, X. He, M. Norgard, E. Blomén, K. Hultenby, G. Andersson and U. Lindgren, Resveratrol-conjugated poly-e-caprolactone facilitates in vitro mineralization and in vivo bone regeneration. *Acta Biomat.* 7 (2011) 751-758.

[53] F. Puoci, F. Iemma, M. Curcio, O.I. Parisi, G. Cirillo, U.G. Spizzirri and N. Picci, Synthesis of Methacrylic-Ferulic Acid Copolymer with Antioxidant Properties by Single-Step Free Radical Polymerization. *J. Agric. Food Chem.* 56 (2008) 10646-10650.

[54] F. Iemma, F. Puoci, M. Curcio, O.I. Parisi, G. Cirillo, U.G. Spizzirri and N. Picci. Ferulic Acid as a Comonomer in the Synthesis of a Novel Polymeric Chain with Biological Properties. *J. Appl. Polym. Sci.* 115 (2010) 784-789.

[55] F. Puoci, C. Morelli, G. Cirillo, M. Curcio, O.I Parisi, P. Maris, D. Sisci and N. Picci. Anticancer Activity of a Quercetin-based Polymer towards HeLa Cancer Cells. *Anticancer Res*. 32 (2012) 2843-2847.
[56] P. Gogoi, S. Hazarika, N.N. Dutta and P.G. Rao, Kinetics and mechanism on laccase catalyzed synthesis of poly(allylamine)–catechin conjugate. *Chem. Eng. J.* 163 (2010) 86-92.
[57] E. I. Chung, M. Kurisawa, Y. Tachibana, H. Uyama and S. Kobayashi, Enzymatic synthesis and antioxidant property of poly(allylamine)–catechin conjugate. *Chem. Lett.* 32 (2003) 620-621.
[58] S. Kim and A. Cavaco-Paulo. Laccase-catalysed protein–flavonoid conjugates for flax fibre modification. *Appl. Microbiol. Biotechnol.* 93 (2012) 585-600.
[59] N. Ihara, S. Schmitz, M. Kurisawa, J.E. Chung, H. Uyama and S. Kobayashi. Amplification of inhibitory activity of catechin against disease-related enzymes by conjugation on poly(ε-lysine). *Biomacromolecules* 5 (2004) 1633-1636.
[60] P. P. Wattamwar, S.S. Hardas, D.A. Butterfield, K.W. Anderson and T.D. Dziubla, Tuning of the pro-oxidant and antioxidant activity of trolox through the controlled release from biodegradable poly(trolox ester) polymers. *J. Biomed. Mat. Res.* A 99A (2011) 184-191.
[61] M. Kakran, N.G. Sahoo, L. Li, Dissolution enhancement of quercetin through nanofabrication, complexation, and solid dispersion. *Col.l Surf. B Bioint.* 88 (2011) 121-130.
[62] M. Kurisawa, J.E. Chung, H. Uyama and S. Kobayashi, Laccase-catalyzed Synthesis and Antioxidant Property of Poly(catechin). *Macromol. Biosci.* 3 (2003) 58-764.
[63] M. Kurisawa, J.E. Chung, H. Uyama and S. Kobayashi, Oxidative coupling of epigallocatechin gallate amplifies antioxidant activity and inhibits xanthine oxidase activity. *Chem. Commun.* 10 (2004) 294-295.
[64] F. F. Bruno, A. Trotta, S. Fossey, S. Nagarajan, R. Nagarajan, L.A. Samuelson and J. Kumar, Enzymatic Synthesis and Characterization of PolyQuercetin. *J. Macromol. Sci.* A 47 (2010) 1191-1196.
[65] M. Kurisawa, J.E. Chung, H. Uyama and S. Kobayashi, Enzymatic synthesis and antioxidant properties of poly(rutin). *Biomacromolecules* 4 (2003) 1394-1399.
[66] H. Uyama, Artificial polymeric flavonoids: synthesis and applications. *Macromol. Biosci.* 7 (2007) 410-422.
[67] Y. Li, X. Li, Y.S. Wong, T. Chen, H. Zhang, C. Liu and W. Zheng, The reversal of cisplatin-induced nephrotoxicity by selenium nanoparticles functionalized with 11-mercapto-1-undecanol by inhibition of ROS-mediated apoptosis. *Biomaterials* 32 (2011) 9068-9076.
[68] N. Ihara, M. Kurisawa, J.E. Chung, H. Uyama and S. Kobayashi, Enzymatic synthesis of a catechin conjugate of polyhedral oligomeric silsesquioxane and evaluation of its antioxidant activity. *Appl. Microbiol. Biotechnol.* 66 (2005) 430-433.
[69] R. Konwarh, J. Prasad Saikia, N. Karak, B. Kumar Konwar, Poly(ethylene glycol)magnetic nanoparticles curcumin' trio: Directed morphogenesis and synergistic free radical scavenging. *Coll. Surf. B Bioint.* 81 (2010) 578-586.
[70] J. Huang, G. Zhan, B. Zheng, D. Sun, F. Lu, Y. Lin, H. Chen, Z. Zheng, Y. Zheng and Q. Li, Biogenic Silver Nanoparticles by Cacumen Platycladi Extract: Synthesis,

Formation Mechanism, and Antibacterial Activity. *Ind. Eng. Chem. Res.* 50 (2011) 9095-9106.

[71] G. Cirillo, S. Hampel, R. Klingeler, F. Puoci, F. Iemma, M. Curcio, O.I. Parisi, U.G. Spizzirri, N. Picci, A. Leonhardt, M. Ritschel and B. Büchner. Antioxidant multi-walled carbon nanotubes by free radical grafting of gallic acid: new materials for biomedical applications. *J. Pharm. Pharmacol.* 63 (2011) 179-188.

[72] E. Szliszka, W. Krol, The role of dietary polyphenols in tumor necrosis factor-related apoptosis inducing ligand (TRAIL)-induced apoptosis for cancer chemoprevention. *European Journal of Cancer Prevention* 20 (2011) 63–69.

[73] C. L. de Dicastillo, M. del Mar Castro-López, J. M. López-Vilariño, M. V. González-Rodríguez, Immobilization of green tea extract on polypropylene films to control the antioxidant activity in food packaging. *Food Research International* 53 (2013) 522–528.

[74] O. Vittorio, V. Raffa, C. Riggio, A. Pietrabissa, A. Cuschieri, PC12 Interaction with Magnetic Nanotubes: Effects on Viability, Cell Differentiation and Cell Translocation Induced by a Magnetic Field. *Current Nanoscience*, Volume 7 (2011) 337-344.

In: Recent Advances in Drug Delivery Research
Editor: Valerio Voliani
ISBN: 978-1-62948-228-6

Chapter 8

Targeting Drug Delivery Systems: Promises, Promises, and More Promises ... Let's Change the Paradigm

Karel Petrak[*]
Strategic Grants Development, Harris Health System, Holly Hall, Houston, Texas, US

Abstract

Many promises have been and are being made about the potential of various targeting drug delivery systems that do not come to fruition only to be replaced by new promises. A PubMed literature search for "target* and drug and delivery and promis*" delivers over 3,000 publications that appeared in the last 10 years. However, very little progress has been made in this field to date, and no effective site-targeting drug delivery systems are available for clinical, therapeutic use. The same technologies are often used under a different name - for example various previously tested particles and liposomes etc. are being hailed as a new solution when given a new name - nanoparticles, nanomedicine, etc.

In this chapter it is argued that it is not likely that thousands or even hundreds of different reasons exist for the subsequent failure of initially "promising" systems. Instead, it is suggested to be more likely that approaches previously shown to be invalid are being re-examined without sufficient understanding and critical review of *prior* data. This chapter examines critically examples of claims that were made about the potential of various systems for drug delivery and analyzes why such claims were not realistic from the start and hence failed. The review stresses the importance of understanding fully what has already been done, within the context of the selected therapeutic indication (the disease, the target, the drug, etc.). It also outlines how best to approach developing site-targeted drug delivery systems.

(*Disclaimer:* The views and opinions expressed in this article are those of the author and do not necessarily reflect the official policy or position of Harris Health System.)

[*] E-mail: klpetrak@gmail.com.

Keywords: Drug delivery, delivery systems, site-specific, drug targeting, targeting efficacy

Abbreviations

A431 – epidermoid carcinoma cell line
Anti-EGFR – anti-epidermal growth factor receptor
APC – antigen-presenting cells
BCECs – brain capillary endothelial cells
BSA – bovine serum albumin
CHO-FR-beta – Chinese hamster ovary cells
DNA – Deoxyribonucleic acid
DO-FUdR – 3',5'-dioctanoyl-5-fluoro-2'-deoxyuridine
DO-FUdR-SLN – 3',5'-dioctanoyl-5-fluoro-2'-deoxyuridine solid lipid nanoparticles
DOX – Doxorubicin
f-L-DNR – FR-targeted liposomal daunorubicin
FR – folate receptor
FUdR – 5-fluoro-2'-deoxyuridine
HepG2 - human hepatocellular liver carcinoma cell line
IgG2a – mouse IgG2a antibody, isotype control
J774 – murine macrophages cell line
KB – oral carcinoma cells
KG1 - human acute myelogenous leukemia cells
L-DNR – non-targeted liposomal DNR
LEAPT – lectin-directed enzyme-activated pro-drug therapy
MAb – monoclonal antibody
NAPE – N-acyl-phosphatidylethanolamine
NCL – Nanostructured Lipid Carriers
Ni-IgG2a – non-immune IgG2a
OX26 – anti-transferrin receptor antibody IgG2a
PEG – poly(ethylene glycol)
PTX – paclitaxel taxol
Rha – α-L-rhamnosidase
RNA – Ribonucleic acid
scFv – single-chain antibody Fv fragment
SLM – solid lipid microparticles
SLN – solid lipid nanoparticles
SP90 – targeting peptide
TfR – human transferrin receptor
UM-SCC-1 – head & neck squamous cell carcinoma cell line
UM-SCC-6 – head & neck squamous cell carcinoma cell line

Introduction

The focus of this paper is on the development of drug delivery technology for delivering therapeutic agents to specific sites within the body and within cells, i.e., for drug targeting. "Drug targeting" has frequently been euphemistically referred to as the "magic bullet". This term was coined by Dr. Paul Ehrlich in 1906 and referred to an ideal therapeutic agent that would target a highly specific site and treat only that site. This ideal is yet to be achieved in medical practice. In modern immunology, a less stringent definition of "magic bullet" is used and refers to any agent with the specificity of an antibody and lethal potential of a toxin. Drug delivery technology field is more forgiving as far as the use of the term goes. For example, Davis and Robinson (2002) [1] argued that "The specificity of carbohydrate-protein interactions can greatly outstrip that of many other ligand-binding systems;...macromolecules allow for the fine-tuning of active drug delivery..." and postulated that "...these two factors suggest that sugar-macromolecule conjugates, targeted using endogenous carbohydrate binding proteins, are a promising route to the 'magic bullet'". Davis and Robinson concept was not new even in 2002. Gregoriadis, for example considered this approach in 1975 [2] and on several other occasions [3]. The fact remains that Ehrlich's concept now more than 100-years old remains unrealized.

Pharmacokinetic Considerations

There are clear reasons why it remains so. Pharmacokinetic considerations for drug targeting have been well documented [4, 5, 6] but are rarely taken into account by material-science approaches predominantly used to develop drug delivery systems.

Several requirements for a targeted drug delivery system must be satisfied for the system to have any chance of returning the 'wished for' performance [7].

- Rate of elimination of drug–carrier conjugate

It is essential that the drug–carrier conjugate is not removed too rapidly from circulation. If it is eliminated from systemic circulation more rapidly than it is delivered to the target site, the amount of conjugate at the target site might never be enough to provide the required concentration of free (unbound) drug.

- Rate of release of free drug at the non-target site

Depending on the amount of drug, the release of drug away from the target site could nullify any benefits that might potentially come from delivering the drug to the target site.

- Rate of delivery of drug–carrier conjugate to the target site

If the drug conjugate reaches the target site too slowly, the supply of free drug (as governed by its rate of release at the site from its conjugate) might never be sufficient to generate the concentration required to elicit the desired therapeutic effect at the site of action.

The total amount of drug delivered (i.e., the area under the curve in a drug-concentration versus time plot for the target site) is irrelevant if, at any time, the free-drug concentration at the target site does not reach its pharmacologically effective level.

- Rate of release of free drug at the target site

The capacity of the system selected for the release of free drug from the conjugate should be considered. It needs to be suitable for processing the entirety of the drug–carrier conjugate arriving at the target site, doing so at a rate that also ensures drug accumulation at this site.

- Rate of removal of free drug from the target site

Drugs that benefit most from target-selective delivery are those that are retained at the site while acting on their target of action. Most existing drugs would have a tendency to diffuse away from the site when converted into their free, unconjugated from. Therefore, drugs may need to be specifically designed to be used with target-selective delivery systems.

- Rate of elimination of the drug–carrier conjugate and free drug from the body

For optimal targeting, systemic elimination of the complete drug–carrier conjugate should be minimal. These systems are frequently too large to be eliminated via the kidneys [8]. Consequently, the liver is mainly responsible for the removal of drug conjugates from circulation. The rate of elimination of free drug from the systemic circulation should be rapid relative to its rate of transfer from the target site to the central compartment of the body. This way, the drug delivery system will at least achieve a decrease in the drug-associated toxicity (in cases when the site of toxicity is different from the site of therapeutic effect).

It should be also noted that site-targeting of conventional drugs that typically reach their targets of action via absorption across biological membranes is unlikely to be effective. The reason is that these drugs can equally well diffuse away after their release at the site. Instead, efforts should focus on target delivery of macromolecular therapeutic entities such as DNA and RNA since these "drugs" cannot reach their intra-cellular targets by simple diffusion, and equally are less likely to diffuse away from the target site after their release from the delivery vehicle. Details of these brief conclusions, derived using the tools of mathematical modeling, can be found in publication by Boddy et al. [9]. It would be prudent to pay attention to these considerations at the start of any drug–carrier system development.

Some "Promising" Delivery Systems

Instead it would appear that in blissful disregard of key principles, many promises continue to be made about the "potential" of various targeting drug delivery systems that do not come to fruition only to be replaced by new promises. A PubMed literature search for "target* and drug and delivery and promis*" delivers over 3,000 publications that appeared in the last 10 years. However, very little progress has been made in this field to date, and no effective site-targeting drug delivery systems are available for clinical, therapeutic use. The same technologies are often used under a different name - for example various previously tested particles and liposomes etc. are being hailed as a new solution when given a new name - nanoparticles, nanomedicine, etc.

Let us examine the possibility that the criteria by which new approaches are classified as "promising" are inappropriate when one considers the technology for use in treating human disease. Building on the possibilities outlined by Davis and Robinson (2002) [1], lectin-directed enzyme-activated pro-drug therapy (LEAPT) was designed and tested [10]. *In vivo* targeting efficacy and the ability of the delivered, glycosylated α-L-rhamnosidase enzyme to selectively cleave a Rha-capped pro-drug (Rha-capped, DOX-conjugate pro-drug DOX-Rha; DOX = Doxorubicin) to release an active drug molecule to complete the LEAPT strategy was demonstrated. In order to establish *in vivo* therapeutic efficacy, nude (nu/nu) athymic mice, three trial groups (n = 13) were given intra-splenic injection of the human hepatocellular liver carcinoma cell line HepG2 and treated with the complete LEAPT system (pro-drug plus enzyme) or dosed with the individual components alone (enzyme or pro-drug, respectively) as controls. The authors reported that even using an un-optimized dosing regimen achieved a near-halving in total tumor burden (from 690 to 370) and a slightly greater than halving of total tumor foci in the treated group as compared with the control group of un-activated pro-drug alone (from 23 to 11). No significant difference was seen between the two control groups of capped un-activated pro-drug alone and enzyme without drug alone. Unfortunately, a group of animals treated with the drug (DOX) alone was not reported by the authors and hence it is not possible to make a conclusion about the "promise" of the approach as compared to the current therapy. Subsequent publication on this [11] was "consistent with the proposed mode of action and efficacy in models of liver cancer, and confirm modular flexibility in the drugs that may be used in LEAPT", without providing fresh data on the actual "promise" of the approach in terms of *in vivo* efficacy.

Targeting of drugs using mannose receptor has been contemplated for at least 30 years [12]. Robbins et al. reported in an article published in 1981 that "Mammalian macrophages contain a transport system that binds and internalizes glycoproteins with exposed mannose residues", and that this "... may be useful in targeting pharmacologic agents to macrophages, and analogous compounds may target such agents to other types of cell". Similar sentiment was expressed 30 years later by D'Addio et al. [13] when describing a new assembly process to produce nano-carriers with variable surface densities of mannose-targeting ligands in a single step, using kinetically-controlled, block-copolymer-directed assembly. They examined nano-carrier association with murine macrophage J774 cells expressing mannose receptor as a function of incubation time and temperature, nano-carrier size, dose, and PEG-corona properties. Characterizing nano-carriers in terms of mannose densities only, and without presenting any data on drug delivery as such, they never-the-less concluded that "This characterization of nano-carrier uptake and targeting provides promise for optimizing drug delivery to macrophages...". No consideration was given to the pharmacokinetics of the potentially released drug.

Safavy et al. [14] suggested in early 2000's that tumor-targeted drug delivery is an attractive strategy in cancer treatment. They reported a paclitaxel model conjugate using a bombesin receptor-recognizing peptide, and paclitaxel (PTX, taxol) conjugated to the anti-epidermal growth factor receptor (anti-EGFR) monoclonal antibody (MAb) Erbitux (C225) to serve as a model MAb-mediated drug delivery compound. Cytotoxicity screening of the drug-antibody conjugate against A431, UM-SCC-1, and UM-SCC-6 cells indicated an enhancement in cytocidal effect of paclitaxel as compared to those of the free drug, the intact antibody, and a physical mixture of the two (the controls). In A431 cells, the conjugates showed 25.2% +/- 2.2% of apoptosis induction as compared to little or no apoptosis caused by the controls. In A431-implanted nude mice, the conjugate and C225 showed tumor-growth inhibition effects of 57.2% and 41.2%, respectively, against a saline-treated control, which were not significantly different from each other. Authors attributed this lack of difference in the *in vivo* antitumor activity of the MAb-delivered drug and free PTX as possibly being due to either a relatively low dose of the antibody-delivered drug (346 μg/kg), or an untimely release of it, or both. Regardless, the authors concluded that "these preliminary results demonstrate the potential of tumor-targeted delivery of taxol as a promising strategy in cancer treatment and warrant further work to develop more suitable drug-MAb linkers as well as improved dosage and treatment protocols", without recognizing that the pharmacokinetics of the drug itself may not favour "targeting". No further progress with these conjugates has been reported by the authors to date.

Since the time of their invention by Horne and Bangham in 1961 [15, 16, 17], liposomes have been hailed as "the answer" to drug delivery problems. Indeed, a number of liposomal drug formulations have been approved and used in clinical practice; however, liposomes have as yet contributed very little to achieving the goals of site-selective, targeted delivery of drugs. For example, the group of Vermehren et al. has published much on how to make and characterize various types of liposomes. The group reported on *in vitro* and *in vivo* aspects of N-acyl-phosphatidylethanolamine-containing liposomes [18], stating that incorporation of the phospholipid, N-acyl-phosphatidylethanolamine (NAPE), had shown to increase the liposomal stability towards plasma components *in vitro*. Besides increasing the circulation time, they showed NAPE to impart liposomes with fusogenic properties. The authors suggested that "fusion between NAPE-liposomes and target cells may be expected, resulting in a favorable delivery of drug to the target cell" and that liposomes containing high percentage of NAPE may be a promising candidate for long-circulating liposomes, possibly in combination with other stabilizing components, e.g., cholesterol. Alas, their subsequent application of liposomes demonstrated that delivering drugs "close" to the intended molecular and disease target is no guarantee of success. They studied the uptake of a potential drug vector (OX26, or anti-transferrin receptor antibody IgG2a) conjugated to polyethyleneglycol-coated liposomes by brain capillary endothelial cells (BCECs; cells that express transferrin receptors) using *in situ* perfusion in 18-day-old rats [19]. Uptake of radio-labeled OX26 by BCECs after 15-minute perfusion was approximately 16-times higher than that of non-immune IgG2a (Ni-IgG2a). OX26 and OX26-conjugated liposomes selectively distributed to BCECs, leaving choroid plexus epithelium, neurons, and glia unlabeled. The failure to label neurons and glia showed that OX26 and OX26-conjugated liposomes did not pass through BCECs. Still, the authors maintained that "the expression of transferrin receptors by endothelial cells selective to the brain qualifies OX26 as a candidate for blood-to-endothelium transport", and postulated that a "specifically designed formulation of liposomes may allow for their degradation within BCECs, leading to subsequent transport of liposomal cargo further into the brain". No justification was offered as to why drugs released at the endothelial surface should preferentially travel into the brain. Lack of subsequent publications on this suggests that progress in this direction has not yet been made.

Based on polymer research of the time, Ringsdorf developed in early 1970s a conceptual model [20] of using pharmacologically active macromolecular compounds as drugs. Although much effort has been expended since that time by many on putting the concept into practice, the model has also been questioned by some for both theoretical and practical reasons. The rationale for using polymers, macromolecules, has been that by attaching drugs to large molecules, specific properties of polymeric materials could be imparted onto low-molecular-weight drugs without changing their structure and hence their specific activity. Since the properties of such "macromolecular drugs" would then depend on the structure of the polymer used, properties of macromolecular drugs could be varied over a large range and could include targeting drugs by their release from polymeric carrier at specific sites. Ringsdorf's model for pharmacologically active polymers incorporated the possibility for continuous variation in (a) solubility and toxicity, (b) fixation and removal of active material, and (c) body distribution.

Some 30 years later, according to Maier et al. [21], carrier-mediated delivery still held great promise for significantly improving the cellular uptake and therefore the therapeutic efficacy of therapeutic agents, in this case of antisense oligonucleotides *in vivo*. They designed a multivalent carbohydrate-recognition motif for the asialoglycoprotein receptor for tissue- and cell-specific delivery of antisense drugs to parenchymal liver cells. They achieved a low-molecular-weight of the conjugate with high receptor affinity be generating a synthetic ligand containing three galactosyl residues attached to a cholane scaffold via epsilon-aminocapramide linkers. According to their three-dimensional structural calculations, this unique design was to provide proper spacing and orientation of the three galactosyl residues to accomplish high-affinity binding to the receptor and thus delivering covalently conjugated oligonucleotides to their intended target. No progress has apparently been reported on this as yet, some 10 years later.

Similarly and at around the same time, Xu et al. [22] stated that "an ideal therapeutic for cancer would be one that selectively targets to tumor cells, is nontoxic to normal cells, and that could be systemically delivered, thereby reaching metastases as well as primary tumor", and that "immunoliposomes directed by monoclonal antibody or its fragments are promising vehicles for tumor-targeted drug delivery". That "promise" has yet come to pass. When extending such methodology to gene delivery, they examined a cationic immunoliposome system directed by a lipid-tagged, single-chain antibody Fv fragment (scFv) against the human transferrin receptor (TfR) [23] only to find that "an extremely low yield of this lipid-tagged scFv limited further downstream development and studies". Adopting a different strategy, they employed covalent conjugation of scFv to the liposome via a cysteine at the 3'-end of the protein and a maleimide group on the liposome, claiming that this scFv-immunoliposome can deliver the complexed gene systemically to tumors *in vivo*, where it is efficiently expressed, and that this "new approach provides a promising system for tumor-targeted gene delivery that may have potential for systemic gene therapy of various human cancers". Unfortunately, while a number of publications have been generated by the authors over time repeatedly applying the same general approach to various delivery applications, for example by Yang et al. [24], now adding the term "nano" to the approach, the "promise" of their work is yet to be fulfilled.

Despite the lack of success with such and similar targeting approaches, the concept remains popular even in 2013. Lu et al. [25] still believe that "development of novel tumor-specific ligands or pharmaceutical nano-carriers is highly desirable". They utilized phage display to identify a new targeting peptide, SP90, which specifically binds to breast-cancer cells, and recognizes tumor tissues from breast-cancer patients. Conjugation of SP90 with liposomes reportedly enabled efficient delivery of drugs into cancer cells through endocytosis. *In vivo* fluorescent imaging demonstrated that SP90-conjugated quantum dots possess tumor-targeting properties. In tumor xenograft and orthotopic models, SP90-conjugated liposomal doxorubicin was reported to improve the drug's therapeutic index. The authors concluded that the targeting peptide SP90 has significant potential in improving the clinical benefits of chemotherapy in the treatment and the diagnosis of breast cancer. Let's hope that future clinical results will indeed confirm this prediction.

Blood-brain barrier is notorious for limiting access of material to the brain. So as to overcome the limited access of the drug 5-fluoro-2'-deoxyuridine (FUdR) to the brain, 3',5'-dioctanoyl-5-fluoro-2'-deoxyuridine (DO-FUdR) was synthesized and incorporated into solid lipid nanoparticles (DO-FUdR-SLN) in 2002 by Wang et al. [26]. The median particle size of DO-FUdR-SLN was 76 nm with drug loading of 29.02% and entrapment efficiency of 96.62%. The brain area under the concentration-time curve of DO-FUdR-SLN and DO-FUdR were 10.97-fold and 5.32-fold higher than that of FUdR, respectively. These results indicated to the authors a good brain-targeting efficiency of DO-FUdR-SLN *in vivo*. The authors concluded that SLN can improve the ability of the drug to penetrate through the blood-brain barrier and that it is a promising drug-targeting system for the treatment of central nervous system disorders. There appear to be no follow-up publications by these authors reporting further development of this "promising" approach.

It is fascinating to observe how particulate form has in itself attracted researches in drug delivery for several decades now. For example, Erni et al. [27] stated in 2002 that "biodegradable microparticles represent a promising carrier system for the efficient delivery of therapeutic macromolecules to phagocytic professional antigen-presenting cells (APC)". In this case, solid lipid microparticles (SLM) consisting of a tripalmitin matrix were prepared using a novel micromixer-based solvent extraction process. A positive surface charge was introduced by the incorporation of cationic lipids into the formulation. Not surprisingly, these "foreign to the body" SLM were efficiently phagocytosed by primary macrophages *in vitro*. Complete intracellular degradation was observed already within 24 h, making the authors to conclude that SLM would be a suitable carrier for the immediate delivery of therapeutics to APC. Cationic SLM with adsorbed plasmid DNA and bovine serum albumin (BSA) were used as a model system, and triggered cellular internalization of the macromolecules by phagocytic macrophages. The authors, while expressing caution that SLM may accentuate cytotoxic effects in the phagocytic cells, concluded that SLM may provide a "new, efficient means for the immediate intracellular delivery of therapeutic macromolecules into APC". While SLM may be finding application in controlled release of drugs, their utility in targeted delivery of drugs remains a speculative promise. In a 2012 review, Selvamuthukumar et al. [28] when discussing trendily named "solid lipid nanoparticles" (SLN) listed a range of shortcomings that need to be considered and resolved when developing delivery systems for anti-cancer drugs: "poor solubility, normal tissue toxicity, poor specificity and steadiness, high incidence rate of pharmaceutical resistance and rapid degradation, need of large-scale output procedures, a fast release of the pharmaceutical from its carrier scheme, steadiness troubles, the residues of the organic solvents utilized in the output method and the toxicity from the polymer with esteem to the carrier scheme", and anticipated that these "shortcomings" will be overcome through the use of the Nanostructured Lipid Carriers (NCL). Here again, solutions are sought in realm of material science without due consideration being given to the pharmacology of the drug and other biologically relevant issues.

The folate receptor (FR) is amplified in a wide variety of human tumors [29], often by as much as some 20+-fold excess over normal cells. This has led many investigators to explore targeting cytotoxic therapies to FR as a "promising" strategy for chemotherapy.

For example, Ni et al. [30] FR-targeted liposomal daunorubicin (f-L-DNR) was compared to non-targeted liposomal DNR (L-DNR) for cellular uptake and cytotoxicity in FR-expressing cells. *In vitro*, cellular uptake of f-L-DNR in KB oral carcinoma cells, Chinese hamster ovary (CHO-FR-beta), and KG-1 human acute myelogenous leukemia cells were 9.4, 40, and 4,6-fold higher than non-targeted L-DNR, respectively. Cytotoxicity of f-L-DNR in KB and CHO-FR-beta cells was 18-times and 49-times higher than L-DNR, respectively, suggesting that FR-mediated delivery of liposomal DNR to FR-expressing cells increases DNR cellular uptake and cytotoxicity. Authors concluded that therapeutic evaluation in relevant animal models was warranted. Although results of any such evaluation are yet to be reported by the authors, it is appropriate to acknowledge that liposomes in general have been developed and are being used in drug products approved for therapeutic use. According to Huwyler et al. [31], approved drugs utilizing liposome formulations include pegylated liposomal doxorubicin (Doxil/Caelyx by Alza/Johnson and Johnson in the US and Schering-Plough outside the US), non-pegylated liposomal doxorubicin (Myocet by Elan), liposomal daunorubicin (DaunoXome by Gilead), liposomal cytarabine (DepoCyte by Skye Pharma/Enzon/Mundipharma) and liposomal cisplatin (Lipoplatin by Regulon). Liposomal formulations of anthracyclines are used for the treatment of ovarian and breast cancer or HIV associated Kaposi's sarcoma. DepoCyte was approved for the treatment of lymphomas with meningeal spread and is the only liposomal drug administered by intrathecal infusion. Lipoplatin is used for the treatment of epithelial malignancies (Stathopoulos et al. [32]).

Yet another particle - dendritic system - has been labeled as "promising" without evidence-based justification that this particle lacks the same fundamental drawbacks as other particles tried for drug delivery. Ihre et al. [33] using the old claim that "attachment of drugs to high-molecular-weight polymers can significantly improve both tumor targeting and therapeutic efficacy due to the enhanced permeability and retention effect observed in tumor tissue" investigated dendritic polymers as promising scaffolds for the preparation of new soluble polymeric-drug carriers. Using dendritic polyester systems based on the monomer unit 2,2-bis-(hydroxymethyl) propanoic acid, they attached to it anticancer drug doxorubicin via a pH-sensitive linkage demonstrating (their claim) the feasibility of using these polyester dendritic structures to prepare a viable polymer-drug conjugate. The authors subsequently evaluated various dendritic architectures composed of a polyester dendritic scaffold based on 2,2-is(hydroxymethyl)propanoic acid for their suitability as carriers for anticancer drug, doxorubicin both *in vitro* and *in vivo* [34]. They reported that cytotoxicity of the DOX-polymer conjugate measured on multiple cancer lines *in vitro* was reduced but not eliminated, indicating that some active doxorubicin was released from the drug polymer conjugate under physiological conditions. Furthermore, biodistribution experiments showed little accumulation of the DOX-polymer conjugate in vital organs, and the serum half-life of doxorubicin attached to an appropriate high-molecular-weight polymer has been significantly increased when compared to the free drug.

It is not clear how this information alone might justify their claim that "this new macromolecular system exhibits promising characteristics for the development of new polymeric drug carriers". It is clear, however that "…increasing our understanding of the impact of chemistry and architecture on polymer pharmacokinetics is essential for improving the design of polymer drug carriers and furthering their progress in clinical trials" [35], and it is even far clearer that developing carriers that meet the demands of drug pharmacokinetics is of the utmost importance in developing therapeutically effective drug delivery systems.

Conclusion and Recommendations

So why has not this been happening? Let me argue that it is not likely that thousands or even hundreds of different reasons exist for the subsequent failure of initially "promising" systems. Instead, I suggest that it is more likely that approaches previously shown to be invalid are being re-examined without sufficient understanding and critical review of prior data. In this chapter I have critically examined several examples of claims that were made about the potential of various systems for drug delivery and attempted to point out why such claims were not realistic from the start and hence failed.

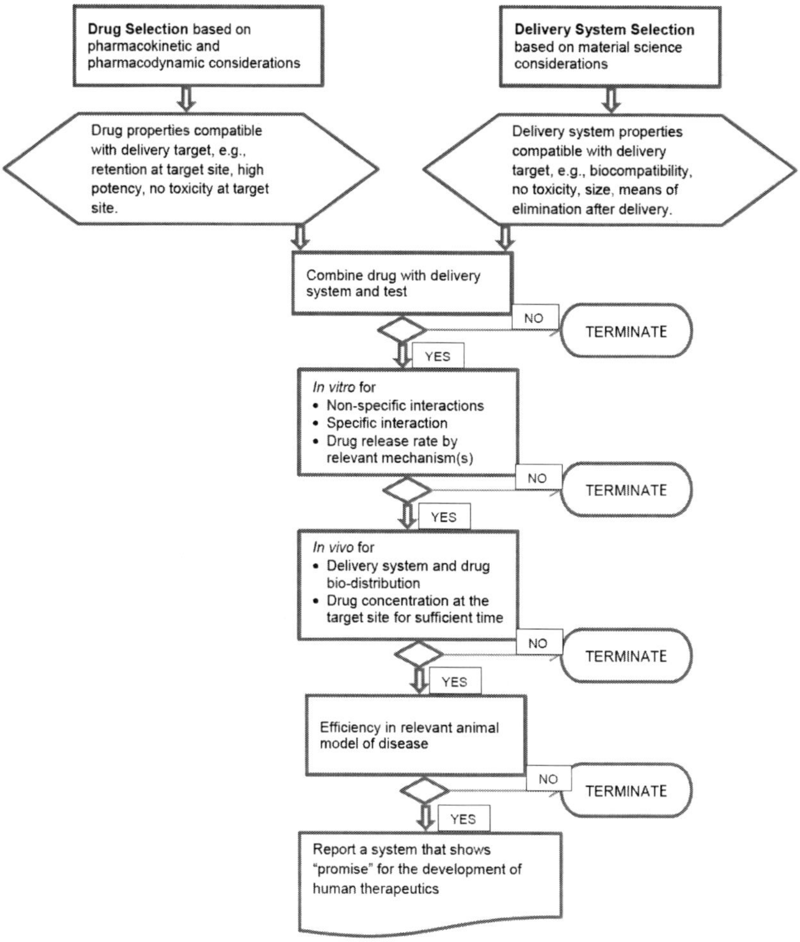

Figure 1. Structured process for the development of drug delivery systems.

The key points to stress are that:

- the starting point for developing effective drug targeting for human therapy needs to be a comprehensive understanding of what has already been done, and that
- full considerations must be given to the context of the selected therapeutic indication (the disease, the target, the drug, etc.).

Future efforts in this area would no doubt benefit from following a structured process briefly outlined in Figure 1.

It is only after due considerations have been given to the drug and delivery materials to be used, and after relevant *in vitro* and *in vivo* testing have been carried out with the selected delivery system in therapeutically relevant model and showed positive results should the researchers conclude that their system is promising to be tested in the context of developing human therapeutics. It should also be encouraged that negative data resulting from well-designed and correctly performed experiments are published so that repeating such experiments by others could be avoided.

References

[1] Davis BG, Robinson MA. Drug delivery systems based on sugar-macromolecule conjugates. *Curr. Opin Drug Discov Devel.* 2002 Mar;5(2):279-88.

[2] Gregoriadis G. Homing of Liposomes to Target Cells. *Biochem. Soc. Trans* (1975) 3, 613-618.

[3] Gregoriadis G, Weissig V, Tan L and Xiao Q. A novel method for the covalent coupling of sugars to liposomes. *Biochem. Soc. Trans* (1989) 17, 128-129.

[4] Stella, V.J. and Himmelstein, K.J. (1985) Prodrugs: a chemical approach to targeted drug delivery. In *Directed Drug Delivery* (Borchardt, R.T. et al., eds), pp. 247–267, Humana Press.

[5] Smits, J.F.M. and Thijssen, H.H.W. (1986) Spatial control of drug action: theoretical considerations on the pharmacokinetics of target-aimed drug delivery. In Rate-*Controlled Drug Administration and Action* (Struyker-Boudier, H.A.J. ed.), pp. 83–104, CRC Press.

[6] Hunt, C.A., MacGregor RD and Sieger RA (1986) Engineering targeted in vivo drug delivery. I. The physiological and physicochemical principles governing opportunities and limitations. *Pharm. Res.* 3, 333–344.

[7] Petrak K. Essential properties of drug-targeting delivery systems. *Drug Discov Today.* 2005 Dec;10(23-24):1667-73.

[8] Petrak, K. and Goddard, P. (1989) Transport of macromolecules across the capillary walls. *Adv. Drug Deliv. Rev.* 3, 191–214.

[9] Boddy, A., Aarons L, and Petrak K (1989) Efficiency of drug targeting: steady-state considerations using a three-compartment model. *Pharm. Res.* 6, 367–372.

[10] Robinson MA, Charlton ST, Garnier P, Wang X, Davis SS, Perkins AC, Frier M, Duncan R, Savage TJ, Wyatt DA, Watson SA, and Davis BG. LEAPT: Lectin-directed

enzyme-activated prodrug therapy. *Proceedings of the National Academy of Sciences of the United States of America*, vol. 101 no. 40, 14527–14532, October 5, 2004.

[11] Garnier P, Wang XT, Robinson MA, van Kasteren S, Perkins AC, Frier M, Fairbanks AJ, Davis BG. Lectin-directed enzyme activated prodrug therapy (LEAPT): Synthesis and evaluation of rhamnose-capped prodrugs. *J. Drug Target.* 2010 Dec;18(10):794-802.

[12] Robbins JC, Lam MH, Tripp CS, Bugianesi RL, Ponpipom MM, Shen TY. Synthetic glycopeptide substrates for receptor-mediated endocytosis by macrophages. *Proc. Natl Acad. Sci. USA*. 1981 Dec;78(12):7294-8.

[13] D'Addio SM, Baldassano S, Shi L, Cheung L, Adamson DH, Bruzek M, Anthony JE, Laskin DL, Sinko PJ, Prud'homme RK. Optimization of cell receptor-specific targeting through multivalent surface decoration of polymeric nanocarriers. *J. Control Release.* 2013 Feb 16. pii: S0168-3659(13)00078-3. doi:10.1016/j.jconrel.2013.02.004.

[14] Safavy A, Bonner JA, Waksal HW, Buchsbaum DJ, Gillespie GY, Khazaeli MB, Arani R, Chen DT, Carpenter M, Raisch KP. Synthesis and biological evaluation of paclitaxel-C225 conjugate as a model for targeted drug delivery. *Bioconjug Chem.* 2003 Mar-Apr;14(2):302-10.

[15] Bangham, A. D.; Horne, R. W. (1964). "Negative Staining of Phospholipids and Their Structural Modification by Surface-Active Agents As Observed in the Electron Microscope". *Journal of Molecular Biology* 8: 660–668. doi:10.1016/S0022-2836(64)80115-7. PMID 14187392.

[16] Horne, R. W.; Bangham, A. D.; Whittaker, V. P. (1963). "Negatively Stained Lipoprotein Membranes". Nature 200: 1340.doi:10.1038/2001340a0. PMID 14098499.

[17] Bangham, A. D.; Horne, R. W.; Glauert, A. M.; Dingle, J. T.; Lucy, J. A. (1962). "Action of saponin on biological cell membranes". *Nature* 196: 952–955. doi:10.1038/196952a0. PMID 13966357.

[18] Vermehren C, Hansen HS, Clausen-Beck B, Frøkjaer S. In vitro and in vivo aspects of N-acyl-phosphatidylethanolamine-containing liposomes. *Int J Pharm.* 2003 Mar 18;254(1):49-53.

[19] Gosk S, Vermehren C, Storm G, Moos T. Targeting anti-transferrin receptor antibody (OX26) and OX26-conjugated liposomes to brain capillary endothelial cells using in situ perfusion. *J. Cereb Blood Flow Metab.* 2004 Nov;24(11):1193-204.

[20] Ringsdorf H., Structure and properties of pharmacologically active polymers. Journal of Polymer Science: *Polymer Symposia* Volume 51, Issue 1, pages 135–153, 1975.

[21] Maier MA, Yannopoulos CG, Mohamed N, Roland A, Fritz H, Mohan V, Just G, Manoharan M. Synthesis of antisense oligonucleotides conjugated to a multivalent carbohydrate cluster for cellular targeting. *Bioconjug Chem.* 2003Jan-Feb;14(1):18-29.

[22] Xu L, Huang CC, Huang W, Tang WH, Rait A, Yin YZ, Cruz I, Xiang LM, Pirollo KF, Chang EH. Systemic tumor-targeted gene delivery by anti-transferrin receptor scFv-immunoliposomes. *Mol Cancer Ther.* 2002 Mar;1(5):337-46.

[23] Xu L, W. H. Tang, C. C. Huang, W. Alexander, L. M. Xiang, K. F. Pirollo, A. Rait, E. H. Chang. Systemic p53 gene therapy of cancer with immunolipoplexes targeted by anti-transferrin receptor scFv. *Mol. Med.* 2001 October; 7(10): 723–734.

[24] Yang C, Rait A, Pirollo KF, Dagata JA, Farkas N, Chang EH. Nanoimmunoliposome Delivery of Superparamagnetic Iron Oxide Markedly Enhances Targeting and Uptake in Human Cancer Cells In Vitro and In Vivo. *Nanomedicine.* Author manuscript;

available in PMC 2009 December 1. Published in final edited form as: Nanomedicine. 2008 December; 4(4): 318–329. Published online 2008 July 26. doi: 10.1016/j.nano.2008.05.004 PMCID: PMC2670493.

[25] Lu R-M, Chen M-S, Chang D-K, Chiu C-Y, Lin W-C, et al. (2013) Targeted Drug Delivery Systems Mediated by a Novel Peptide in Breast Cancer Therapy and Imaging. *PLoS ONE* 8(6): e66128. doi:10.1371/journal.pone.0066128.

[26] Wang JX, Sun X, Zhang ZR. Enhanced brain targeting by synthesis of 3',5'-dioctanoyl-5-fluoro-2'-deoxyuridine and incorporation into solid lipid nanoparticles. *Eur. J. Pharm Biopharm*. 2002 Nov;54(3):285-90.

[27] Erni C, Suard C, Freitas S, Dreher D, Merkle HP, Walter E. Evaluation of cationic solid lipid microparticles as synthetic carriers for the targeted delivery of macromolecules to phagocytic antigen-presenting cells. *Biomaterials*. 2002 Dec;23(23):4667-76.

[28] Selvamuthukumar S, Velmurugan R. Nanostructured Lipid Carriers: A potential drug carrier for cancer chemotherapy. *Lipids Health Dis*. 2012; 11: 159. Published online 2012 November 20. doi: 10.1186/1476-511X-11-159 PMCID: PMC3561225.

[29] Weitman SD, Lark RH, Coney LR, Fort DW, Frasca V, Zurawski Jr VR., and Kamen BA. Distribution of the Folate Receptor GP38 in Normal and Malignant Cell Lines and Tissues. *Cancer Res June* 15, 1992 52; 3396.

[30] Ni S, Stephenson SM, Lee RJ. Folate receptor targeted delivery of liposomal daunorubicin into tumor cells. *Anticancer Res*. 2002 Jul-Aug;22(4):2131-5.

[31] Huwyler J, Drewe J, and Krähenbühl S. Tumor targeting using liposomal antineoplastic drugs. *Int. J. Nanomedicine*. 2008 March; 3(1): 21–29. PMCID: PMC2526358.

[32] Stathopoulos GP, Boulikas T, Vougiouka M, Deliconstantinos G, Rigatos S, Darli E, Viliotou V, Stathopoulos JG. Pharmacokinetics and adverse reactions of a new liposomal cisplatin (Lipoplatin): phase I study. *Oncol Rep*. 2005;13:589–95.

[33] Ihre HR, Padilla De Jesús OL, Szoka FC Jr, Fréchet JM. Polyester dendritic systems for drug delivery applications: design, synthesis, and characterization. *Bioconjug Chem*. 2002 May-Jun;13(3):443-52.

[34] Padilla De Jesús OL, Ihre HR, Gagne L, Fréchet JM, Szoka FC Jr. Polyester dendritic systems for drug delivery applications: in vitro and in vivo evaluation. *Bioconjug Chem*. 2002 May-Jun;13(3):453-61.

[35] Fox ME, Szoka FC, and Fréchet JM. Soluble Polymer Carriers for the Treatment of Cancer: The Importance of Molecular Architecture. *Acc. Chem. Res*. 2009 August 18; 42(8): 1141–1151.

Editor Contact Information

Dr. Valerio Voliani
Universidad de Valencia
Istituto Ciencia Molecular (ICMOL)
Catedratico Jose Beltran 2
4698 Paterna Valencia (Spain)
Tel: + 3496 3544 315
v.voliani@sns.it

And

NEST – Scuola Normale Superiore
P.zza San Silvestro, 12
56100, Pisa (Italy)

Index

A

B

C

D

E

F

I

J

K

L

M

N

O

P

Q

R

S

T

U

V

W

X

Y